HAND-BOOK

OF

SURGICAL OPERATIONS

HAND-BOOK

OF

SURGICAL OPERATIONS

BY

STEPHEN SMITH, M.D.

GYAN

Published by

GYAN

Gyan Publishing House
5, Ansari Road
Daryaganj, New Delhi-110002
Phone: 011-47034999, 9811692060
E-mail: books@gyanbooks.com

Distribution Network
gyanbooks.com
India, USA, Canada, UK, Australia, France

ISBN : 978-81-212-9783-7 (PB)
First Published, 1862

2nd Impression 2023

Printed at: Gyan Press, Delhi.

HAND-BOOK OF SURGICAL OPERATIONS
Author:STEPHEN SMITH

HAND-BOOK

OF

SURGICAL OPERATIONS.

BY

STEPHEN SMITH, M.D.,

SURGEON TO BELLEVUE HOSPITAL.

SECOND EDITION.

1862.

PREFACE.

This Hand-Book of Surgical Operations has been prepared at the suggestion of several professional friends, who early entered the medical staff of the Volunteer Army. It was alleged that the military surgeon of this country had no small and convenient work suitable for a pocket companion, containing the details of the more common as well as the important operations in surgery. He must either encumber himself with the large treatises on general and operative surgery, or rely upon his unaided memory in the emergencies of the service.

In its scope the work is limited to those branches of operative surgery which are of the most importance to the military surgeon. This was deemed advisable, in order to render the volume as convenient and portable as possible. Within these limits the constant effort has been to embrace the greatest number of subjects, to arrange them in the best form for reference, and to give the largest amount of practical details, anatomical and operative.

As the value of such a work is much enhanced by engravings, care has been taken to illustrate every subject to the fullest extent. For this purpose works on operative surgery have been largely consulted, and such illustrations selected as were deemed most valuable. To avoid frequent repetitions, no mention is made in the text of the source from which they have been derived, and this occasion is taken to make proper acknowledgment. In the chapter on Minor Surgery, the illustrations are copied from English surgical treatises, Sédillot's *Traité de Med. Operat.*, and Jamain's *Manuel de Petit Chir.*; the illustrations of the Operations on Arteries are from Sédillot (*op.*

cit.) and Guérin's *Elem. de Chir. Operat.*; in the chapter on Amputations, the illustrations are from English works, viz. Skey, Fergusson, Liston, Guthrie, and Druitt, and from Guérin (*op. cit.*), Chassaignac's *Traité Clinique et Pratique des Operations Chirurgicales, &c.*, and Bernard and Huette's *Illustrated Manual of Operative Surgery and Surgical Anatomy*; in the chapter on Resections, the illustrations of operations are from Chassaignac (*op. cit.*), Guthrie, Heyfelder's *Operationslehre und Statistic der Resectionen*, Erichsen, and Bernard and Huette (*op. cit.*). The illustrations of instruments through the volume have been selected by Tiemann & Co., and Wade & Ford, Instrument Makers, of this city, and generally represent the latest improvements.

Although this work is limited, as stated above, yet the subjects treated are, with the exception of Gunshot Wounds, such as constantly engage the attention of the surgeon in civil and hospital practice, and it is believed that it will prove to this class of practitioners a useful and acceptable aid to the memory. To the students of Operative Surgery, it presents in sufficient detail for the purposes of study and practice, the methods of performing the ordinary operations in Surgery.

MAY 15, 1862.

CONTENTS.

CHAPTER I.

MINOR SURGERY.

CHAPTER II.

ON THE ARTERIES.

CHAPTER III.

ON THE VEINS.

CHAPTER IV.

ON AMPUTATIONS.

CHAPTER V.

ON RESECTIONS.

CHAPTER VI.

ON GUNSHOT WOUNDS.

HAND-BOOK

OF

OPERATIVE SURGERY.

CHAPTER I.

MINOR SURGERY.

INSTRUMENTS.

Pocket Case.—Pocket cases are of various sizes, according to the number and kind of instruments which they contain. They may be divided into, 1st. The complete; and 2d. The select case. The complete case usually contains the following instruments, arranged in four folds:—A large and small scalpel; a straight and curved scissors; an artery, dissecting, and dressing forceps; a sharp and probe-pointed bistoury; tenaculum; an abscess, gum, and common lancet; an exploring and seton needle; spatula; probes; director; male and female catheter; surgeon's needles.

Select cases are made to suit the wishes of individual surgeons, and generally contain a limited number of instruments in a compact form. The case may consist of several folds, or a single fold. The following select cases of well known surgeons are now much used, and may be given as illustrations:—

Contents of Dr. Willard Parker's Pocket Case, of two folds.—One scalpel and blunt bistoury, spring back; one tenotomy knife, and small curved bistoury, spring back; one gum lancet and tenaculum, double spring back; one pair scissors; one pair of silver probes; one silver director; one artery forceps; one double catheter and caustic holder; needles, silk, silver wire in pocket of fold. Dimensions, five inches long, two and a half inches wide.

Contents of Dr. Wm. H. Van Buren's Pocket Case, of two folds.—One scalpel and sharp bistoury, spring back; one scalpel and blunt bistoury, spring back; one tenaculum and tenotomy knife, spring back; one double catheter; one pair silver probes; one exploring needle; one pair straight scissors; one artery forceps; one silver director with spoon; needles, silk, and silver wire in the pocket. Dimensions, five inches long, two and a half inches wide.

The regimental surgeon of the U. S. Army is provided with the following list of instruments in his pocket case:—

One large scalpel; one small scalpel; one artery forceps; one bull-dog forceps; one curved forceps; one dressing forceps; one needle; one sharp-pointed bistoury; one probe-pointed bistoury; one long probe-pointed bistoury; one straight scissors; one knee scissors; one flat-curved scissors; one gum lancet; one tenaculum; one tenotomy knife; one abscess lancet; one exploring needle; one exploring trocar; one seton needle; one spatula; two probes; one director; one double canula; one compound silver catheter; six surgeon's needles; one artery needle.

The pocket case of the surgeons of the U. S. Navy contains the following instruments:—

Scalpels, two; bistouries, curved shape, one; bistouries, curved, probe-pointed, one; finger-knife, one; scissors, straight, one; tenaculum, one; abscess lancet, one; thumb lancet, one; artery forceps, one; director, one; probes, two; small needles, two; ligatures.

A case may be selected which contains all the instruments ordinarily required in every-day practice, and which occupies so little space in the pocket as to become a constant companion without the slightest inconvenience. The author has prepared a case which contains in a single fold (Fig. 1) the following instruments:—

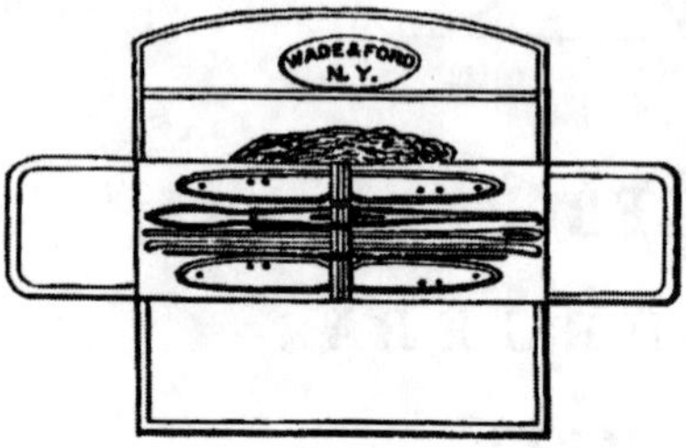

FIG 1.

One scalpel and small sharp bistoury, spring back; one gum lancet and probe bistoury, spring back; one silver director and probes; one pair slide artery forceps; male and female catheters; needles; silk in the pocket of the case. Dimensions, four inches long, one inch and a half wide.

The General Case.—This case contains a variety of instruments sufficient for any emergency in practice. A well appointed case should have instruments for amputating; for trephining; for hernia; for lithotomy, etc., etc. Various general cases are now in use, manufactured by instrument makers according to the plans of different surgeons. The following are given in illustration:—

Contents of Dr. James R. Wood's General Operating Case **(Fig. 2).—One long amputating knife; one catling; one circular knife; one large amputating saw; one amputating and trephining scalpel; one metacarpal saw; one pair fine bone forceps; one tourniquet; one pair trephines; one Hey's skull saw; one elevator; one brush; two minor operating scalpels; one blunt and one sharp bistoury; one straight scissors; one tenaculum; one aneurism needle; one artery forceps; two couching needles, straight and curved; one Beer's bone knife; one bullet forceps; one strabismus hook; one curved eye forceps; one pair eye scissors; one steel director; one pair silver probes; two steel sounds, assorted; two silver catheters; two English gum elastic bougies; silver wire, needles, and ligatures. Dimensions of case, fifteen and three-quarter inches long, six inches wide, three inches deep.**

Contents of the Compact Case of Dr. Willard Parker of New York. **—One capital saw; one metacarpal saw; one amputating knife; one catling, handle to change; one small amputating knife; one bone forceps; one spring catch artery forceps; one artery forceps; one large artery forceps; one tenaculum; one tourniquet; one trephine; one Hey's saw; one elevator; one brush; three scalpels; one curved bistoury, sharp; one curved bistoury, probe; one Cooper's bistoury; one scissors; one polypus forceps; one pessary forceps; one grooved director; two silver probes; one eye needle; one strabismus hook; one Beer's knife; one double tenotomy knife; one hydrocele trocar; one long curved trocar; one exploring trocar; one set aneurism needles, Dr. Mott's; two retractors; one lithotomy forceps; one grooved staff; two steel sounds; one probe-pointed lithotomy knife; two silver male catheters. Dimensions of case, twelve inches long, six inches wide, three and a half inches deep.**

Contents of Field Case of Dr. Frank H. Hamilton, of New York. **—One long amputating knife; one amputating knife; one catling; two small amputating knives; one metacarpal saw; one large saw; one bone forceps; one tenaculum; one short bistoury, sharp; one pair slide artery-forceps; one pair bull-dog artery forceps; one pair large scissors; one pair small scissors; one pair dressing forceps; one long silver bullet probe; one whalebone bullet probe; one small silver probe; two doz. serrefines; two doz. needles; one tourniquet, screw; one tourniquet, field; one director; one conical**

trephine; one necrosis trephine; one elevator; one Hey's saw; one brush; three bullet forceps; two retractors; one needle forceps; one plain aneurism needle; one set Dr. Mott's needles; silk and silver wire. Dimensions, seventeen inches long, nine inches wide, and two and a half inches deep.

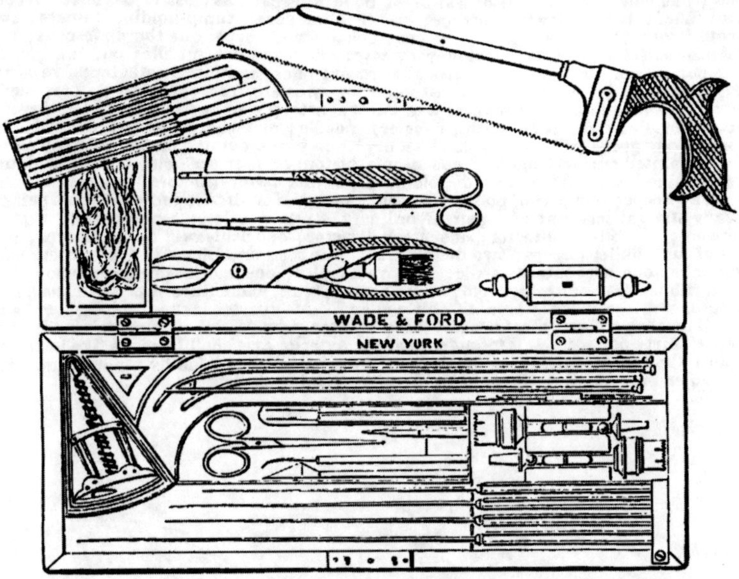

FIG. 2.—DR. WOOD'S CASE.

The regimental surgeon in the U. S. Army is provided with a general operating case, in addition to special cases for amputation, trephining, and exsection, containing the following instruments:

One small amputating knife; one small catling; three bistouries; one hernia knife; three scalpels; one cataract knife; one cataract needle; one tenaculum; one double hook; six steel bougies, silver, double curve, Nos. 1 and 2, 3 and 4, 5 and 6, 7 and 8, 9 and 10, 11, 12; six wax bougies, Nos. 2, 4, 6, 8, 10; three silver catheters, Nos. 3, 6, 9; six gum elastic catheters, Nos. 1, 3, 5, 7, 9, 11; two mahogany cases, brass bound; one gutta percha pouch; one metacarpal saw; one trocar; one ball forceps; one gullet forceps; one artery forceps; one dressing forceps; two scissors, straight and curved; one artery needle, with four points; twelve surgeon's needles; one tourniquet.

The surgeon in the U. S. N. is provided with two cases, as follows:

CASE, No. 1.—FIXED CONTENTS.—*Lid.* Plated dilators, six, and Nos. from 1 to 12, graduated; silver catheters, two, Nos. 4 and 6. *Upper Compartment.*—Stomach-pump and self-injecting apparatus. *Lower Compartment (Upper Tray).*—One probang; trocars, curved, one; trocars, straight, one; ear and hydrocele syringe, one; bullet forceps, one; hone, one. *Minor Surgery Tray, containing*—Scalpels, four; bistoury, sharp-pointed, one; bistoury, blunt-pointed, one; aneurism needle, one; artery forceps, one; tenaculum, one; scissors, one; tongue depressor, one; *Lower Tray.*—Amputating set, consisting of.—Two amputating knives; one catling; one metacarpal saw; one tenaculum; one bone forceps; six needles; one scalpel; one artery forceps; one tourniquet; one capital saw. *Trephining.*—Two trephines; one elevator; one brush; one Hey's saw.

CASE No. 2.—*Amputating.*—Two amputating knives; one catling; capital saw; one metacarpal; one tenaculum; six needles; one scalpel; one artery forceps; one bone forceps; one tourniquet. *Trephining.*—One trephine; one Hey's saw; one elevator; one brush. *Dental.*—Two forceps; one key, with three claws, assorted; one gum lancet.

Dr. Henry S. Hewitt, brigade surgeon, U. S. Army, has devised a "brigade case," containing the following assortment of instruments:

Four amputating knives; two amputating scalpels; one amputating tenaculum; one capital saw; one finger saw; two spiral tourniquets; two trephines; one Hey's saw; one elevator; one Liston's straight bone forceps; one Isaac's bayonet forceps; two Lüer's bone gnawing forceps; one Strohmeyer's stump-holding forceps; two tooth forceps; two Lüer's artery forceps; one torsion forceps; one thumb forceps; one mouse-tooth forceps: one Strohmeyer's saw; one saw à dos mobile; one saw guard; one curved rectum trocar; one straight trocar; one partitioned catheter; five silver catheters, 1, 3, 5, 7, 9; one silver catheter for prostate, 12; one steel staff grooved; twelve English flexible catheters; one Mott's artery needle; one right Deschamps' artery needle; one left Deschamps' artery needle; one sharp-pointed straight bistoury; one probe-pointed straight bistoury; one probe-pointed curved bistoury; one sharp-pointed curved bistoury; one hernia bistoury; four scalpels; one tenaculum; two double hooks, sharp; two double hooks, blunt; two retractors; one pair of Museux's forceps; one pair of polypus forceps; one pair of dressing forceps; one pair of heavy straight scissors; one pair of ordinary straight scissors: one pair of curved scissors; one silver director; one steel director; one Schleswig bullet forceps; one Hamilton's bullet forceps; two double trachea tubes; one Lüer's articulated œsophagus tube; one wire suture needle; two eye needles; one vaccinating scarificator; one hard rubber four-ounce syringe; silver probes, wire, and suture silk. Dimensions—length, eighteen inches; breadth, thirteen and three quarter inches; depth, two and a half inches; weight, nineteen and three-quarter pounds, and with containing leather valise, thirty pounds. It is intended that the exterior case shall be made five inches in depth, the lid to contain two rollers two and a half inches wide by seven yards long, placed on end, and lint, cerate, oil, chloroform, and sponges.

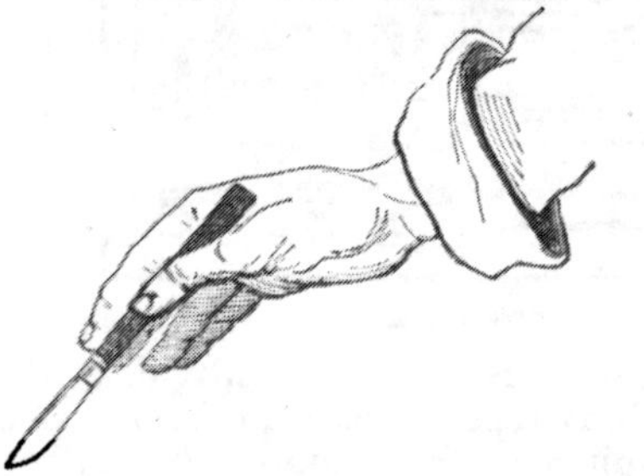

FIG. 3.

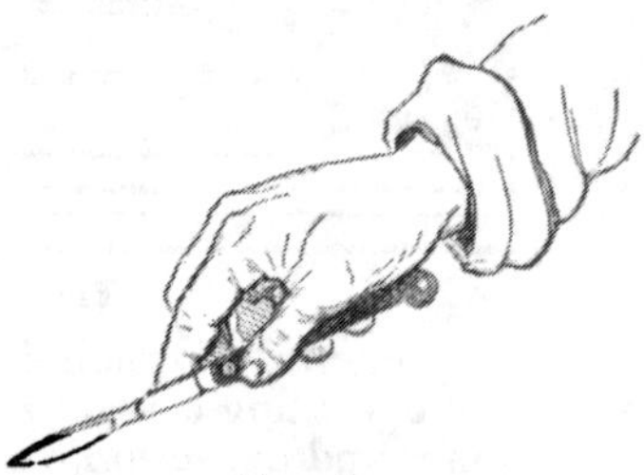

FIG. 4.

Positions of the Scalpel and Bistoury.—Authors generally describe several different positions in which the cutting instrument is held, but they may be reduced to the following:—

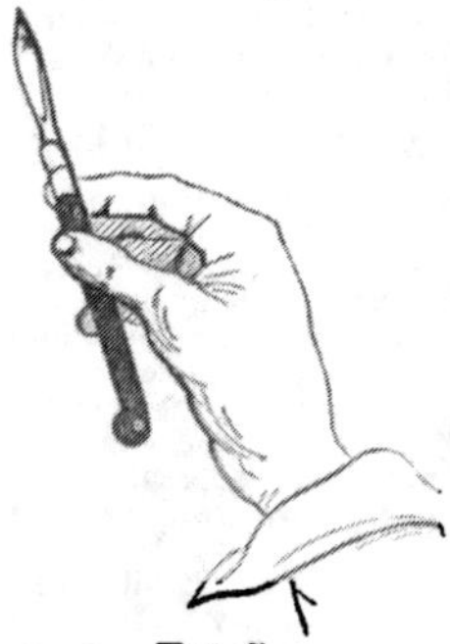

FIG. 5.

Position of the Scalpel.—In all ordinary operations the scalpel is used as a pen (Fig. 3); or, the handle resting in the palm, is firmly grasped by the thumb and the first and second fingers, and lightly supported by the third and fourth fingers (Fig. 4). The edge of the blade may in either case be turned upwards, and in the second position (Fig. 4) the index finger may be applied to the back of the blade. By a slight depression of the extremity of the handle, in the second position, the scalpel will be held very much as the bow of a violin (Fig. 5). The first position is adapted to nice dissections and limited incisions, the little finger being placed firmly upon the adjoining parts to give steadiness; the second position is adopted when long incisions are required; the edge of the instrument is turned upwards in the first position for dissection, and in the second when it is desired to puncture; the position assumed in Fig. 5 is designed for very delicate dissections.

Position of the Bistoury.—The bistoury is generally held like a pen (Fig. 6), but it may be substituted for the scalpel in any of the various positions already given; thus it may be used for penetration or incision, with the edge of the blade turned upwards or downwards, forwards or backwards, in any of these positions; or it may be employed on the director (Fig. 7), in laying open sinuses, and in very minute dissections.

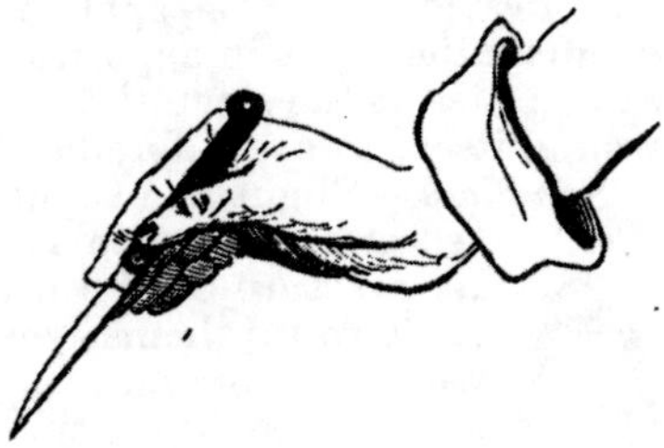

FIG. 6.

Incisions.—Incisions may be made from without inwards, or from within outwards. They should generally be made in the course of the vessels, nerves, and muscles, and when one is above the other the lower should be made first. They are divided into simple and compound:—

Simple Incision.—This is a single incision, whether straight or curved. It is made thus: the skin is first put on the stretch by the fingers of the left hand, then the scalpel or bistoury, held in one of the positions given (Figs. 3, 4), is entered nearly at right angles to the surface and to a sufficient depth; the handle is then depressed to an angle of about forty-five degrees, and the incision made of the requisite length; it is completed by again elevating the handle perpendicularly to give an abrupt termination.

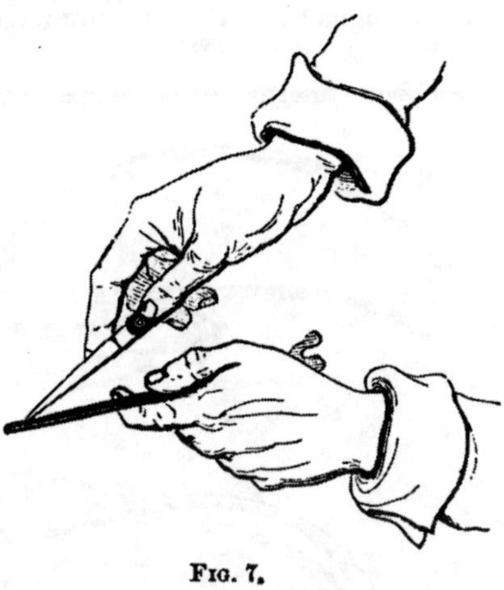

FIG. 7.

Compound Incisions.—These incisions are of various kinds, and consist of the intersection of one or more single incisions. Thus, two straight incisions meeting at an acute angle make the letter V; meeting at right angles they make one of the following letters, L, H, or T, or the crucial incision, +. Again, incisions may meet so as to make an ellipsis ⬭, or ⌣, or O.

UNION OF WOUNDS.

Adhesive Plaster.—The edges of wounds may often be so firmly maintained in apposition by adhesive strips as to obtain immediate union. The plaster should be sufficiently long to reach two to four inches beyond the margin of the wound, but not to extend around the limb; in its application the sides of the wound should be firmly supported, the first end being applied to the most yielding part. In general the straps should not be more than half an inch in width, and be applied so close to each other as to firmly maintain the edges in apposition. To remove the straps, raise both extremities at the same time, and withdraw them equally from the wound itself, to avoid forcibly separating the edges.

Serrefines.—Slight and superficial wounds may be united by the self-closing French forceps, known as serrefines (Fig. 8). By pressure on the sides, the teeth separate, and may be made to fix themselves upon both lips of the wound, and when the pressure is removed they close with sufficient firmness to bring the edges of the wound together, and maintain them in apposition.

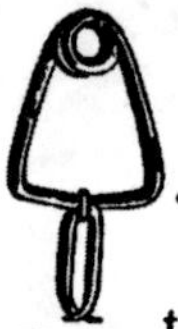

FIG. 8.

SUTURES.—In the application of the suture the needle and thread are employed. The best form of needle for general use is about two inches in length, and straight two-thirds of its length, the remaining third being gently curved, with two cutting edges (Fig. 9). In some cases a needle curved throughout its entire length (Fig. 9) will be found useful, as where the wound is deeply seated; finally, the straight needle, with sharp point and three cutting edges, is the most serviceable form in wounds on a slightly elevated surface. In some deeply-seated wounds, a needle with a handle (Fig. 10)

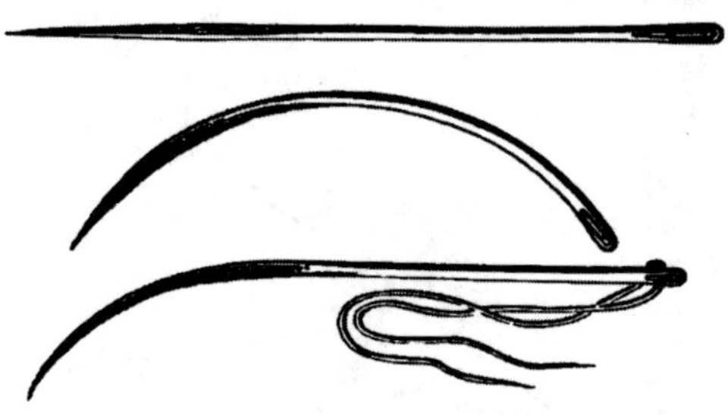

FIG. 9.

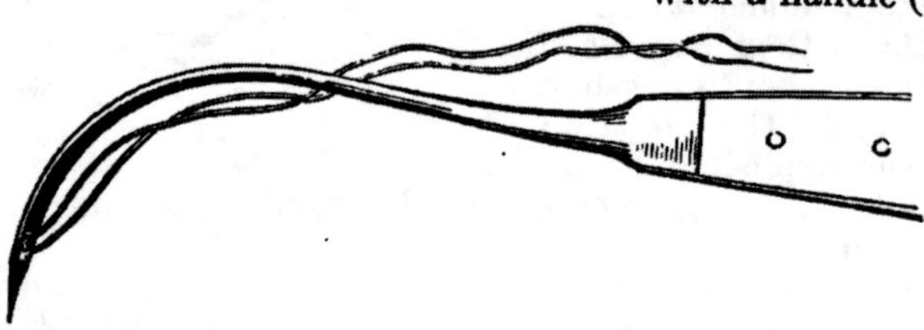

FIG. 10.

either fixed or attached by a screw, will answer a better purpose than either of those described.

Material for Sutures.—The material used for sutures may be animal, vegetable, or metallic. Of the *first*, catgut has been most frequently employed; it has, however, never proved reliable. Of the *second*, silk is almost universally selected, and still maintains its supremacy as a suture and a ligature. What is known as dentists' silk, with three threads, is the best form. Of the *third*, the silver wire is preferred, as combining the least irritating properties with great flexibility. It may be obtained of different sizes, and the larger should generally be preferred, as it is less liable to cut the edges of the wound. The wire suture may be inserted with the common surgical needle, but a needle has been devised by Mr. Lister, having a groove in the shaft from the eye to the butt, in which the wire is completely buried (Fig. 11), and which thus prevents the mass of wire occasioned by its being doubled upon itself at the eye. Another needle answering the same purpose has been invented by Mr. Price

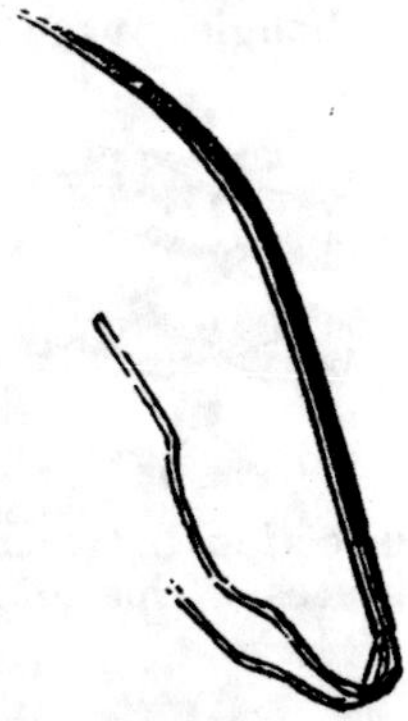

FIG. 11.

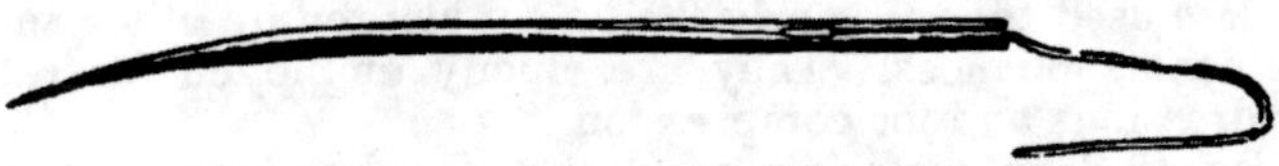

FIG. 12.

(Fig. 12), which has two eyes, and a groove on each surface; the wire is passed from the lower to the upper, and then doubled and twisted.

There are various forms of suture, as follows:—

Interrupted Suture.—A needle of the desired shape, armed with a ligature of the material chosen, is passed from without inwards through the right lip of the wound, at a distance from its margin, varying from a line to one-third of an inch, and being continued, it should be passed through the left lip from within outwards, exactly opposite the point of insertion in the right. All the sutures should be introduced before any are tied; the common reef-knot is then made, and the ends cut off closely (Fig. 13).

Continued Suture.—This suture is that made by the glover, and consists in passing the needle, as in the interrupted suture, diagonally, and leaving the thread uninterrupted; it is used in wounds of the intestines.

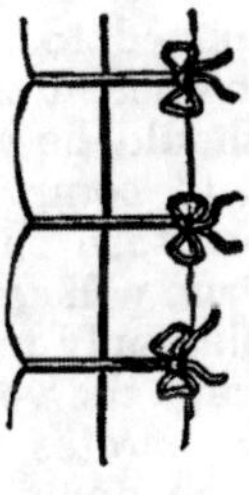

FIG. 13.

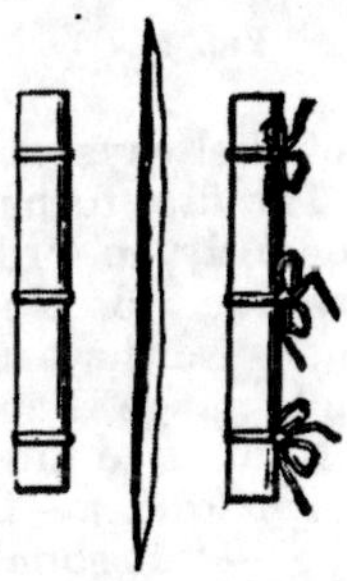

FIG. 14.

Quilled Suture.—In this suture (Fig. 14) the double thread is passed through the lips of the wound, as in the interrupted suture, but at greater distances, and the ends are tied over quills or pieces of bougie cut of the proper length. It is used to close deep wounds.

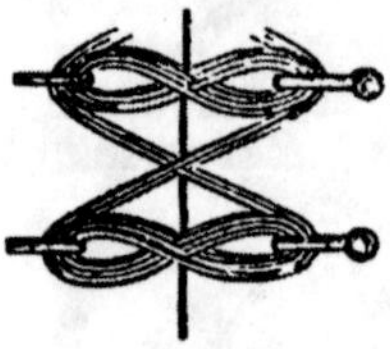

Fig. 15.

Twisted Suture.—This suture is made by introducing a needle of steel, silver, or other unirritating metal through the sides of the wound, as in the uninterrupted suture, and then twisting the thread around the ends in the form of a figure-of-eight (Fig. 15), or directly forming an ellipse. When several needles are required they should all be introduced before the thread is applied, which should then also take a diagonal direction between the pins (Fig. 15) to protect the intervening spaces. This suture is employed after operations for hare-lip.

DRESSINGS.

The Bandage.—Bandages have been employed for uniting, dividing, expelling, retaining, compressing, etc. They are now much less used than formerly, being supplanted by other and more convenient appliances. They are chiefly employed for retaining other dressings and for compression.

Material.—The materials employed for bandages are muslin, flannel, linen, calico, or gum elastic cloth. Muslin is generally selected of a coarse, unglazed quality. Flannel is useful when it is desirable to secure warmth.

Form.—When the material is selected, it should be cut or torn into strips of one, two, or three inches in width, according to the part to which it is to be applied. The bandage may be simple or compound; simple, when it consists of a single piece (Fig. 16); compound, when it is composed of two or more pieces, as in the T bandage (Fig. 24). It may have a single head (Fig. 16), or a double head (Fig. 22).

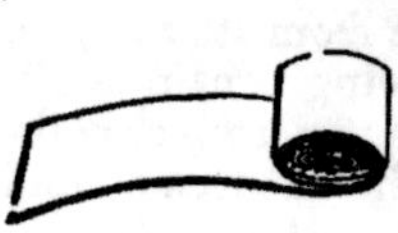

Fig. 16.

General Rules.—1. When the bandage is applied to a limb, especially for compression, it should always commence at the extremity, and proceed upwards. 2. The first turns should be *more* firmly applied than those subsequently, in order to compress the superficial veins from below upwards. 3. No one turn should be more firm than those below, otherwise the bandage will act as a ligature to the part. 4. When the bandage is applied only to a part of the limb, it should not be so tight as to interrupt the venous circulation.

Application.—Hippocrates says of the application of the bandage:—"It should be done quickly, without pain, with ease, and with elegance." Take the cylinder in the palm of the right hand, and with the thumb and fingers of the left, seize the free extremity, drawing the roller out six to ten inches between the thumb and fingers of the right hand, the cylinder unrolling in its palm; place the external surface upon the limb, and retaining it with the *first* and *second* fingers of the left hand, pass the cylinder under the limb, and by the aid of the third and fourth fingers of the left hand, make a turn or two to fix the initial extremity of the bandage. In continuing the application have but little of the bandage unrolled, keep the cylinder close to the limb, and pass it from one hand to the other without reaching with the respective hands beyond the centre of the limb. The following special forms of bandages require separate consideration:—

Circular.—The turns of this bandage pass nearly horizontally around portions of the limb, of equal diameter, one turn overlapping the other at fixed intervals (Fig. 17).

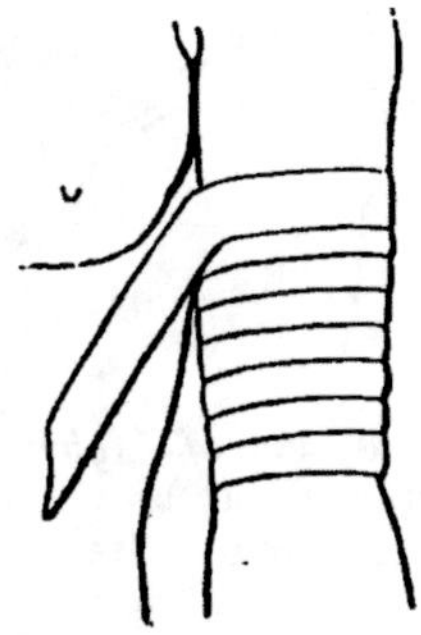

Fig. 17.

Spiral.—This bandage ascends a more or less conical portion of the limb, each succeeding turn partially overlapping the other. To apply the spiral bandage smoothly it is necessary to reverse the turns on the more conical parts. This is done as follows:—At the point where the roller ascends the limb so rapidly as to be irregularly applied, press the ends of the two fore-fingers of the left hand upon the upper fourth of the bandage, and retain it firmly at that point; then relaxing the bandage, turn the cylinder held between the fingers of the right hand, quickly, and completely over, by pronating the right hand, thus applying the upper surface in turn to the limb (Fig. 18).

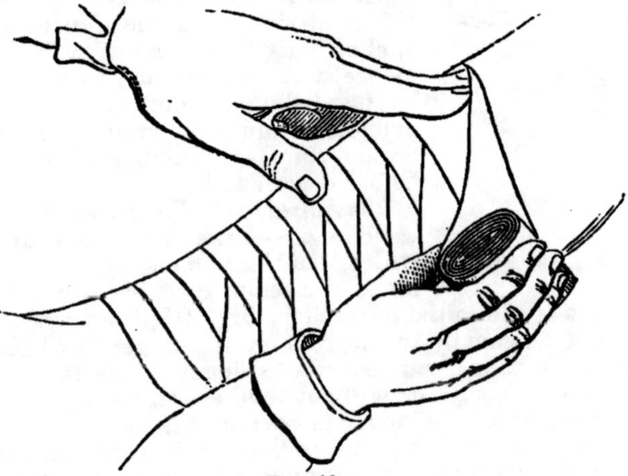

Fig. 18.

The Spica.—This bandage is named from the resemblance of the turns to the position of the grains on an ear of wheat. It is

applied on the upper part of the arm and thorax, of the thigh and pelvis, and of the thumb. In applying it to the groin (Fig. 19), stand in front of the patient, place the initial extremity on his right side, and carry the cylinder circularly around tbe body twice, then carry it downwards and around the thigh, passing from the inside to the outside of the limb, then upwards around the body, crossing the downward turn in the groin. The first turn around the thigh should be as low as its upper fourth, and the subsequent turns should ascend regularly until the requisite pressure is attained. The spica may be applied to the shoulder.

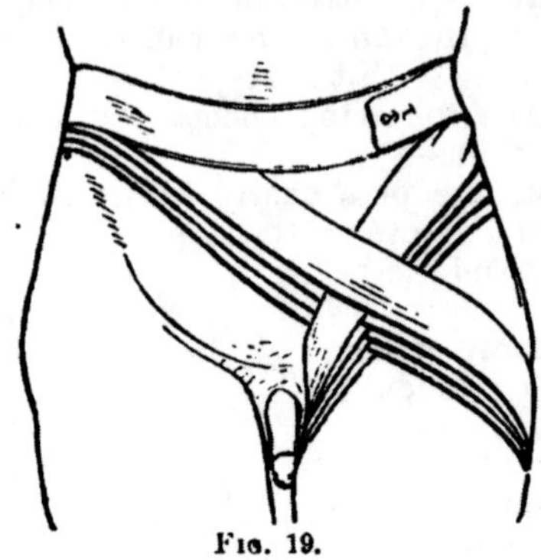

Fig. 19.

Figure-of-Eight.—This bandage is generally applied about the joints. If at the knee, continue the bandage of the leg, after it has reached the lower border of the joint, by passing the cylinder behind the knee, obliquely across the ham to the opposite side of the limb, arouud the thigh, and downwards again obliquely across the ham to the point of departure; each successive turn should overlap the other until the knee is covered, or the object attained. If the figure-of-eight is applied only to the knee (Fig. 20), commence with two circular turns around the leg just below the joint, and then carry the cylinder obliquely upwards across the ham, around the thigh, and again downwards as before described.

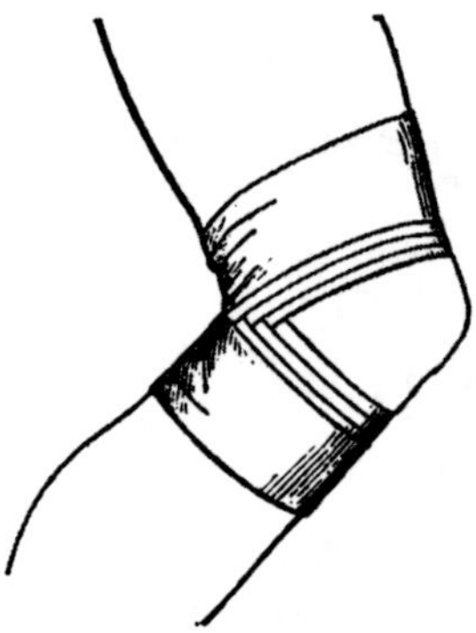

Fig. 20.

The Spiral of the Fingers.—This is applied as follows:—Take a bandage an inch in width, and commencing at the wrist make a circular turn, leaving free two or three inches at the initial extremity (Fig. 21); then cross the back of the hand diagonally to the root of the finger to be bandaged; then along the palmar surface of the finger to its tip, where the spiral commences, with or without reverses according to the shape of the finger; when the finger is covered the bandage should pass to the side of the wrist opposite to that where it began, and be tied to the initial extremity. If it is required to bandage other fingers, instead of tying the two extremities, the bandage should pass around the wrist and across the back of the hand to the root of the finger, and be applied as above described. In this manner all the fingers may be bandaged with a single roller.

Double-headed Bandage.—This bandage (Fig. 22) may be applied to the limbs or the head. In its application take the two cylinders in the hands, and placing the outer surface of the central portion upon the anterior part, carry the two cylinders to the back part and exchange, then bring them forward (Fig. 23), and reverse, if necessary.

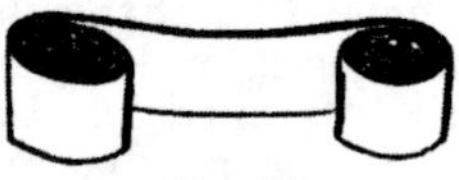

Fig. 22.

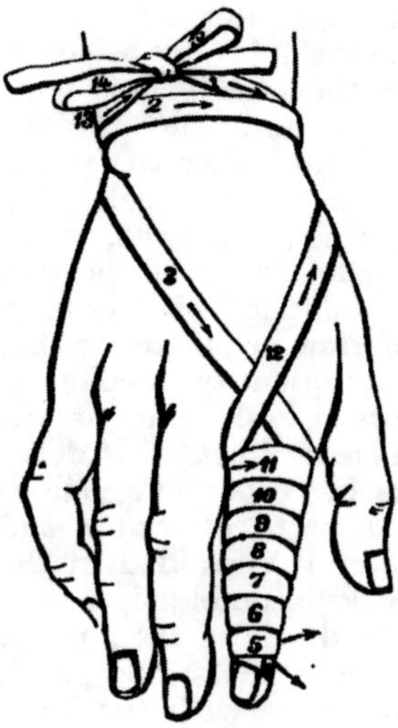

Fig. 21.

The T *Bandage.*—This bandage consists of the simple bandage with one or two pieces added at right angles (Fig. 24). It is employed in the diseases of the region of the perineum and anus. It is applied by carrying the horizontal portion around the pelvis and firmly securing the vertical strips behind, after being passed under the perineum and the dressings.

The Recurrent Bandage.—This bandage should be five yards long and two inches wide; it is applied to the head as follows:—The roller is first passed two or three times around the head in a line running just above the eyebrows, the ears, and below the occipital protuberance; next, at the centre of the forehead, the cylinder is reversed and

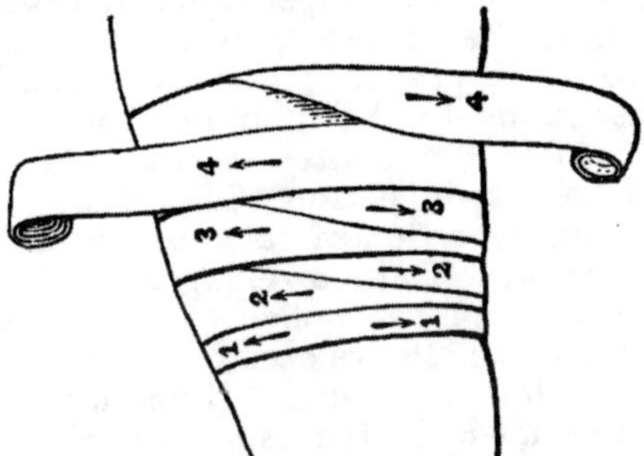

Fig. 23.

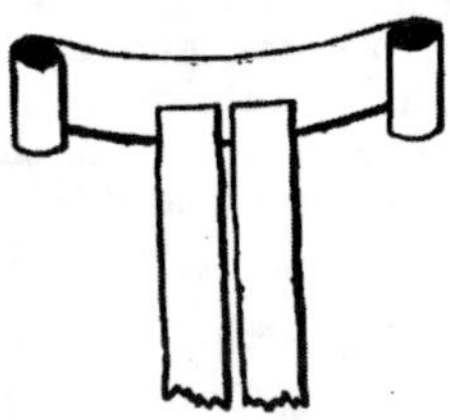

Fig. 24.

carried directly over the head to the circular turns behind, where it is again reversed, and carried back to the forehead, overlapping the former about one-third, as usual; these reverses to be continued until first one and then the other side of the head is covered; and the whole is completed by two or three firm circular turns, as at the commencement. The reverses are to be held by the fingers of an assistant.

Plaster of Paris.—The following description of the method of application of this dressing is given by Dr. James L. Little, House Surgeon to the New York Hospital:—The limb is first shaven or slightly oiled; a piece of old coarse washed muslin is next selected, of a size so that when folded about four thicknesses it is wide enough to envelop more than half of the circumference of the limb, and long enough to extend from a little below the under surface of the knee to about five inches below the heel. The solution of plaster is then to be prepared. Fine, well dried, white plaster should be selected, and, before using, a small portion should be mixed with water in a spoon and allowed "to set," with a view of ascertaining the length of time requisite for that process. If it is over five minutes, a small quantity of common salt may be dissolved in the water before adding the plaster. The more salt added, the sooner will the plaster "set." If delay be necessary, the addition of a few drops of carpenter's glue or mucilage will subserve that end. Equal parts of water and plaster are the best proportions. The plaster is sprinkled in the water and gradually mixed with it. The cloth, unfolded, is then immersed in the solution and well saturated; it is then to be quickly folded as before arranged, and laid on a flat surface, such as a board or a table, and smoothed once or twice with the hand in order to remove any irregularities of its surface, and then, with the help of an assistant, applied to the posterior surface of the limb. The portion extending below the heel is turned up on the sole of the foot, and the sides folded over the dorsum and a fold made at the ankle on either side, and a roller bandage applied pretty firmly over all. The limb is then to be held in a proper position (extension being made, if necessary, by the surgeon), until the plaster becomes hard. The time required in preparing the cloth, mixing the plaster, and applying the casing to the limb, need not take more than fifteen minutes. After the plaster is firm and the bandage removed, there will be a solid plaster of Paris case partially enveloping the limb, leaving a portion of its anterior surface exposed to view. If any swelling occurs, evaporating lotions can be applied to the exposed surface, and we can always easily determine the relation of the fractured ends. If necessary, an anterior splint, made of the same material, can be applied, and then both bound together with adhesive plaster, and if desirable a roller bandage over all.

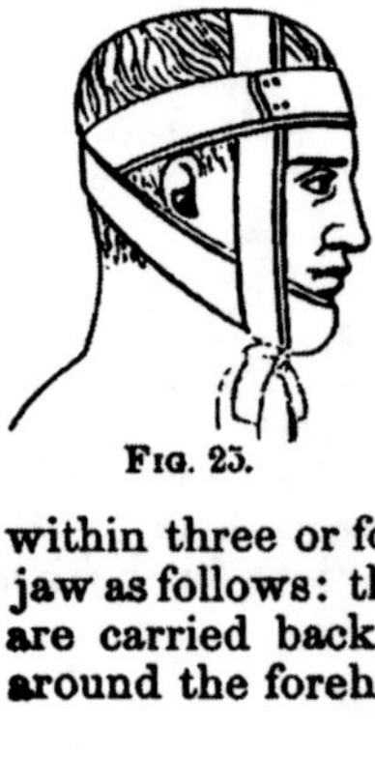

FIG. 25.

The Four-tailed Bandage.—This consists of a piece of muslin, six or eight inches wide, and a yard or more in length, torn at either extremity, to within three or four inches of the centre. It is applied to the lower jaw as follows: the centre being placed over the chin, the upper slips are carried back behind the neck and tied, or crossed and passed around the forehead once or twice, and secured by pins at the side;

the lower strip is passed directly up to the vertex, where it is tied, or again brought down and tied under the chin (Fig. 25).

Starch Bandage.—Take common starch, a sufficient quantity, and boil it in water a few minutes. In its application, 1. Envelop the limb with cotton wadding, so thickly applied as to cover all the prominences and fill the cavities; 2. Over this apply a roller well saturated with the starch; 3. Along the sides of the limb apply pasteboard splints of proper thickness, soaked in hot water, and nicely shaped to the limb; 4. Repeat the bandage twice, and saturate the whole with starch, rubbed in with the hands or a brush; 5. When the starch is completely dry, cut out a portion of its body, and bring the edges together with strong tapes, or leather straps with buckles.

STRAPPING.—Various kinds of plaster are in use, but the common adhesive strap is generally preferred. It should always be cut in the length of the material, to prevent the yielding which takes place in the width.

Strapping the Breast.—The straps should be cut sufficiently long to pass from the opposite shoulder, under the breast, to the point of starting, and in width about two inches; having the breast firmly raised, apply the end of the strap over the opposite shoulder, and pass it under the breast and axillæ, and over the back to the place of departure, allowing the ends to overlap (Fig. 26). Each successive strap should overlap the preceding towards the nipple, until the required compression or support is attained.

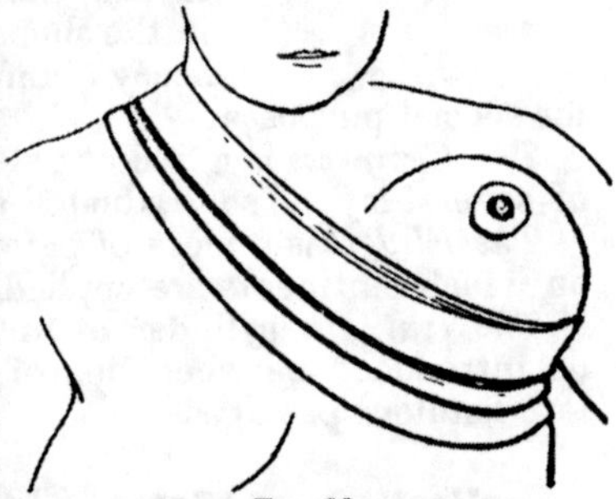

FIG. 26.

Strapping the Testicle.—The patient should first be placed in a recumbent position, to relieve venous congestion; then shave the hair cleanly from the parts; the straps being cut into pieces of one-half or two-thirds of an inch in width, and eight or nine inches long, grasp the testicle with the left hand, and compress it firmly to the bottom of the scrotum; now pass one strip around the gland, at its upper part, as tightly as it can be borne; from this as a basis commence and pass the straps vertically around the organ, overlapping slightly, until it is covered. Mr. Curling gives the following directions:—"The patient being placed in the recumbent position, with the testicle raised, is to remain there three or four minutes, in order to allow the vessels of the gland to become as empty as possible. The parts are to be shaved; and some adhesive plaster or chamois leather must be cut into strips, about three-quarters of an inch in width, and eight or nine inches in length. The opposite testicle and side of the scrotum being drawn away from the diseased one, so as to render the integuments of the latter quite tense, the first strap is to be placed circularly (Fig. 27) around the cord, just above the testicle, as tightly as the patient can bear it. A strip of lint may be placed beneath the edge of the plaster to prevent its irritating the scrotum. The second strap is to be placed in an opposite direction, from behind forwards, at the side of the testicle, near the septum. The third strap is to be applied below the first, so as partly to overlap it; and the fourth in like manner, internal to the second, and so on until the straps meet, and the whole of the testicle is covered and evenly compressed."

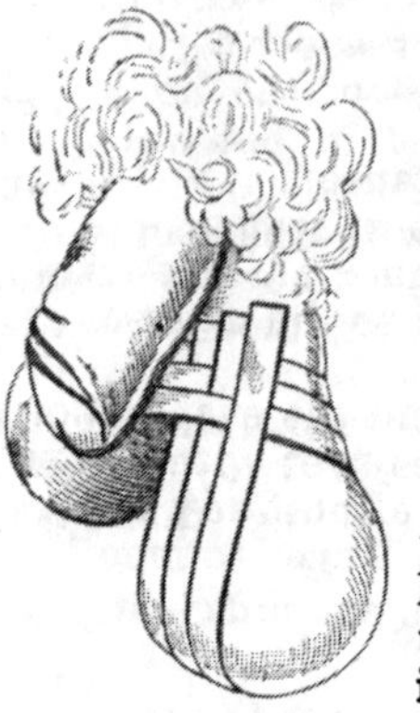
FIG. 27.

Lint.—The material used for dressing is for the most part lint. It is prepared by scraping linen, or by ravelling old linen thread by thread, the French Charpie. It is now found in the shops as *patent* lint, having one surface fleecy. Lint is arranged into different forms for special purposes:—

The Compress is a fold of patent lint or muslin, or it may consist of several layers, so graduated as to make a conical body.

The Pledget is a piece of patent lint, shaped to the wound, and on which ointments are applied.

The Tent is a cylinder of lint of any desired length, designed to be introduced between lips of wounds to prevent adhesion, or into fistulous passages.

Applications of Water.—The employment of water in surgery has been most intelligently discussed by M. Amussat, in his thesis on that subject. We condense the general principles of its application in practice from the translation of Prof. Hamilton.

Water-Dressings.—That these may prove useful, and be exempt from the inconveniences heretofore urged against them, they must fulfil the following indications:—1. They must permit the pus to escape freely as fast as it is formed, and to be absorbed by the dressings. 2. They must be kept constantly moist. 3. Evaporation must be prevented, lest the part should become chilled, or in other words a uniform temperature must be preserved. We have accomplished these several indications by a water dressing, formed of four pieces of different tissues regularly superposed, which pieces may be called respectively the *sifter* (*crible*), the *absorbent*, the *humectant*, and the *inevaporant.*

Sifter.—The sifter is a tissue perforated with a great number of holes, to allow the pus to escape as fast as it is formed, and to separate the wound from the substance which absorbs the purulent matter. Common tulle, with very open tissue, perfectly answers the indication. If tulle cannot be obtained, we may use linen with larger and more frequent perforations, or strips of linen arranged in quadrille form, with larger spaces than are usually left.

Absorbent.—Isolation of the wound being obtained, the best means of absorbing the pus as fast as it is formed, are old rags from linen or cotton, sufficiently worn; place a disk of proper size, after having moistened it with tepid water, over the sifter. This piece of dressing has received the name of *absorbent.*

Humectation.—The best humectant, or substance for retaining moisture, is punk (*amadou*), prepared without saltpetre or gunpowder. This substance, with very little volume, absorbs much water, is soft to the touch, and yields its water to the sifter more easily than sponge, flannel, lint, or cotton.

Inevaporant or Impermeable Tissue.—To prevent the evaporation of the liquid as much as possible, the compresses, wet with water, must be covered with an impermeable tissue. Almost any impermeable tissue will answer the purpose, but it is proper to mention that as in the country the means are not always so abundant, a hog's bladder soaked in oil does very well. If we desire to prevent the evaporation completely, we must not neglect to make this cover larger than the other portions of the dressing, otherwise there will be along the borders of the dressing a slow evaporation, producing a coldness, especially in winter. Dressings of the fingers, of the great toes, and of the penis, ought to be completely enveloped in the impermeable tissue so as to form a sac within which the moisture shall be retained. A piece of intestine, caoutchouc, or oiled silk, made into a sac, and placed over the member, will serve an excellent purpose. An emollient effect being that which we wish generally to produce, we ordinarily use in these cases soft and tepid water at a temperature of 64° or 77° F. The liquid acquires soon the temperature of the part, especially if the impermeable tissue completely envelops the dressings; but if it does not, evaporation occurs, and a sense of chilliness results.

The time during which the application is to be continued without renewal, must vary according to the effects which we wish to obtain, and according to the state of the parts. If the inflammation is active, the dressing should be often renewed, and so also if the production of pus is very abundant. In simple cases, however, it will be sufficient to change the dressing every four or six hours. When we wish to discontinue the water-dressing, it must not be done suddenly, but gradually, so as not to incur the hazard of a return of accidents. We must begin by diminishing the quantity of water employed in moistening the dressings, and then little by little make it cease altogether.

Compared with other modes of dressing, the water-dressing is infinitely superior to cataplasms. We observe that in the great majority of cases it possesses all their advantages without their inconveniences, and as it can be easily maintained without being disturbed, it saves much pain to the patients.

Irrigation.—Irrigation is the uniform flow of liquids over tissues.

Amussat gives the following rules:—A sufficiently large vessel, of zinc or earthenware, is placed upon an elevated piece of furniture, near the bed; an elastic syphon, furnished with a stopcock, guides the water from the reservoir upon the tissues. The part undergoing irrigation is quite insulated by the aid of a gutter, or of impermeable cloth so arranged as that the water does not moisten the neighboring parts, and escapes freely into a vessel placed near. A compress placed upon the member, serves to disperse the water uniformly. Ordinarily we adapt to the extremity of the syphon tubes, a strip of linen divided into bandalets which serve not only to direct the liquid, but principally to obviate its dynamic effect. Once mounted, this apparatus works of itself, provided that care is taken to prevent the vessel from becoming empty, so that the flow of water may not be intermittent. We ought also to be particular in relation to the cleanliness and especially the temperature of the water, which should always be uniform, and not cause any disagreeable sensation to the patient. When we wish to submit an extensive surface to continued and abundant irrigation, we ought to employ an apparatus which discharges its water in several streams, rather than one which is furnished with a single large conductor. In fact, when the water flows in a large stream it becomes warmer as it passes over the tissues, and the whole surface is not submitted to a uniform temperature. If continued irrigations are to be made in any case with cold or iced water, it will be best to commence with tepid water, and gradually lower the temperature. In pursuance of the principle which we have sought to establish, we ought to be exceedingly careful that the temperature of the water is not suddenly changed, and especially that its current is not interrupted, for a severe inflammatory reaction might result. When it is thought proper to suspend the water, its temperature should be gradually raised, and we ought even, as Cloquet advises, to apply it for only a few hours each day before withholding it completely. The quantity of water should be regulated by the degree of inflammation; that is to say, if it is feeble a continued moisture will suffice; if very intense, on the contrary, the fluid should be poured upon it very rapidly, inundating, so to speak, the part, especially if the water used has a temperature of 64° or 68° F. This liquid placed in contact with the tissues subtracts morbid caloric, and the more there is developed, the more water should be poured on, taking care, however, that the temperature is not too much below the standard of health. The irrigation ought to be made not only upon the part wounded, but also upon a considerable extent of surface about; without this precaution, serious accidents may occur, in parts supposed to be at first sound, and when no inflammation is developed at the point of injury which is submitted to the action of the water.

It is difficult to fix the proper duration of irrigations, for it must depend upon the nature of the affection, the temperament of the patient, the stage, whether acute or chronic, of the malady.

Those who employ cold or iced water, are in the habit of suspending it when the patient complains of a feeling of cold in the part submitted to its action; but we must not be too hasty, for M. Josse tells us "that under these circumstances he had but too often seen the inflammation reproduced in all its former intensity;" and we have ourselves often verified the justness of this remark. It will be advisable, then, not to suspend the application of the water, but gradually to raise its temperature until the patient no longer experiences any disagreeable sensation, and not to change the treatment until all chance of inflammation has disappeared. When we use tepid water we may continue the irrigation a much longer time, since the process of reparation of traumatic lesions goes on very regularly under its influence.

Immersion.—Immersion is the act of plunging the body, or some portion of it, into a liquid; in a word, it is a bath, either general or local. This method of applying water is exceedingly simple for lesions of the forearm or hand, and for the leg or foot. It is only necessary to place near the patient a vessel containing water of a mild and agreeable temperature, into which the part may be completely plunged. Care must be taken that the temperature of the liquid does not sensibly vary, and that it is renewed sufficiently often to keep it clean. In order to determine the variations of temperature of the water, so that it may be renewed at the proper moment, we should use a thermometer; and for the greater convenience we may adapt two tubes to the bath, the one for the admission and the other for the escape of the fluid. As to the position of the part undergoing an immersion, we can only say that we must always have regard to the escape of the pus and the return of the venous blood. Water at 64° or 68° F., more or less, is generally preferable to cold water.

The duration of the immersions must vary much, according to the degree, extent, and depth of the inflammation, and it is impossible to establish precise rules; nevertheless, they ought to be prolonged sufficiently to insure against a return of the inflammation, and then they should be discontinued gradually, replacing them at first with water dressings. To avoid the inconvenience of absolute confinement of the patient, we may in certain cases, as in lesions of the fingers and penis for example, use a pig's bladder or a caoutchouc bag, filled with water, into which the part may be immersed and secured. In the most severe surgical accidents, we should commence, if possible, with immersions or irrigations, or both, and terminate with water-dressings.

In comparing the three principal modes, we observe that the *water-dressing*, if properly made and often renewed, is generally more simple, and more easily applied, than immersion or irrigation; that it has, moreover, the advantage of taking off at each dressing the pus and the stratum formed by a mixture of the purulent matter and the substances contained in the water; the granulations are thus kept always red, &c. *Irrigation* is more powerful than water-dressing, but more difficult, and sometimes even impossible to apply. *Immersion* is more powerful than either, more prompt, and in all respects superior whenever it can be properly applied.

HÆMORRHAGE.

Hæmorrhage must be guarded against before, and suppressed during and after operations.

Prevention.—Hæmorrhage is prevented before operations by controlling the circulation in the arteries leading to the part. This may be accomplished by ligating the vessel, as hereafter described, or by pressure by the following means:—

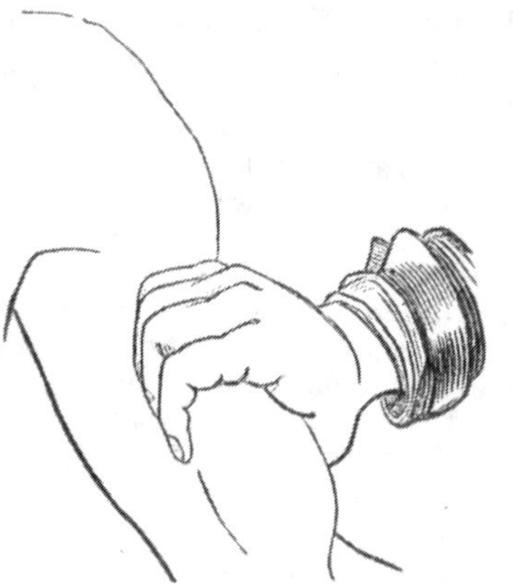

FIG. 28.

Manual Pressure. — Pressure may be made in the course of the vessel with the fingers. They are to be accurately applied, and the artery must be compressed steadily against a bone (Fig. 28); if the thumb is used, it must be laid flat upon the vessel; in either case the pressure must not be relaxed; if the vessel slips from the grasp it should be instantly compressed again upon the bone by the fingers or thumb, but not by grasping the limb. The fingers are best employed in compression of the brachial, the radial, and the ulnar arteries; the thumb in compressing the abdominal against the vertebræ, the external iliac against the brim of the pelvis, the femoral against the pubes, or in the upper part of the thigh.

The Key.—A common door key is sometimes used, the ring being so padded as to make a hard mass. It is chiefly used in compression of the subclavian above the clavicle.

The Tourniquet.—The tourniquet is an instrument designed to make such pressure over an artery, at some point in its course, as to control the circulation. There are many varieties, which differ principally in the extent to which they affect the venous circulation. In some, as that of Signorini, pressure is made only at two points, the intervening part of the leg being free. The old tourniquet of Petit (Fig. 29), however, has never been surpassed in reliability. In its application it is usual to put several turns of a roller around the limb at the point where it is applied, terminating with placing the cylinder of the roller over the artery; the tourniquet should now be applied, but the screw should not be placed over the cylinder lest the ball roll from the artery when the screw is worked. The screw being placed at one side of the limb (Fig.

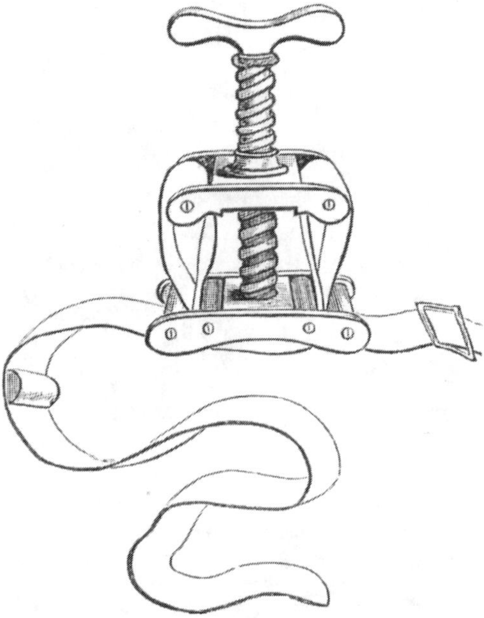

FIG. 29.

30), the strap should be buckled tightly, and the screw gradually turned to the necessary tightness.

Twisted Handkerchief.—If a tourniquet is not at hand, as in military practice, and the fingers cannot be used, a handkerchief or cord cast around the limb and tied, may be sufficiently twisted with a stick to answer the purpose. In the Prussian service, simple tourniquets, without a pad, and consisting of only a strap and buckle to hold it, as in the upper figure (Fig. 31), are supplied to the troops in great numbers, and answer an admirable purpose. A more complete form used in the same service, is represented in the two lower illustrations (Fig. 31).

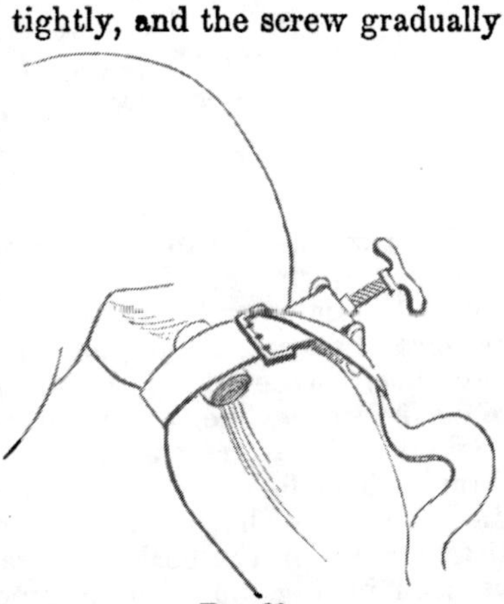

FIG. 30.

The tourniquet can be applied only to the femoral and brachial arteries, but in these positions it cannot be surpassed in efficiency.

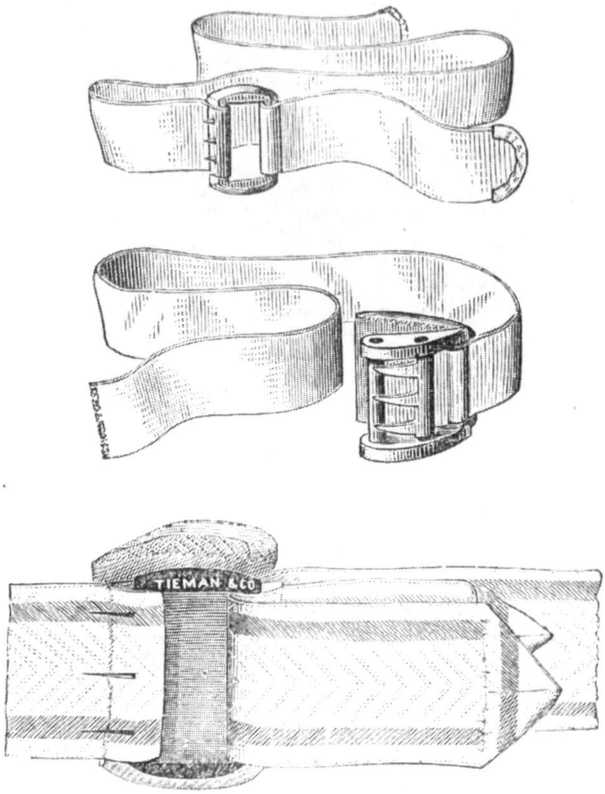

Fig. 31.

Suppression.—During an operation hæmorrhage is most promptly and directly suppressed by the fingers of an assistant. They should follow the knife, and make firm pressure upon the bleeding points, or seize the vessel, especially if an artery. Various instruments have been invented for this purpose, consisting for the most part of small forceps, like the serrefines (Fig. 8). One of the most convenient is the artery clamp of Dr. Stearns, surgeon in the U. S. Army. The following is a description of this instrument (*Am. Med. Times*):—The instrument resembles a slender pair of dentists' forceps, in the beak or jaws of which are two short grooves, as seen in Fig. 33. These grooves are designed to hold little horse-shoe shaped clamps, of any convenient size, *c′ c″ c‴* (Fig.

34.) The clamps are made of annealed or passive iron wire (gauge, 15, 16, or 17). Between the handles of the forceps there is a spring, *s s′* (Fig. 32), the action of which is to draw the handles together, and so prevent the clamp from falling out of its place, without the necessity of constant pressure on the handles by the hand of the operator. The forceps with a wire clamp in its jaws (Fig. 32) is ready for use; and may be applied instantaneously to a bleeding vessel. By simply thrusting the points of the clamp astride of the open mouth of the artery, and *then* compressing the handles of the forceps with a *moderate* force, the artery becomes securely gripped between the points of the wire clamp. Then by expanding the handles of the forceps, the wire clamp (as seen in Fig. 34, *C*) is left tightly clinging to the closed mouth of the artery. The annealed iron wire used for the clamps, is wholly devoid of elasticity, and makes what would be called in mechanical phrase, a "dead pinch" on any substance on which it is compressed. Dentists and jewellers make frequent use of this sort of wire clamp to hold their work together while soldering under the blow-pipe. These clamps, therefore, have no resemblance to the "serrefines" or to Liston's elastic figure-8-shaped wire instruments.

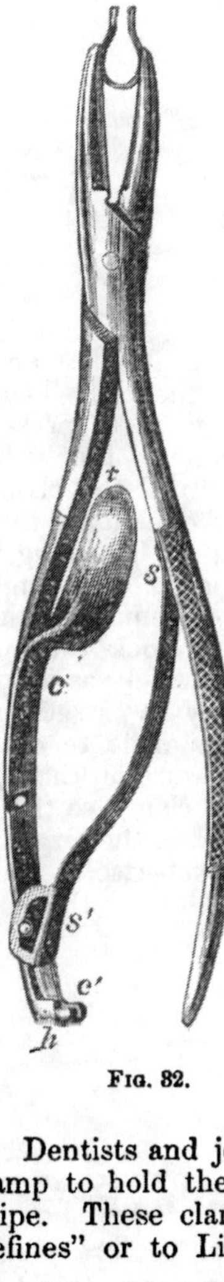

FIG. 32.

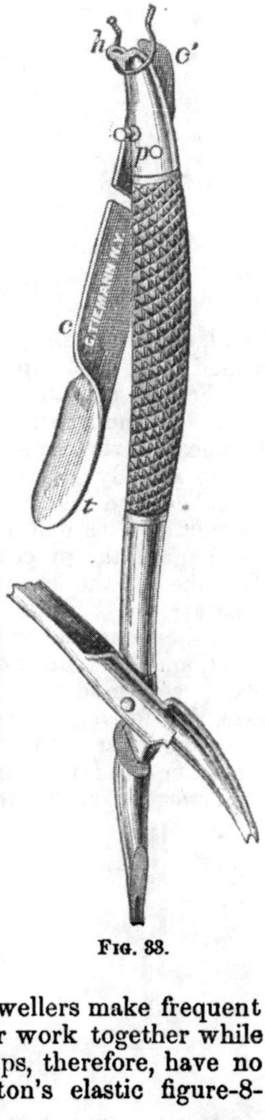

FIG. 33.

To the inside of one of the handles of the forceps (as seen in Fig. 33), is added a contrivance for *removing* the clamp, when necessary. It is a lever, *c c′*, moving on a pivot, *p*, with a thumb-piece, *t*, at one end, and a blunt hook, *h*, paired with a similar blunt hook at the end of the handle, and which, when closed, may be hooked within the loop of the clamp, and then by pressure on the thumb-piece, *t*, the two hooks separate and force open the clamp, so that it loses its hold on the flesh, and can be drawn away. Surgeons can, in a few minutes, accustom themselves to the use of this instrument, by compressing the clamps on the fold of the skin between the thumb and forefinger of the left hand; or by practising upon a bit of small-sized rubber tubing; or, what is better still, by partially clenching the left hand, so as to form a conical hollow, and then taking the fōrceps, armed with a clamp, in the right hand, pass it down deep into the hollow of the left, so as to press strongly against the skin over the metacarpal bone of the little finger, and compress the handles of the forceps, until the clamp is felt to bite or pinch pretty smartly; then, by expanding the handles, the instrument is detached, and the clamp is left, clinging firmly to a fold of the palmar skin, as will be seen on opening the hand. Closing the hand again, the process of removing the clamp may be practised. To take off the clamp, unhook the end of the spring at *s*, and separate the handles as widely as they can be; then that handle with the thumb lever may be passed down into the hollow of the hand, and the blunt hooks made to enter the loop of the adhering clamp, with moderate pressure on the thumb-piece the hooks separate, thus forcing open the clamp, so that it can be withdrawn. The instruments are of two sizes, the larger for the operating case, and a smaller size for the pocket-case.

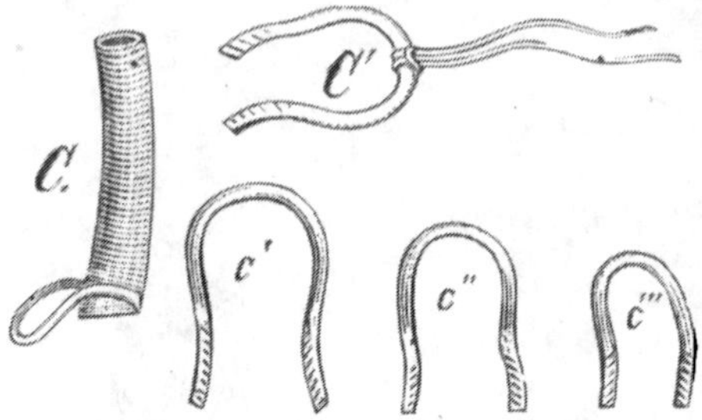

FIG. 34.

Torsion.—Arteries which have their coats lacerated do not bleed.

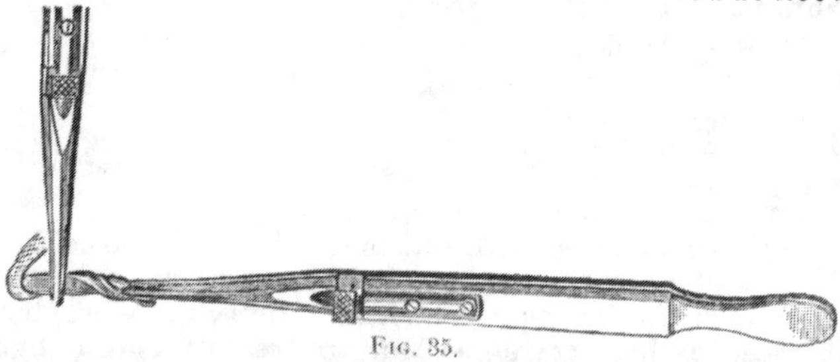

FIG. 35.

By torsion we design to effect this laceration of the coats of an artery. It is accomplished by seizing the vessel with one pair of forceps, and dragging it down an inch or more; with a second pair of forceps it is separated from the surrounding parts; the vessel is then grasped firmly as high up as possible, transversely to its diameter, with well grooved sliding forceps, and with another pair its extremity is seized and rotated upon its axis, three to eight times, according to its size (Fig. 35). It is always necessary to hold the artery firmly at a given point above the extremity, otherwise the coats may not be lacerated.

Ligature.—The ligature is used to control arterial hæmorrhage. It is made of silk, linen, hemp, or it may be metallic, as silver wire. The silk ligature is generally used, and the best is that known as dentists' silk; for larger arteries it should be three-threaded, and so strong as to bear the full force of the fingers in tightening the knot, without yielding; hemp and linen make excellent ligatures; silver wire has also been used, and the ends cut off close, with good results. When the common ligature is applied the artery may be hooked up with the tenaculum (Fig. 36) and drawn

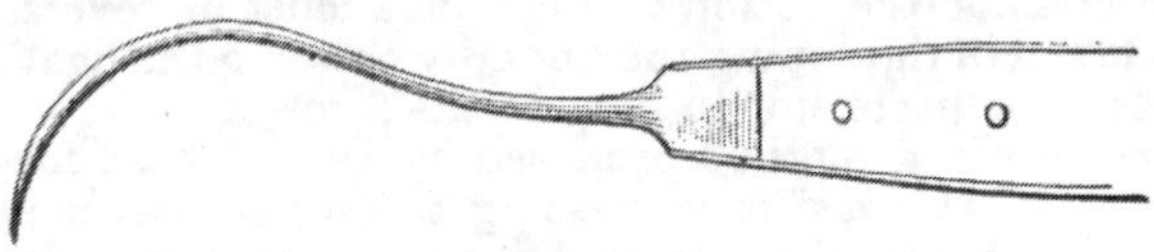

FIG. 36.

out from the surface of the wound; or the artery forceps (Fig. 37)

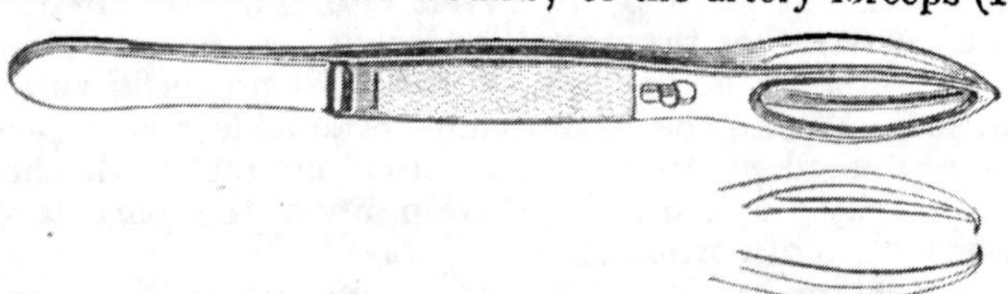

FIG. 37.

having rounded blades, and a pair of small forceps with dog-teeth, and having a slide or catch by which they can be maintained closed, will be found useful. Whatever instrument is used, the artery

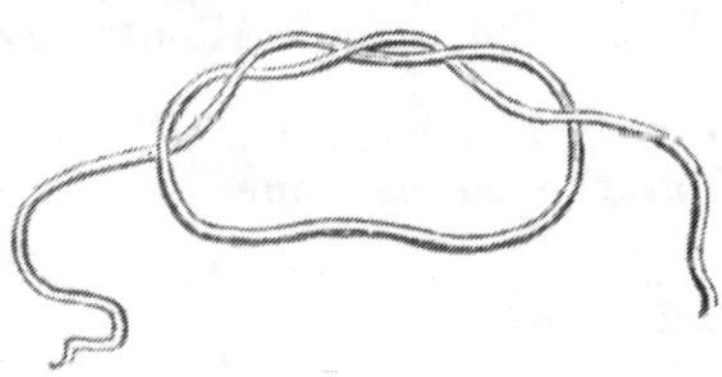

FIG. 38.

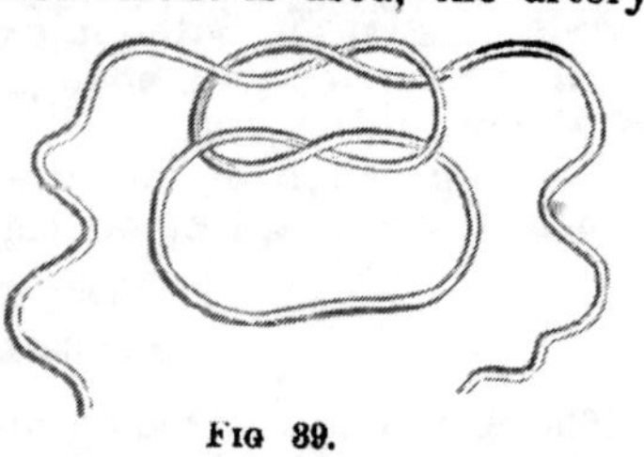

FIG 39.

should be seized, drawn out, and separated from surrounding tissues, and the ligature applied. There are two kinds of knots, called the surgeon's (Fig. 38), and the reef or sailor's knot (Fig. 39). The surgeon's knot has the advantage of not loosening while the second knot is being tied, but is liable not to be tightly applied when the knot is completed. The reef knot is generally to be preferred. It will be noticed that this knot differs from the ordinary knot in this, that both ends of the thread pass over or under the respective loop, while in the ordinary knot one passes over and the other under. To tie the reef knot readily observe the following rules:—Holding the ligature between the thumb and finger of the right hand, throw the end around the forceps, and seize the body of the ligature between the middle and ring finger of the left hand, in a prone position, the end being grasped between the thumb and index finger; then draw the thread in the right hand over the end of the left index finger and the extremity of the ligature, and pass it between the ends of the index and middle fingers; now taking the end of the ligature from the grasp of the left index finger and thumb with the right index finger and thumb, the knot is completed by drawing out the portion passed between the left index and middle finger. In tying the second knot the action of the hands must be reversed. Care must be taken in tightening the knot, by pressing the ligature firmly down upon the parts, not to include the forceps.

Acupressure is a method proposed by Dr. Simpson for arresting hæmorrhage. It consists in passing a long slender needle under the artery and into the tissues beyond, in such a manner as by the elasticity of the needle to exert sufficient pressure to control the circulation. It is to be removed after two or three days, or when it is certain that the vessel is closed.

Cold may be regarded as one of the most powerful and reliable hæmostatics. Where the hæmorrhage is considerable ice should be used, so protected as to prevent actual contact with the parts. Iced water may be allowed to drain upon the part through a syphon or a strip of porous cloth.

Styptics.—Alum, matico, gallic acid, tincture of the sesquichloride of iron, nitrate of silver, turpentine, and other similar agents are employed for this purpose. But that which is now most relied on is the persulphate of iron, or Monsel's salt, which has the power of controlling hæmorrhages by its local application, and by its internal administration, without exciting any inflammatory action. It should be applied with sponge or lint. The surgeon should never be without this agent.

The application of the *actual cautery* has been a most reliable means of arresting hæmorrhage from the earliest time.

BLOODLETTING.

The abstraction of blood is divided into general and local bleeding.

General Bleeding.—In general bleeding, blood may be drawr from the veins, when the operation is called *venesection*; or fron the arteries, when it is known as *arteriotomy*.

Lancets differ as to their points; some are very blunt, others are very acute; the more obtuse are generally used when the vessel is superficial, and the more acute when it is deeply seated.

VENESECTION.—Blood may be taken from any of the superficial veins, but those of the neck, the bend of the arm, and at the ankle, are generally selected. The patient may be seated or recumbent, but in general the position should be chosen which most enlarges the vessels. The operation should commence by stopping the flow of blood to the heart by a ligature applied around the part on the proximal side of the point selected for the operation, sufficiently firm to close the veins and still leave the arteries unobstructed. The veins now become prominent unless the person is very fleshy, when the position of the vein must be determined by its corded feel. The operation is performed by placing the thumb of the left hand firmly on the vein (Fig. 40), a little to the distal side, to prevent the vessel from rolling aside on the attempt to puncture it. The lancet, held between the thumb and index finger of the right hand, the blade at an obtuse angle with the hand, is plunged into the vein obliquely to its transverse diameter, and the hand being fixed, the point of the lancet is elevated so as to cut its way out.

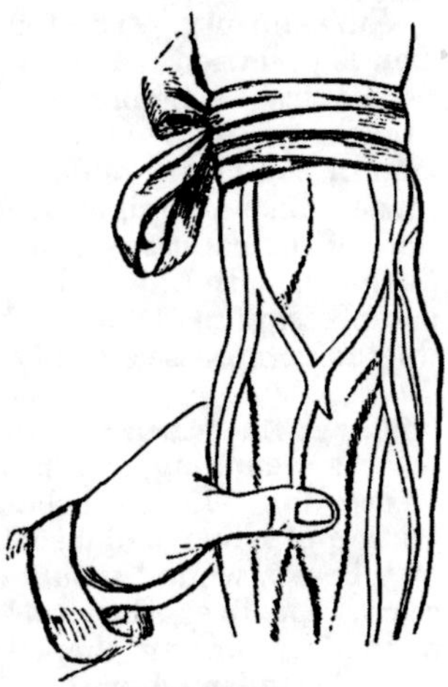

FIG. 40.

The success of the operation is determined by the flow; if this should be slight, it may be due to too small an orifice, which should then be enlarged; or to a mass of protruding fat, which may be pushed aside. If an increased flow is required the patient should be directed to grasp repeatedly the staff, or the operator may rub the limb from the wrist towards the elbow.

When the proper amount of blood is drawn the band should be removed, and a small compress being placed over the wound, a figure-of-eight bandage is applied; to prevent air entering the circulation in bleeding from the jugular, pressure on the wound should be made before the compress is removed.

Venesection is generally performed either on the external jugular, the median basilic or cephalic, or the internal saphena.

External Jugular.—A compress is placed over the vein in the supra-clavicular fossa, and firmly retained by a bandage passed over it and under the opposite axilla; the index finger of the left hand is placed upon the vein above, and the incision is made upwards and outwards across the platysma myoides.

Median Basilic and Cephalic.—The cephalic vein may be selected on account of its isolation. The basilic is the largest, but the brachial artery passing directly under it is in danger of being wounded. The position of the artery must first be determined. A band is then passed firmly around the arm, above the elbow, and with his hand the patient grasps a staff. The operator, standing in front of the patient, grasps the arm with the left hand, placing the thumb on the distended vein, and the fingers on the back of the elbow, and holding the lancet in the right, opens the vessel.

Internal Saphena.—The foot is first placed in a vessel of warm water to distend the veins; a band is then passed around the leg, just above the malleoli; the thumb being placed on the vein it is opened just above the inner ankle, with an oblique incision.

Arteriotomy.—The temporal artery is that on which this operation is practised. It may be opened just over the zygoma, in front of the tragus, before its division into the anterior and posterior branches, but the anterior branch is generally selected. The position of the artery is determined by its pulsations; the skin being made tense a straight incision is made with a scalpel, involving a part of the calibre of the vessel; when a sufficient amount of blood has been withdrawn the artery should be completely divided, and compression made on either side of the incision with small graduated compresses, firmly retained with a bandage.

Local Bleeding.—The local abstraction of blood is effected by leeching, cupping, scarification, and punctures.

Leeching.—Leeches should not be applied to parts liable to infiltration of blood, and discoloration, as the eyelids, scrotum, prepuce, or where a wound would disfigure, as their bites sometimes leave scars, nor over the track of a superficial vein. They are best applied by placing them in a small glass vessel, and inverting it over the inflamed part; blood, or sweetened milk, is often put on the skin. A single leech can take about an ounce of blood. When removed, the parts may be fomented to increase the flow; if it is desired to stop the blood the bites may be sprinkled with flour, starch, or other absorbent material; if the flow of blood continues astringents are used, of which the best is the persulphate of iron.

Cupping.—Cupping requires a scarificator and cupping-glass. The scarificator is an instrument containing eight or twelve blades, moved by a single spring, and so arranged as to be readily graduated as to the depth which they shall penetrate. They cover but the small space of an inch and a half or two inches square, and make eight, twelve, or more parallel cuts. The cupping-glass may be simple tin or glass, of the proper size and shape, and applied by exhausting the air within by burning a few drops of alcohol; or it may have an exhausting pump attached to the top; or, finally, it may have an india-rubber top, which requires only to be squeezed to produce a vacuum. The latter cups have but lately come into use, and are preferable to any other.

Scarification.—In making scarifications, the lancet, scalpel, or bistoury should be used, and the cuts should be made only partially or entirely through the skin, as may be necessary to promote the local abstraction of blood. The incisions should generally be made the entire length of the inflamed part, and within an inch of each other. The flow of blood may be greatly increased by warm fomentations.

Puncturing.—Punctures are made with a straight sharp-pointed bistoury, or a common lancet. The instrument is thrust into the inflamed tissues, to a depth varying from an eighth of an inch to an inch, carefully avoiding vessels and nerves. They should be repeated until the entire surface is relieved of tension. Warm fomentations will increase the depleting effect.

COUNTER-IRRITANTS.

Seton.—The seton may consist of a few threads or a full skein of silk, according to the effects desired; or a piece of tape, or, what is now more frequently used, on account of cleanliness, a strip of india-rubber cloth. The instruments required for its introduction are either the seton needle (Fig. 41) or a straight bistoury, with a probe having an eye. The skin being pinched up in a fold corresponding with the direction of the muscles of the part, or vertical with the body, the seton needle, armed with the seton, is passed deeply through the parts, but without involving tendons or muscles; the seton drawn through should be tied loosely.

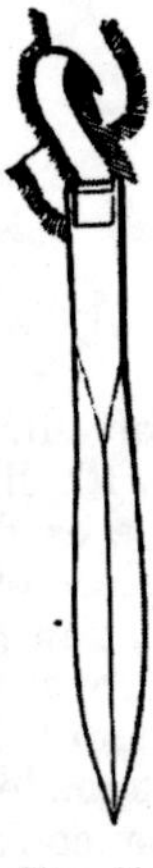

FIG. 41.

If the bistoury and eyed-probe are used, the integuments are first pinched up and transfixed with the bistoury (Fig. 42); the probe having the seton passed through the eye, or attached by a thread (Fig. 43), is then passed through the wound, and the seton is tied. The subsequent dressings consist of either a common poultice at once, or a simple fold of greased lint, and a bandage around the part to be exchanged for a poultice when suppuration commences.

Issue.—An issue, being an ulcer produced by the surgeon, may be made with caustics, or with an incision kept open by irritating applications to the part. The caustic may be the actual cautery, or Vienna paste, or other powerful escharotics. In shape the iron cautery should have a more or less flattened surface, when it is required to produce a superficial slough, or conical when it is required to penetrate more deeply (Fig. 44). If it is applied at a white heat, and firmly pressed upon the part until an eschar is formed, although not severely painful, anæsthetics are very often used; cold water dressings should be applied for several hours, followed by moist warm applications, as a poultice, until the slough separates.

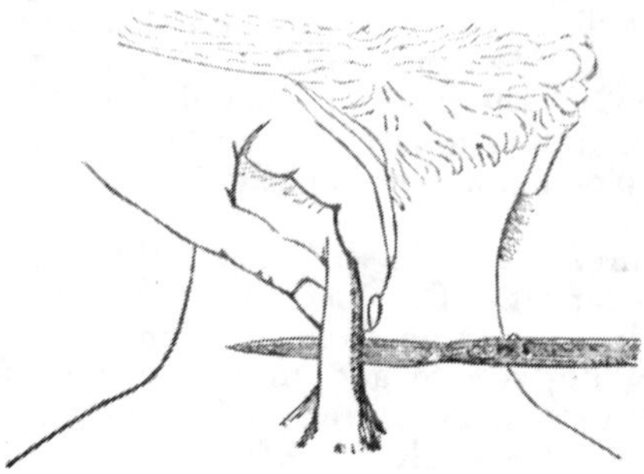

FIG. 42.

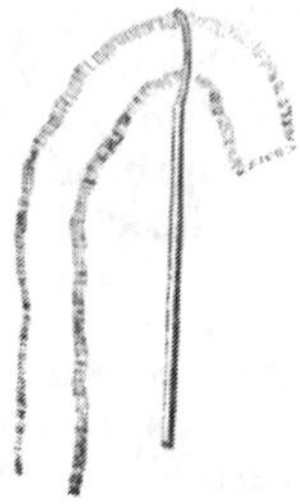

FIG. 43.

Of escharotics the Vienna paste, prepared by triturating equal parts of quicklime and caustic potassa, is generally used; it is applied to the part, of the required size, and allowed to remain ten

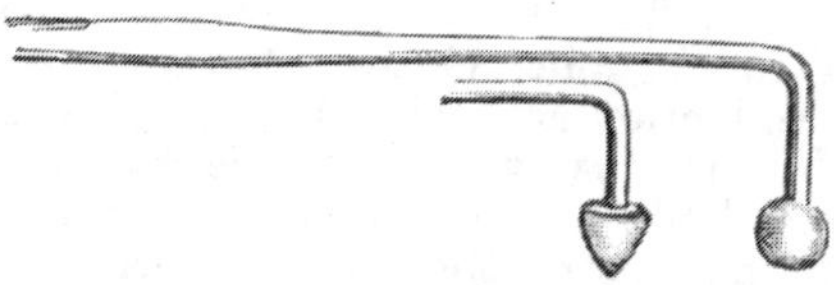

FIG. 44.

or fifteen minutes, when it is removed, and the surface washed with diluted vinegar, to counteract its action. Caustic potassa may be used in a similar manner, the parts being circumscribed by a piece of adhesive plaster, through an opening in which the application is made. Strong sulphuric acid also makes an issue of the proper depth, its effect being controlled by an alkali. The subsequent dressings are poultices, already described. When an issue is made with the knife, the incision must penetrate into the subcutaneous cellular tissue, and a foreign body, as a pea, or a grain of corn, is introduced and retained by adhesive straps until suppuration is established.

Moxa.—The moxa is a combustible substance, which is burned upon the surface of the body, for the purpose of counter-irritation. It may be composed of lint, carded cotton, hemp, agaric, &c., or the lint may be saturated with the nitrate of potassa. Whatever substance is selected should be firmly rolled into a pyramidal form, and held together by threads, or a solution of gum arabic; it should be an inch or an inch and a half long, and of a diameter at the base corresponding with the size of the proposed eschar. The moxa is held in position with forceps or wire, and is ignited at the top; as it burns down, any desired degree of irritation can be obtained from a simple redness to a deep eschar, according to the time it is maintained in contact with the skin. The combustion can be intensified with the blowpipe. The resulting pain may be mitigated by the application of aqua ammonia, or cold. The eschar which follows the complete combustion of the moxa upon the surface separates under the poultice in about a week.

Acupuncture.—This is a method of counter-irritation effected by passing slender needles into the part, and allowing them to remain from a few minutes to several hours. The needle should be of steel, from two to four inches in length, polished, very sharp-pointed, flexible, and soft, having a metallic head (Fig. 45). They are inserted by making the skin tense with the left hand, and with the right introducing the needle, with a rotatory motion, to the required depth, avoiding joints and viscera. They may safely penetrate several inches, and have even been introduced into viscera without ill effects. They are liable to become oxidized, and on removing them pressure should be made upon the adjoining surface, while the needle is rotated slightly.

Electro- and Galvano-Puncture.—The design of this operation is to introduce electricity and galvanism to deep tissues. The needles used have a small ring (Fig. 45) to which the wire of the pole of the battery is attached. In their application two needles are introduced, one at either extremity of the organ, and the two are then connected with the poles of the battery.

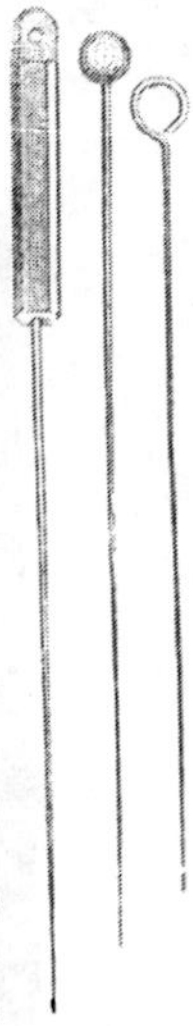

FIG. 45.

VACCINATION.

The following description of the various instruments employed in vaccination, was drawn up by Dr. Loines, House Physician of the Eastern Dispensary, New York, whose familiarity with this practice entitles his advice to confidence:

"The rationale of vaccination is as follows, viz. Vaccine virus should be exposed to the absorbent vessels when they are in a proper state for absorption: to produce this state, or to open these vessels, that instrument which causes the least irritation, and the least flow of blood, is by far the best, as both the flow of blood and the irritation of the skin are likely to carry off the virus before it can be properly taken up; moreover, that which causes the least pain is preferable.

"*The Narrow Bladed Lancet* (Fig. 46).—This is a lancet of peculiar construction, somewhat resembling the common exploring needle, narrow, pointed, and sharp, convex on one side of the cutting part of the blade, and plane on the other. This instrument may be used like the common lancet in introducing any kind of vaccine to the absorbents. In employing dried lymph in vaccination, such as is usually supplied upon a section of a quill or a piece of ivory, proceed with the point of this lancet to pick out ten or twelve minute particles of cuticle from the arm, in a circle of not more than one third of an inch in diameter, so as to expose the true skin, and in the fluid which exudes therefrom dissolve and commingle the dried lymph by gentle friction over the punctured surface. Many persons will acquire such dexterity with this instru-

*Instruments for Vaccination.**

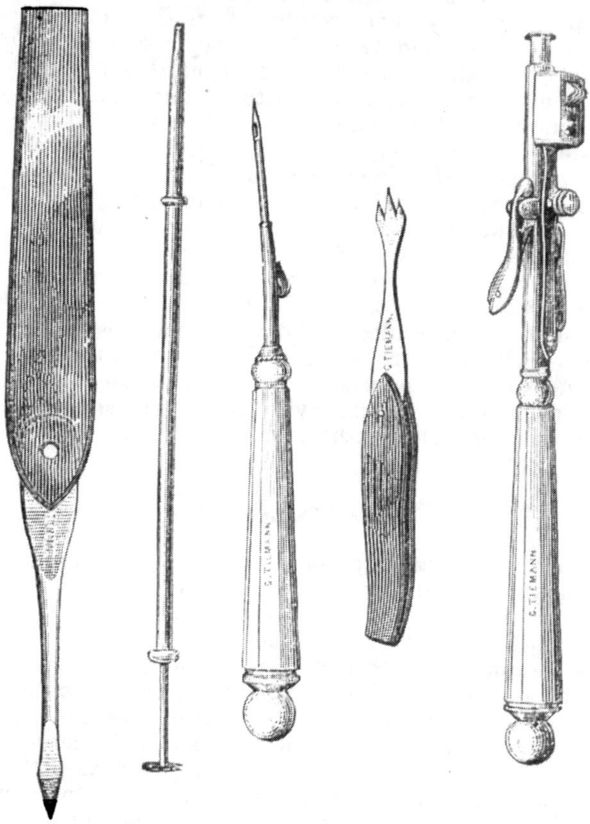

FIG. 46. FIG. 47. FIG. 48. FIG. 49. FIG. 50.

ment, that by a single gentle push, with its convex side next to the skin, they will be able to lay over, as it were, a furrow of cuticle, and thus, with but little cutting and with scarcely any

* The two first instruments are shown in the engravings of their actual size, the remaining three are but two-thirds of it.

danger of puncturing too deeply, expose a comparatively large absorbent surface. This instrument may also be advantageously used by those who do not possess the Syringe Self-Vaccinator (Fig. 48), to make a valvular incision under the skin, into which a minute piece of scab may be inserted by means of a needle or a probe, or by means of what is better, the instrument to be next described.

" *The Syringe Vaccinator* (Fig. 47).—This consists of a cylinder of metal, three inches long, with a closely fitting piston, which, when pushed its whole length through, it projects an eighth of an inch from the cylinder itself. By means of this instrument, a small piece of the vaccine scab, or a small quantity of the same pulverized or fluid lymph with which the cylinder is to be first charged, can be pushed into the valvular openings or cuts in the arm, previously made for it.

" *The Syringe Self-Vaccinator* (Fig. 48).—In its uses this instrument presents a combination of the two previous instruments, and is sufficiently well explained in the descriptions already given of them, and by reference to the accompanying engraving. It is apparent that the open side should be introduced downwards, and that the push by which the scab is inserted, should be made very suddenly. In the handle of this instrument is a cavity, to hold vaccine material, secured by a screw top.

" *The Trident Lancet* (Fig. 49).—This lancet is a labor-saving one, for introducing vaccine lymph in either a fluid or a dried state, by the same process as that described for the Narrow-Bladed Lancet (Fig. 46).

" *The Vaccine Scarificator* (Fig. 50).—This is another labor-saving instrument, by the use of which five incisions are simultaneously made in the arm of the patient. It has the advantage of requiring neither skill nor steadiness of hand in its employment, while it makes the most imposing appearance of any instrument used in vaccination, in the eyes of the patient, or in those of the witness of the operation. Lymph is introduced into the incisions, drawn open or pressed apart by the fingers of the operator, in the same manner as is explained in describing the Narrow-Bladed Lancet (Fig. 46). A skilful person, in using any of these vaccinating instruments, need not, generally, cause sufficient pain to awaken a sleeping infant. It is proper to mention in this connexion, that the best part of the surface of the body for vaccination lies directly over the place of the insertion of the deltoid muscle of the left arm.

" *The best kind of Vaccine, the best instruments, and the best modes of using them.*—It is self-evident that fluid lymph transferred directly from an eighth day vesicle to any kind of incision made in the arm, is the most certain to infect. The best instrument to use in such a case is the Vaccinating Scarificator (Fig. 50). It is assumed that every one knows that none of the instruments here described are intended to be dipped into fluid vaccine, unless it be the Syringe Vaccinator, which has no cutting edge; as scarcely anything is more corrosive to a sharp-edged instrument than this material. The Vaccine crust, or scab, can be best used by introducing a small piece of it with the Syringe Self-Vaccinator (Fig. 49). In selecting the part of the scab to be used, choose only a fragment of the hard interior part, as that is the best and most reliable. Fluid lymph, preserved in glass capillary tubes, is best used by first breaking the tube at the point to which the fluid ascended in charging it, and then drawing the fractured end through or over the incision made by the Vaccinating Scarificator (Fig. 50). The scab, in a finely powdered form, may be successfully used by dropping a small quantity of it into the incisions made by the instrument just named; or, if it be previously dissolved in a small quantity of glycerine, the fluid may be applied to the absorbents through similar incisions. Water may also be used instead of glycerine as a moistener, with the same mode of use in view. Dried lymph, on a pointed quill, is best used by introducing it into a valvular cut made by the Narrow-Bladed Lancet (Fig. 46), and holding it there a minute or two."

ANÆSTHETICS.

THE anæsthetics in general use are sulphuric ether and chloroform.

Sulphuric Ether.—This agent is liable to adulteration, by sulphurous acid, alcohol, volatile oils, and by oxydation; it may be rendered purer by agitation with lime water, and afterwards separating it by decanting.

Method of Administration.—The following practical remarks on the administration of ether were made by a Committee appointed by the Boston Society for Medical Improvement to investigate the alleged dangers from inhalation of ether:—"Ether should never be given from any inhaling apparatus. The best medium of its administration is a bell-shaped sponge, large enough to cover in the nose, mouth, and chin; but it is difficult to find one of sufficient size and close enough in texture, or without such numerous apertures at the root as to admit too freely the atmospheric air. A sponge of this sort, moreover, being as expensive as rare, is seldom used outside of hospitals. A stiff towel, properly folded, may be substituted, and has the advantage of being always at hand; as it may be left behind, the surgeon does not carry away with him the annoying odor of an impregnated sponge. It is desirable that the towel should be a new one, and of pretty good size. It is to be taken just as it comes from the laundry, and not unfolded further than to display it in the dimensions of about ten inches by five; by folding down two of the corners in such a way that they shall lap over each other a little, and securing them by stout pins, a cone will be made which fits the face admirably. The thick layers of towelling will hold sufficient ether, and its texture will prevent a too free dilution of the anæsthetic by the atmospheric air, provided the apex and seam of the cone are carefully and tightly closed, either by pins or the fingers. As the cone becomes collapsed by saturation, it should from time to time be opened, and kept in shape by distending it with the hand. Unless these details are attended to, and especially the closure of the apex of the cone, the induction of anæsthesia will be uncertain and protracted. In anything so porous as a towel or sponge, the difficulty is to exclude enough air; for while its adequate admission to the lungs during etherization is essential to the life of the patient, its too free entrance not only delays anæsthesia, but induces a condition of excitement, both mental and physical. The importance of excluding the air, as above stated, is a point not generally appreciated, but the necessity of it has long been known to those most accustomed to the use of ether, as shown by the "chemise" with which, in hospital practice, a too porous sponge is often covered to expedite the etherization of a rebellious patient. Ether should be poured lavishly on the towel or sponge, an ounce or two at a time, especially at the commencement of inhalation. Although it may be wasted, too much, as far as safety is concerned, cannot be used. A small quantity poured on hesitatingly and timidly, as is sometimes done, has the same effect as a too free dilution of the vapor with air, producing simply intoxication and its accompanying excitement without anæsthesia; whereas a large amount, though the cough and choking sensation which the greater volume of vapor produces may cause the patient to resist and struggle, is certain to bring about a satisfactory condition of insensibility.

"*Phenomena of Etherization.*—A strong, full-blooded man is pretty sure to resist the approaches of anæsthesia under any circumstances. This may sometimes be overcome by warning him beforehand of such a possibility, and inducing him to resolve not to struggle; the last impression on his mind influences him even in his stupor. The same thing is liable also to happen with almost all patients just before complete anæsthesia takes place, but the ether rarely requires to be suspended. Occasionally the respiration becomes embarrassed during the period of excitement, partly from the struggle itself, and partly perhaps from the increased flow of saliva, which is a common phenomenon of etherization, or from the position of the tongue or head of the patient, and a condition may sometimes show itself characterized by lividity, rigidity, and convulsive motions of the extremities. Although alarming to the inexperienced, the state is in fact devoid of danger, provided the ether be momentarily suspended; this being done, the refusal to breathe soon gives place to a long-drawn inspiration, and in most instances complete insensibility immediately ensues. In such a case it is interesting to observe how readily the spasm yields, and how complete is the muscular relaxation which follows the free respiration of air unmixed with ether. It should therefore be

3*

borne in mind, that when there is muscular rigidity with lividity, the suspension of etherization will transform this into the relaxation of anæsthesia. Persons of intemperate habits succumb to ether slowly, and with greater reluctance and more opposition than persons unused to intoxication. The pulse should be watched by a competent person from the outset, and its failure, either in strength or frequency, lead to more cautious use of the ether. It must, however, be remembered, that in experiments with anæsthetics upon animals, the heart has been found to be the *ultimum moriens;* the respiratory movements, therefore, should not be forgotten or neglected, but any slowness or irregularity in the performance should at once receive attention. Ether is not to be withheld from a patient to be operated on, even in a state of collapse after severe accident, but great caution is demanded in its use with patients who are near death from chronic and exhausting disease, and who require operations. The best test of complete etherization is the snoring of the patient; and no operation, unless slight, should be undertaken until this symptom presents itself. The relaxation of the muscles of the extremities may occur without insensibility. The important distinction between *snoring* and *stertor* is, however, to be borne in mind. Whilst the former is caused only by the relaxation of the muscles of the palate, the latter arises from spasm of the vocal cords and partial closure of the rima glottidis, and thus becomes the immediate forerunner of the train of symptoms already referred to as indicative of partial asphyxia. Stertorous respiration demands, therefore, a brief suspension of inhalation; one or two inspirations of fresh air will, as already mentioned, almost instantly dispel the symptom. Ether may be administered to persons of all ages, from the new-born infant to the octogenarian. There is, however, a condition prone to manifest itself with children, especially those who are weak, strumous, or overgrown, which is due to its cumulative properties. It may show itself after almost any degree of etherization, and is characterized by a feeble pulse and slow respiration, not passing off with the readiness usually marking the phenomena of etherization. With young persons a cautious inhalation of five minutes will often induce an anæsthesia of half an hour, an effect wholly out of proportion to what the same amount of ether would produce in an adult. This state is not a dangerous one, and only requires time to dissipate its symptoms. Compression of the chest will expel the fumes of ether being eliminated from the pulmonary surface, and permit the entrance of a fresh supply of oxygen to stimulate the circulation. The inhalation should therefore be suspended at short intervals with children, and but little ether given at a time."

Chloroform.—Chloroform may be adulterated with alcohol, oils, and ether. Alcohol can be added without being detected by the smell, but may be detected by dropping the chloroform into water, when it assumes a milky appearance. Oils are detected by strong sulphuric acid, which gives a yellowish or reddish brown color; the presence of ether is detected by its readily burning when exposed to a flame. Pure chloroform may be thus tested:—When dropped on the hand it evaporates without leaving the least smell or moisture behind; it is free from color or opacity; it does not redden or bleach litmus paper; it does not become opaque when dropped into water; it does not coagulate the white of egg.

Administration.—In the administration of chloroform great care must be exercised. The following judicious rules by Prof. Gross (*System of Surgery*) cannot be too carefully followed:—

"1st. During etherization the patient may sit up with impunity, but this is not the case during the inhalation of chloroform, owing, apparently, to the greater relaxation of the muscles, and consequently, to the greater difficulty in maintaining the circulation of the brain through the influence of the heart's action. Not only should the body be recumbent, but care should be taken to depress the head and shoulders, bringing them nearly to a level with the trunk.

"2d. An empty state of the stomach is desirable for two reasons; first, because if chloroform be given soon after a hearty meal it will be almost certain to induce vomiting; and, secondly, because a crowded condition of the organ interferes materially with the movements of the diaphragm. Food must not be taken for at least four hours before the exhibition; but, on the other hand, the interval should not be too protracted, lest serious exhaustion result from the want of the necessary stimulus.

"3d. Care must be taken, before the inhalation is commenced, that the patient's clothes are sufficiently loose to prevent constriction of the chest and abdomen. Any compression from this source would necessarily impede the action of the diaphragm, and might thus become a cause of mischief.

"4th. The importance of having an abundance of atmospheric air during the inhalation of an article so potent as chloroform, is self-evident; in etherization this is of comparatively little consequence, but in the exhibition of chloroform for surgical and obstetrical purposes, it is absolutely indispensable to the safety of the patient.

"5th. The inhalation must be effected gradually, not hurriedly, time being allowed to the system to accommodate itself to the influence of the remedy, thus avoiding the shock which might otherwise result to the heart and brain. From six to eight minutes should usually be spent in producing the full effects of the anæsthetic.

"When the patient is very feeble, or pale and timid, it will be advisable to give him, immediately before the operation, from half an ounce to an ounce of brandy; and the dose may afterwards be repeated, if the effect is obliged to be maintained for an unusual length of time. sufficient consciousness being permitted for the performance of deglutition. The best mode of administering chloroform is to pour the fluid upon a napkin or handkerchief, previously folded into a kind of cup-shaped hollow, and held securely in the hand. Or, instead of this, a small, hollow sponge may be used. As to the various inhalers that have been devised for the purpose, they are all objectionable on account of their inconvenience and the difficulty of obtaining a sufficiency of atmospheric air. The patient having taken his place upon the table, and emptied his lungs by a deep and protracted expiration, the napkin, impregnated with a drachm of chloroform, is held over the mouth and nose, at a distance of about two inches, being gradually brought nearer and nearer until it is within half an inch, beyond which it should not be carried, the chest being at the same time regularly and powerfully distended. On no account should the liquid be permitted to come in contact with the surface, as it might thus cause vesication. All unnecessary conversation is avoided, lest the attention of the patient should thereby be unduly distracted. The assistant having charge of the administration gives it his earnest and undivided care; wetting the napkin from time to time with the fluid, and seeing that the patient gets an abundance of air, his vigilance increasing as the effects of the medicine become more and more apparent. As soon as the sensibility is completely abolished, the operation is commenced, a return to consciousness being prevented by holding the napkin, wet with a small quantity of the vapor, occasionally before the nose; and thus the impression is maintained, steadily and cautiously, not only until the knife has fully accomplished its object, but until the principal arteries have been secured, and, in some cases, even until the dressings have been applied.

"As soon as the inhalation has been fairly entered upon, one of the attendants should sedulously watch the state of the pulse, of the respiration, and of the countenance. Any sudden failure in any one of these should at once create alarm, and induce a suspension of the operation, or provision for the admission of a greater quantity of atmospheric air. I do not deem it necessary that a finger should be constantly kept upon the pulse; for the color of the face and the nature of the breathing will always sufficiently indicate the effects which the anæsthetic is exerting upon the system, and thus afford abundant opportunity for preventing any unpleasant occurrence.

"The *quantity* of chloroform required during an operation, and the time during which its effects may be safely maintained, must, of course, vary according to the exigencies of each particular case. In general, from half an ounce to an ounce may be regarded as a fair average, but very frequently it takes three or even five times that amount, depending upon the severity and duration of the operation, and the susceptibility of the individual. In some instances almost an incredibly small portion answers the purpose. Children usually require comparatively little; and it is well known that women are, as a general rule, more susceptible to its influence than men. Persons exhausted by hæmorrhage are very easily affected by it, owing to the rapidity of its absorption, and hence it should always be administered to them with unusual care."

Dr. Simpson has advised that chloroform be given by laying a handkerchief over the face, and letting the chloroform fall on it drop by drop.

Resuscitation.—The towel or inhaler being removed, the patient's tongue should be drawn forward with forceps or a tenaculum, fresh air admitted from the door or windows, or induced by a fan, and artificial respiration instituted. Stimulating applications to the surface, cold douche to the head, and stimulating injections may be added. The main reliance is on artificial respiration, and this is best kept up by Marshall Hall's method as follows: "Turn the body gently, and completely, *on the side and a little beyond*, and then on the face, alternately; repeating these measures deliberately, efficiently, and perseveringly, fifteen times in a minute, *only* [when the patient reposes on the thorax, this cavity is *compressed* by the weight of the body, and *ex*piration takes place; when he is turned on the side, this pressure is removed and *in*spiration occurs]. When the *prone* position is resumed, make equable but efficient *pressure along* the spine; removing it immediately before rotation on the side [the first measure augments the *ex*piration, the second commences *in*spiration]." As soon as the patient can swallow, give brandy and ammonia. Efforts at resuscitation should not cease until death is evident.

A method of producing artificial respiration has been introduced by Dr. Sylvester; it consists in laying the patient on his back, drawing the tongue forward, then carrying the arms slowly upwards over the head, thus elevating the ribs by means of the pectoral muscles, and inducing respiration; the arms are then brought down to the side of the chest and slightly compressed against it; these movements are to be repeated slowly as by the other method.

If a galvanic battery is at hand it should be resorted to among other possible means of restoring animation.

CHAPTER II.

ON THE ARTERIES.

WOUNDS OF ARTERIES.

Arteries may be contused, lacerated, punctured, and incised.

Contused Wounds.—An artery may, without any apparent lesion of its coats, be so contused as to lead to its permanent contraction; this injury is liable, in connexion with concurrent injuries, to terminate in gangrene. Sloughing of the coats may occur.

Lacerated Wounds.—Lacerated wounds of arteries are met with under the following forms:—1. The internal coats of an artery may be ruptured without a lesion of the external coat; 2. The external coats may be lacerated without a lesion of the internal coat; 3. All the coats may be torn through. The two first accidents to arteries may lead to the following results:—1. To the obliteration of the vessel in the same manner as when the ligature is applied; 2. Severe hæmorrhage from the sloughing of the remaining coat; 3. To an aneurismal tumor formed by the gradual yielding of the remaining coat; 4. To immediate obliteration of the artery and gangrene of the limb. The third lesion, or rupture of all the coats, is liable to be followed by gangrene, especially when the accompanying vein is also involved; hæmorrhage seldom occurs.

Punctured Wounds.—Arteries may be penetrated by large or small instruments; when the instrument is very small, as a needle, the wound may heal without any hæmorrhage or other symptom; if the instrument is larger, hæmorrhage may be immediate, or the elasticity of the coats may close the wound temporarily, and subsequent ulceration reopen it, resulting in free bleeding.

Incised Wounds.—The incised wound may partially or wholly divide the vessel; it may be transverse, oblique, or longitudinal to the axis of the vessel. When the vessel is completely divided it is much less liable to continued and repeated hæmorrhage than when partly divided, as it is capable of contraction and retraction, which favors the formation of a clot. Partial division of an artery by a transverse or oblique wound is constantly liable to hæmorrhage; if the clot forms externally, which is always the case, it is readily displaced and the bleeding is renewed. Longitudinal wounds are capable of spontaneous cure.

Treatment.—The following general and special rules in the treatment of wounded arteries, are principally from Mr. Guthrie; slight modifications have been made:—

General Rules.—1. If the wounded artery is in an extremity, the hæmorrhage may be temporarily controlled, either by strongly flexing, or by very forcibly extending the limb (in the former case the artery is compressed at the bend of the limb, and in the latter compression is made in its course by the muscles and the fasciæ).

2. In general, no operation ought to be performed on a wounded artery unless it bleed.

3. No operation is to be done for a wounded artery in the first instance but at the spot injured, unless such operation not only appears to be, but is, impracticable.

4. If the artery is small, like the temporal, the practice to be pursued is to divide the vessel, when it will be enabled to retract and contract; and the bleeding will in general permanently cease under pressure, especially when it can be applied against the bone.

5. If the artery is of a larger class, and continues to bleed, it should be sufficiently exposed by enlarging the wound; a ligature should be applied above and below the opening in the vessel, which may or may not be divided between them at the pleasure of the surgeon.

6. When the external wound closes under pressure, and blood is extravasated in such quantity under the fascia, and between the muscular structures, as is not likely to be removed by absorption under general pressure, the wounded artery should by incision be laid bare and be secured in a similar manner, even at the expense of any muscular fibre which may intervene.

7. When an aneurismal tumor forms *some time* after such an accident, in the upper part of the forearm in particular, the application of a ligature on the brachial artery is admissible on the Hunterian principle.

8. Whenever the main artery of a limb is injured by a musket-ball, mortification of the extremity will frequently be the result, particularly if it be the femoral artery; it will be of certain occurrence if both artery and vein are injured, although they may not be either torn or divided. Immediate amputation at the seat of injury is not advised. Wait with the hope that the mortification will not extend, provided there are no constitutional symptoms; but, if they should present themselves, or the discoloration of the skin should appear to spread, amputation should be performed forthwith, immediately below the knee. A wound of the axillary artery rarely leads to mortification of the fingers or hand. If it should do so, the principle of treatment should be similar.

9. In all cases of punctured wounds, when pressure can be effectually made, and especially against a bone, it should be tried by graduated compression over the part injured, in the course of the artery above and below the wound; if in an extremity, over the whole limb generally, the motions of which should be effectually prevented, and absolute rest must be enjoined, if the artery is of any importance. This should be continued for two, three, or more weeks, according to the nature of the injury.

10. In every case of wounded—not aneurismal—artery in the neck, one ligature should be applied above, and another below the

opening in the injured vessel, and not one alone on the common trunk, even if that should be the part injured.

11. When an artery lying superficially upon one side of a limb is wounded by an instrument penetrating from the opposite side, Mr. South advises to cut directly upon the artery on the uninjured side, and apply the ligatures.

Special Rules.—1. When the internal carotid is wounded through the mouth, Mr. Guthrie advises that a ligature be placed above and below the opening made into it; the rule which generally obtains among surgeons is to apply a ligature to the common carotid.

2. When any one of the branches of the external carotid has been wounded, it ought to be tied at both ends, at the part wounded; if the surgeon cannot do this, and the hæmorrhage demand it, the trunk of the external carotid is the vessel on which the ligature should be placed, not that of the common carotid.

3. The internal carotid artery, when wounded near the bifurcation of the common carotid, is to be secured by two ligatures.

4. A ligature may be placed on the internal or external carotid, close to the bifurcation, with safety; but if the wound of either vessel should encroach on the bifurcation, one ligature should be applied on the common trunk, and another above the part wounded; but as neither of these would control the collateral circulation through the *uninjured* vessel, whichever of the two it might be, a third ligature should be placed on it above the bifurcation.

5. The error of placing a ligature on the subclavian artery above the clavicle, for a wound of the axillary below it, should never be committed.

6. Punctured wounds of the arteries of the arm and forearm ought to be treated by pressure applied especially to the part injured, and to the limb generally; but when the bleeding cannot be restrained in this manner, a ligature should be applied above and below the part injured, whether the artery be radial, ulnar, or interosseal.

7. When the ulnar artery is wounded in the hand, which is comparatively a superficial vessel, two ligatures should be placed upon it; when the opening is small, pressure may be tried.

8. When the radial artery is wounded in the hand, in which situation it is deep seated, and the bleeding end or ends of the artery can be seen, a ligature should be placed on each. If this cannot be done, search should be made by incisions through the fascia, as extensively as the situation of the tendons and nerves in the hand will permit. The bleeding point should be fully exposed, all coagula removed, and a piece of lint, rolled tight and hard, of a size only sufficient to cover the bleeding point, should be laid upon it; a second and larger hard piece should then be placed over it, and so on, until the compresses rise so much above the level of the wound as to allow the pressure to be continued and retained on the proper spot, without including the neighboring parts; a piece

of linen, kept constantly wet and cold, should be applied over the sides of the wound, which should not be closed, so as to allow of any blood being freely evacuated.

9. The anterior tibial artery is to be tied at that part of its course at which it may be wounded. A case has been supposed, in which a knife, a sword, or other narrow instrument, having penetrated the upper part of the leg, has wounded the anterior tibial artery just after it has been given off from the posterior tibial, behind the interosseous space or ligament. The bleeding is free, and from the wound in the front of the leg, although the artery cannot be secured, from the narrowness of the space between the tibia and fibula, behind which space it is situated. This very peculiar injury, which may, however, occur at any time, cannot be known until an incision has been made on the fore part of the leg, and the bleeding point seen so deep between the bones as not to admit of two ligatures being placed on the artery above and below it. In such a case, an incision is to be made through the calf of the leg, when the artery can be secured without difficulty.

10. The posterior tibial, or the peroneal artery, or both, if wounded at the same time, are to be tied through a free incision in the calf.

11. The popliteal artery is never to be secured by ligature, unless wounded and bleeding.

12. An instrument penetrating the thigh two inches below Poupart's ligament, and wounding the superficial femoral artery, will necessitate the application of two ligatures, one above and the other below the wound in the vessel; but as the profunda under ordinary circumstances is given off posteriorly at this spot, it is possible the upper ligature may be placed on the main artery a little above the bifurcation. The result might, and would probably be, on some sudden movement of the patient, a recurrence of the hæmorrhage by regurgitation from the profunda into the main trunk below the ligature; and thus through the wound in the artery, the lower ligature assisting by the obstacle it offers to the passage of blood through it. In such a case, the wound should be reopened, and the profunda sought for and tied.

13. When a wound of the femoral artery or its branches occurs, and the bleeding cannot be *restrained* by a moderate but regulated compression on the trunk of the vessel, and perhaps on the injured part, recourse should be had to an operation, by which both ends of the wounded artery may be secured by ligature; and the *impracticability* of doing this should be ascertained only by the failure of the attempt. If the lower end of the artery cannot be found at the time, the upper only having bled, a gentle compression maintained upon the track of the lower may prevent mischief; but if dark-colored blood should flow from the wound, which may be expected to come from the lower end of the artery, and compression does not suffice to suppress the hæmorrhage, the bleeding end of the vessel must be exposed, and secured near to its extremity.

14. Wounds of the sciatic and internal iliac should be treated by a ligature applied to both cut extremities, and not to the arteries at their origin.

LIGATURE OF ARTERIES.

The object sought in the ligation of an artery is the permanent obstruction of the current of blood by the obliteration of its cavity. To effect this object the internal coats of the vessel should be ruptured by the ligature; the process of obliteration then consists in the organization of the clot in the vessel with the adhesion of the ruptured tunics.

Instruments.—The instruments immediately required are a scalpel, forceps, aneurismal needle, ligature, director, and spatulas.

The Scalpel.—The common scalpel answers the best purpose in this operation. Its blunt, rounded edge, is best adapted to the dissection, and the broad extremity of the handle can be used to advantage in separating layers of fascia, and parts where the cutting edge is not desirable.

The Forceps.—The common dissecting forceps should be selected for the dissection; they should have accurately fitting teeth, and not be liable to open at the extremity when firmly closed; a pair of small forceps may also be required.

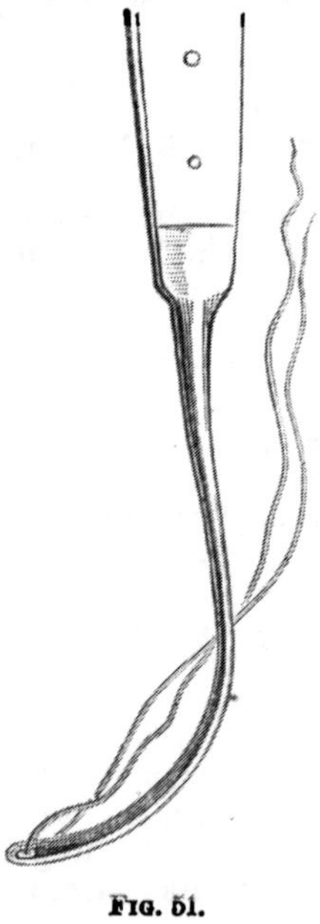

FIG. 51.

The Needle.—The common aneurism needle is a curved blunt instrument, with an eye near the extremity, and firmly fixed in a handle (Fig. 51). When used, the extremity is gently insinuated under the vessel, and as it appears upon the opposite side, the loop of the ligature is seized with the forceps, or a hook, and one end being drawn through, it is held as the instrument is withdrawn, carrying the other end, and thus leaving the ligature under the vessel. Of the different needles invented for this operation, that known as the "American needle," of Dr. Mott, is, perhaps, the most convenient, and is especially well adapted to those cases where the artery lies very deeply. It consists of the handle and hook (Fig. 53), and the blunt needle with two eyes (Fig. 52). The needle is fitted to the shaft (Fig. 53) by a screw. When used, the ligature is first inserted into the second eye; the needle is then passed under the artery, and as the extremity emerges upon the opposite side, the blunt hook is inserted into the eye, and the needle is thus held until the handle is unscrewed, when it is drawn through with the ligature. It is sometimes necessary to include other tissues with the artery, when the sharp-pointed needle (Fig. 52) should be used.

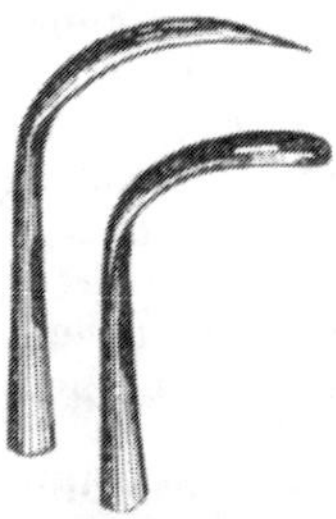

FIG. 52.

The Director.—The director is used in the dissection to raise the fascia before its division; it is sometimes passed under the artery as a guide to the needle.

Spatulas.—Two spatulas are often required, with which assistants separate the sides of the wound, and expose the deep-seated parts; pieces of flexible metal or wood may be used.

The Ligature.—The ligature is generally of the strongest dentists' silk, or of silver wire; its size proportionate to the size of the vessel. In general a large ligature irritates more than a small one, and is longer in separating.

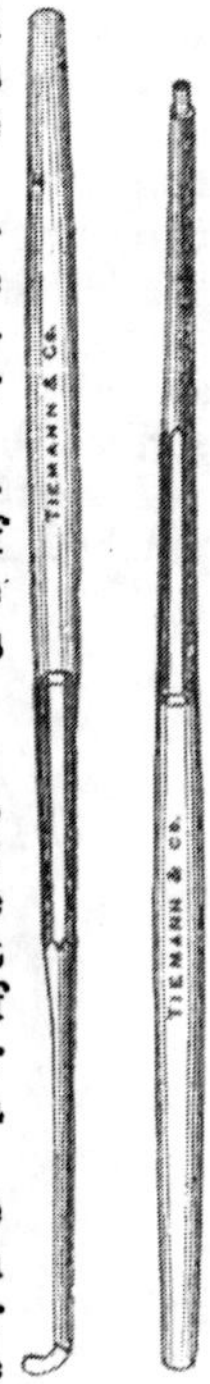

FIG. 53.

Arrangements.—The patient is placed upon a firm bed, or on a table, and the assistant administers the anæsthetic; the surgeon takes his position generally on the outside of the limb which is the seat of the operation; a second assistant takes a position where he can command the artery above if by any accident it is wounded, or if the artery yields under the tightened ligature; a third uses the sponges; and a fourth separates the wound with the spatulas.

Position of the Artery.—The precise location of the artery is determined, 1. By its pulsations; 2. By given anatomical points in the vicinity. To render the former distinct, the limb should be placed in a position favorable to arterial circulation; to render muscles and tendons most distinct the limb should be forcibly extended at the commencement of the operation. When the dissection has proceeded so far as to reach the vicinity of the artery, the operator is aided in detecting its position by flexing the limb so as to relax the muscles and tissues.

Position of Superficial Veins.—It is important, before the first incision is made, to guard against wounding superficial veins. Their position is readily defined by compressing the parts above the point of the proposed operation.

Operative Procedure.—The operation involves several consecutive steps:—

Incision.—When the first incision is about to be made, the skin should be rendered tense by the thumb and fingers of the left hand applied on either side of the vessel, or the fingers applied at the extremity of the proposed incision, parallel to its course; if the first method is chosen, care must be taken not to make more traction on one side than on the other; the second method answers where the skin is naturally tense and but slight traction is necessary. The scalpel should be held in the second or third position (Figs. 4, 5), and the incision should be made directly over and generally parallel to the artery, through the skin only if the artery is superficial, but also through the cellular tissues if it is deep, its length varying with the depth of the vessel and the fleshiness of the subject. The incision is sometimes made in the direction of the fibres of the muscle covering the artery, as where the great pectoral overlies the axillary; at other times it should be curved, so as to raise a flap. The length of the incision cannot be prescribed, but it should always be ample.

Dissection of Fasciæ and Muscles.—The fasciæ are carefully pinched up with the forceps (Fig. 54), and being opened with the scalpel applied horizontally, are incised freely on a director introduced beneath them. In dissecting among muscular structures it is important to enter the muscular interstices, and not wound the substance. These inter-muscular spaces are marked by deposits of fat, especially towards the terminal extremity of the muscles, and hence we should commence the separation of muscles as nearly as possible at their terminal extremity. If there is doubt as to the line of separation, a puncture with the bistoury will disclose adipose or muscular tissue, according to the nature of the underlying structure. If the dissection is made through the body of the muscle, the fibres separate more readily in an inverse direction, viz. from their origin to their attachments. The muscles may be separated with the handle of the scalpel or the finger nail.

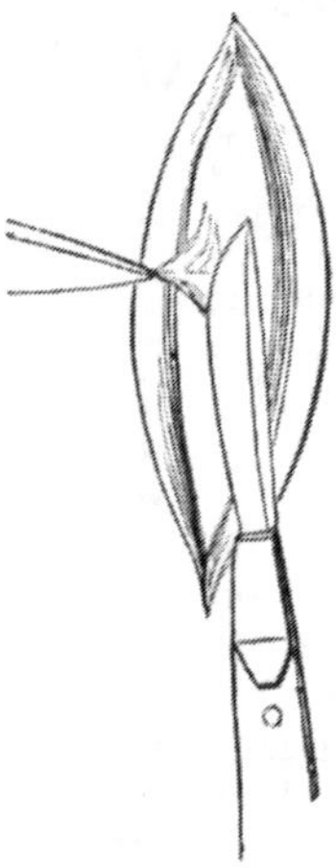

FIG. 54.

Isolation of the Artery.—The larger arteries have firm sheaths, which require to be opened by dissection; the smaller vessels have but slight fibrous investments, and are readily exposed with the point of a director, or the aneurism needle. The true sheath of the artery is opened by pinching up a small portion with the forceps, and nicking it slightly with the scalpel, held as before noticed (Figs. 4, 5); into the opening thus made, the end of a director or the aneurism needle is gently insinuated, and by slight movements of its point, first upon one side and then upon the other, the sheath is separated completely around the vessel, to an extent sufficient to allow simply the passage of the ligature; as the extremity of the instrument emerges on the opposite side, the finger of the left hand, or the thumb and forefinger pressed together, should steady its point as it penetrates the last of the investing sheath.

Passage of the Ligature.—If the artery is small and very superficial, a director may be passed under, and along its groove a blunt needle carrying the ligature. If more deeply situated, the common aneurism needle (Fig. 51), or the American needle (Figs. 52. 53), should be used. In the isolation of the artery the aneurism needle is often used, and the operation is then completed by drawing one end of the ligature out upon the opposite side (Fig. 55). The needle should be passed from the veins; no force should be used, lest the instrument penetrate the coats of the artery.

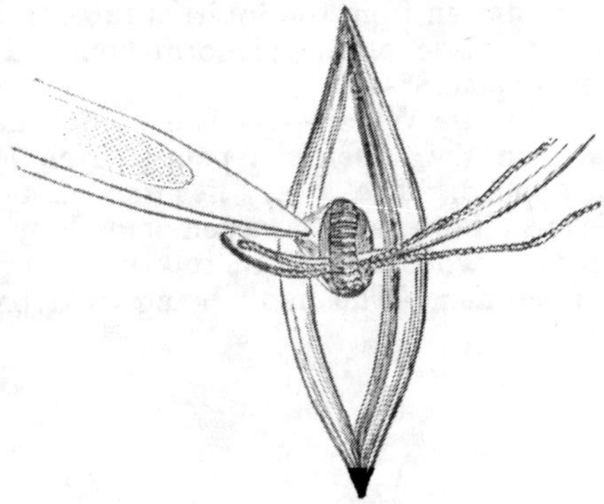

FIG. 55.

Tying the Ligature.—The ligature should be placed at right angles with the long axis of a vessel, and the reef-knot (Fig. 39) tied, unless there are special reasons for adopting the surgeon's knot (Fig. 38). The first knot is tightened around the vessels firmly, on either side of the ligature, near the artery, with the index fingers carried to the bottom of the wound (Fig. 56). The degree of constriction varies with the size of the arteries, but it should always be sufficient to rupture the internal coats, the sensation of which is communicated to the fingers. In tying the second knot care must be taken not to tighten the thread firmly until traction is made on a plane with the first knot, with the fingers again carried down to the vessel.

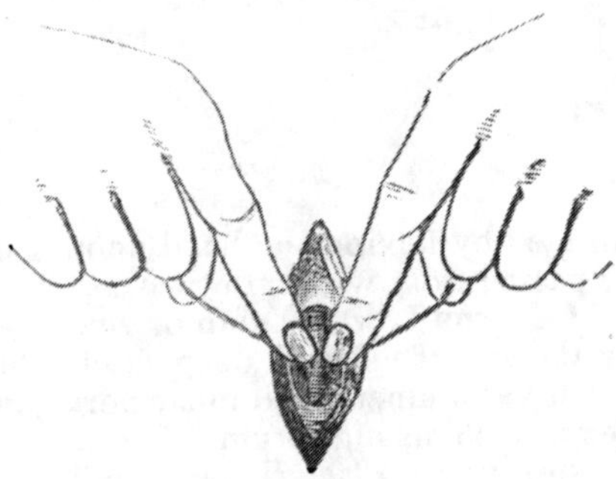

FIG. 56.

Dressings.—The two ends of the ligature are tied together, and being brought out of the wound at its most dependent part, are fastened to the external parts by an adhesive strap; the edges of the wound are brought together by adhesive straps, or if the wound is deep and gaping, sutures are used.

ARTERIES OF THE UPPER EXTREMITIES.

Ulnar Artery.—The ulnar, the larger terminal division of the brachial artery, passes to the inner side of the forearm, at the lower part of its upper third, continues along the ulnar side to the wrist passes over the annular ligament, on the outer side of the pisiform bone, and terminates in the superficial palmar arch. Its course is marked by a line drawn from the internal tuberosity of the os brachii to the external side of the pisiform bone. It may be ligated in the following places:—

I. At the Wrist.—At the point where the ulnar artery terminates in the superficial palmar arch (Fig. 57), the ligature is to be applied. The artery lies immediately to the radial side of the pisiform bone, and is accompanied by its veins, *b*, and the ulnar nerve, *c*, which lies on its internal and posterior aspect.

Operation.—The hand being held back, make a slightly curved incision on the radial side of the pisiform bone, through the skin and adipose tissue of the hypothenar eminence, about three inches in length, its concavity looking inwards; the artery, *a*, is deeply seated in a groove, and the dissection should be continued along the side of the pisiform bone until it is exposed; the latter part of the dissection will be facilitated by flexing the hand upon the forearm; the needle should be passed from within outwards.

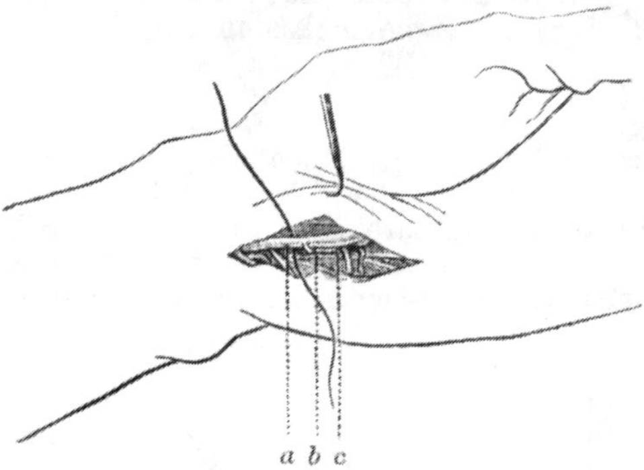

Fig. 57.

II. In the Lower Third of the Forearm.—The artery is covered by the superficial and deep fasciæ, having upon its inner side the flexor carpi ulnaris and ulnar nerve, and upon its external side the flexor sublimis digitorum.

Operation.—Place the arm supine, and extend the hand so as to make prominent the tendon of the flexor carpi ulnaris; then along the internal border of this muscle, *a*, or at the union of the external four-fifths of the arm with the internal fifth, or on a line drawn from the internal condyle to the pisiform bone, make an incision about two inches in length, through the skin, *c*, and subcutaneous cellular tissue,

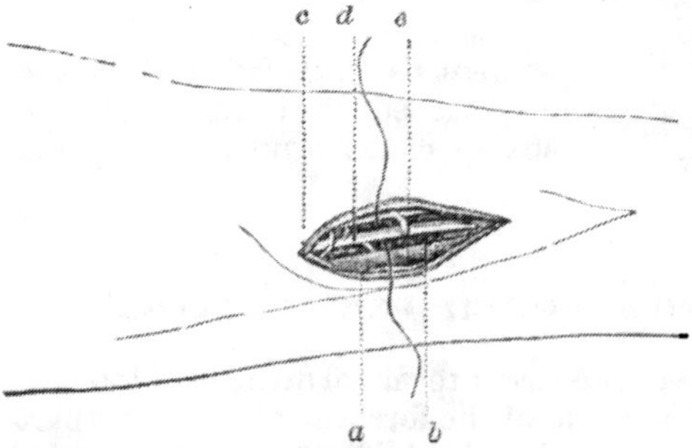

Fig. 58.

e; the deep fascia is raised on a director, or with the forceps, and incised, exposing the tendon of the flexor carpi ulnaris; this should be pressed inwards, and immediately behind it the artery, *d*, will be found with its two accompanying veins and the nerve upon the inside.

III. In the Upper Third.—The ulnar artery, arising from the brachial, curves inwards deeply beneath the flexor muscles, and passes along the ulnar side of the forearm, between and covered by the flexor carpi ulnaris and flexor sublimis digitorum; it is accompanied by two veins, and by the ulnar nerve, which is more superficial and internal.

Operation.—(Fig. 59.) The forearm being supine, the hand is strongly extended and inclined to the radial side; an incision is made on the imaginary line given, three inches in length, and beginning three fingers' breadth below the internal condyle; the incision divides the skin and superficial fasciæ, and exposes the aponeurotic connexion of the flexor carpi ulnaris and flexor sublimis, which is of a yellowish-white color; this is divided with the director from below, where it is the most delicate, carefully avoiding the division of muscular substance; the flexor sublimis, *a*, is drawn outwards, and the deep aponeurosis exposed, under which lies the artery; if the vessel is not seen, press the flexor carpi ulnaris, *c*, inwards, and expose the ulnar nerve, *b*, a little external to which lies the artery, *e*, with its two veins, *d;* the artery is isolated by flexing the arm slightly and the hand strongly, and passing the needle from within outwards.

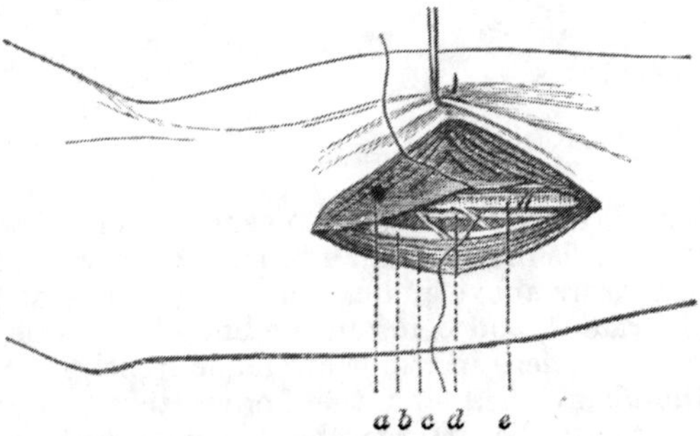

Fig. 59.

Radial Artery.—The radial, though the smaller branch of the brachial artery, lies in the direct course of the latter like a continuation; its course is marked by a line drawn from the centre of the elbow to the inner side of the styloid process of the radius. It is superficial throughout nearly its entire course, but is generally ligated at three points:—

I. On the Dorsum of the Wrist.—(Fig. 60.) The radial artery at this point passes in the groove between the upper extremities of the first metacarpal bones, a fibrous band separating it from the tendons of the thumb; the artery may be tied here, just as it is about to form the palmar arch. Again, as it passes under the extensor muscle of the thumb, and may sometimes be detected pulsating between the extensor ossis metacarpi pollicis, and the extensor secundi metacarpi pollicis, a little below and posterior to the extremity of the styloid process of the radius; at this point the ligature may also be applied.

Operation.—In ligating the artery at the commencement of the palmar arch, an incision of an inch in length is made along the outer borders of the extensor secundi and metacarpi pollicis, at the angle formed by the two first metacarpal bones, care being taken not to wound the superficial veins. The artery is readily exposed and tied. If the point of ligation is higher, the hand is placed between pronation and supination, the thumb strongly abducted so as to render prominent the extensors, and an incision is made an inch in length, between the tendons of the two extensors above indicated, commencing at the lower extremity of the radius, and being in the line of the axis of the first metacarpal bone. These incisions are made lightly, the superficial vein of the thumb avoided, and the fibrous tissues over the artery divided, exposing the artery; the extensor ossis metacarpi pollicis, *a*, is drawn inwards, and the extensor secundi internodii pollicis, *d*, outwards, exposing the artery, *c*, and its accompanying veins, *b*.

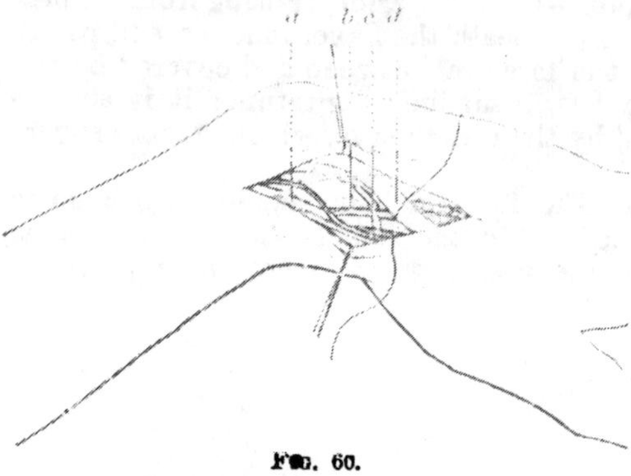

FIG. 60.

II. IN THE LOWER THIRD OF THE ARM.—The artery is situated superficially, lying between the tendons of the supinator longus and the flexor carpi radialis; it is accompanied by venæ comites, and by the radial nerve which lies external; its pulsation is easily detected.

Operation.—(Fig. 61.) The arm is held supine; the hand forcibly extended makes prominent the flexors; the operator standing on the external side of the limb makes a light incision, two inches in length, from half an inch above the articulation of the radius, on the external border of the flexor carpi radialis or on a line joining the external with the three internal

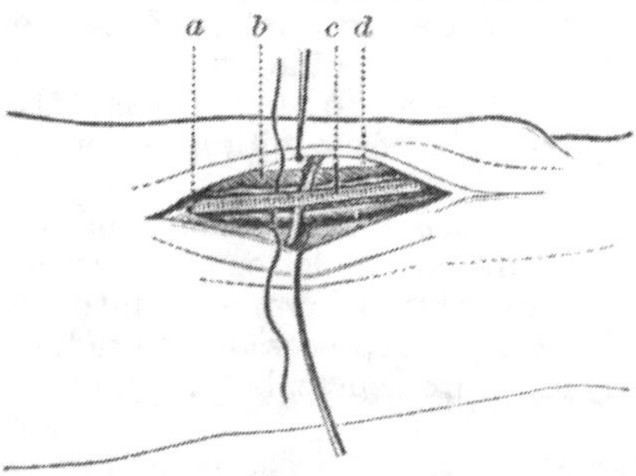

FIG. 61.

fourths of the arm; the deep fascia, *a*, is raised on a director exposing the artery, *c*, with its two veins, *b*, and the nerve, *d*, external and posterior; the needle may be passed in either direction.

III. In the Upper Third of the Arm.—The artery lies between the supinator longus and the pronator radii teres; it has venæ comites; the radial nerve lies immediately on its external side.

Operation.—(Fig. 62.) The limb being extended supine, the superficial veins are defined by pressure of the thumb above; an incision is made, two to three inches in length, on the internal border of the supinator longus, if recognised by the depression, or on a line drawn from the middle of the bend of the elbow to the inner side of the styloid process of the radius, dividing the skin and superficial fasciæ; the deep fascia is divided on a director; the arm is slightly flexed to relax the muscles, and the supinator longus, *a*, being drawn aside, the sheath of the artery, *b*, is exposed. The needle is passed from without inwards.

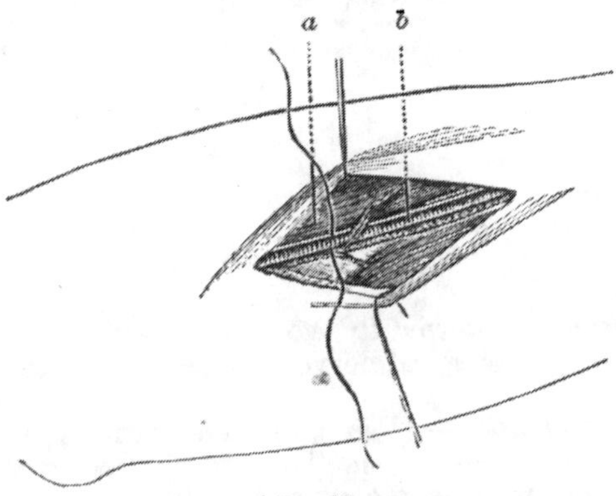

Fig. 62.

Brachial Artery.—The brachial artery extends from the lower margin of the axilla to an inch below the bend of the elbow, in a line drawn from the junction of the anterior with the middle third of the axilla to the middle of the bend of the elbow. The brachial artery is usually ligatured at one of the following points:—

I. At the Elbow.—The brachial artery lies in the centre of a triangular space at the bend of the elbow, formed by the supinator longus, externally, and the pronator radii teres, internally; it rests on the brachialis anticus; the median nerve lies to the inner side half an inch; the tendon of the biceps lies on the outer side; its coverings are the skin, superficial fascia, and the median basilic vein, which is separated by the bicipital fascia.

Operation.—(Fig. 63.) The arm extended and held in a supine position, an oblique incision, two inches and a half in length, is made along the internal edge of the tendon of the biceps, within the median basilic vein, dividing only the skin; push aside the vein and divide the aponeurosis, which is the deep fascia, *e*, on a director; the tendon of the biceps, *c*, is now seen, and on its inside the artery, *a*, with its two veins, and still further inward the median nerve, *b*. The forearm is now slightly flexed, and the needle passed from within outward, carefully avoiding the veins.

II. In the Middle of the Arm.—The brachial descends on the inner side, first of the coraco-brachialis, and afterwards of the biceps; it is covered by the fascia and integuments, and overlapped slightly by the biceps; its sheath contains the two venæ comites; the internal cutaneous nerve lies superficial to it; the median is superficial to it above, and rather to its outer side; about the middle of the arm, it crosses the artery, and inferiorly it is to its ulnar side; the ulnar nerve is internal to the artery, and at some distance from it inferiorly; the spiral nerve is posterior, and separates it above from the triceps.

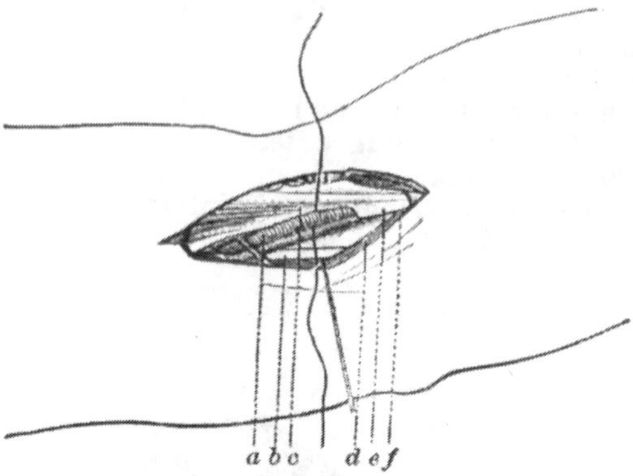

Fig. 63.

Operation.—(Fig. 64.) The arm is extended and carried at right angles to the body, and held supine. The course of the artery may be recognised, 1. By its pulsation; 2. By the internal margin of the biceps and coraco-brachialis; 3. By the median nerve, to the inner side of which it lies; 4. By the line above given. An incision is made two or three inches in length, along the inner border of the biceps, dividing the skin freely down to the fasciæ; this is incised on a director, and the position of the median nerve detected in the wound with the finger; this is exposed, and being pushed aside with the biceps, *d*, and the median nerve, *b*, the artery, *c*, is found immediately behind and inside, accompanied by its venæ comites, *a*. The arm is now flexed, the vessel isolated, and the ligature passed from without inwards.

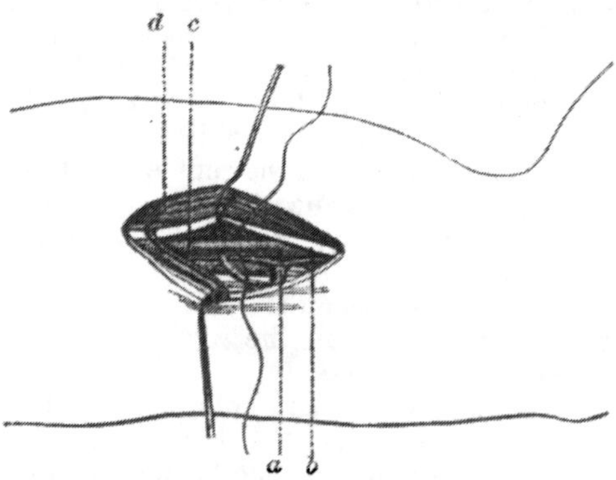

Fig. 64.

Modifications.—If the incision is made a little too far back the ulnar nerve is exposed, and is liable to be mistaken for the median; and this error may be confirmed by the presence of the vein, occupying the same relative position as the brachial to the median, which may be mistaken for the artery. If it is remembered that the ulnar nerve here passes downwards and backwards, the error will be rectified. The brachial may have a high division into the radial and ulnar; or it may have a high division, and the branches again unite in the arm.

III. Operation at the Upper Third.—The arm being extended as before, an incision two inches and a half in length is made along the inner border of the coraco-brachialis; the artery is readily exposed, lying between and behind the median and ulnar nerves, the former to the outside, and the latter to the inside.

Axillary Artery.—This artery extends from the lower border of the first rib to the lower margin of the tendon of the latissimus dorsi, or the inferior boundary of the axilla; its course is in a line dividing the anterior and middle third of the axilla. It may be ligated in two places:—

I. Below the Pectoralis Minor.—In its lower half the artery is superficial, covered only by the integuments and deep fascia; the coraco-brachialis muscle is in contact with the artery, which may be found at its internal and posterior border; the branches of the brachial plexus of nerves surround the artery, the musculo-cutaneous lies along the outer side; the two roots of the median meet in front, at the lower border of the pectoralis minor; the nerve then lies in front and to the outer side of the artery; the internal cutaneous lies in front and to its inner side; the ulnar and radial are still further within and behind; the axillary vein is in front of the artery and nerves, which it partly conceals.

Operation.—(Fig. 65.) The patient is placed on the back, and the arm rotated outwards; the operator stands on the outside if it is the right arm, and on the inner side if the left, and recognising the inner border of the coraco-brachialis muscle, *g*, and the pulsations, makes an incision two or three inches in length, in the line indicated, *b*, dividing only the skin; the fascia is then incised on a director; with the end of the direc-

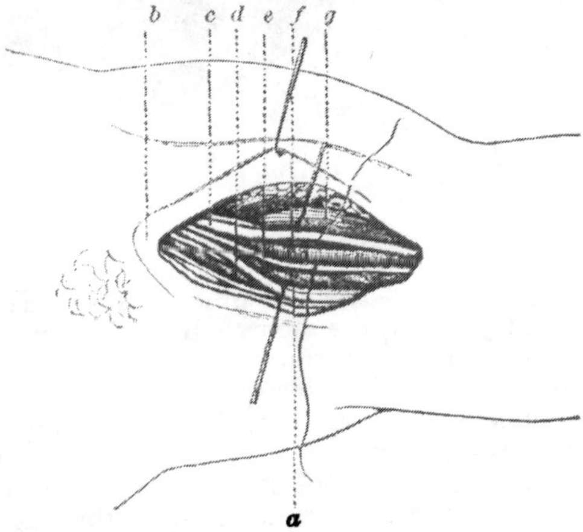

Fig. 65.

tor, the axillary vein, *a*, is first pushed backwards, then the brachial plexus; the median nerve, *c*, is now recognised, and being brought forward, while the internal cutaneous, *e*, and ulnar, *d*, are pushed backwards, the artery, *f*, is exposed. The artery is carefully separated from the vein, which is pushed backwards, and the nerves which surround it, and the needle is passed from behind forwards.

II. Below the Clavicle.—(Fig. 66.) In its upper part the axillary artery is covered successively by the insertion of the pectoralis minor, *j*; higher up by the pectoralis major muscle, *i*, from which it is separated by a layer of adipose tissue, containing numerous small veins and arteries; and finally by the fasciæ and the skin; the suprascapular artery, *a*, crosses the base of the neck just above the clavicle; the axillary vein, *h*, in front and to the inner side of the artery, is not in immediate contact with it; the cephalic vein passes upwards in the interspace between the deltoid and pectoralis major muscles, crosses the axillary artery above the pectoralis minor, and empties into the axillary vein; the nerves, *b*, of the brachial plexus, *c*, lie behind and above; a thoracic branch often crosses the artery, sometimes in front, and sometimes behind it.

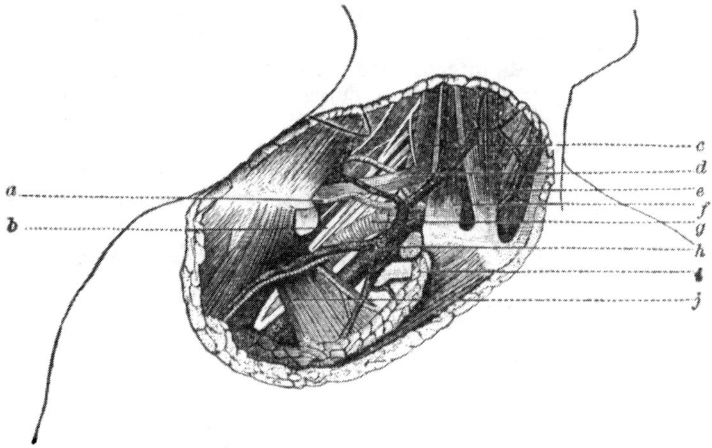

Fig. 66.

Operation.—The patient is placed on his back, with his shoulders slightly raised, the elbow a little separated from the body, and the head inclined to the opposite side; an incision is made three inches in length, three quarters of an inch below the clavicle, and commencing about two inches outside of the sterno-clavicular articulation, through the skin, platysma, and subcutaneous cellular tissue; the fibres of the pectoralis major are separated gradually until the posterior investment of this muscle, like an aponeurosis, appears; the shoulder is now depressed and this fascia torn by the point of the director; the upper border of the pectoralis minor is now pressed downwards and outwards with the finger, when the axillary vein is brought to view; this is drawn gently forward with a blunt hook, and behind it the artery is found, with the nerves of the brachial plexus still further behind and above. The needle is passed from within outwards.

Method with a Flap.—(Fig. 67.) The following method, known as Chamberlaine's, has many obvious advantages. A transverse incision is made, three inches in length, through the skin and platysma, along and upon the lower edge of the clavicle, three fingers' breadth from the sternal extremity of that bone, and terminating an inch from the acromion process of the scapula; a second incision, three inches in length, is made obliquely through the integuments,

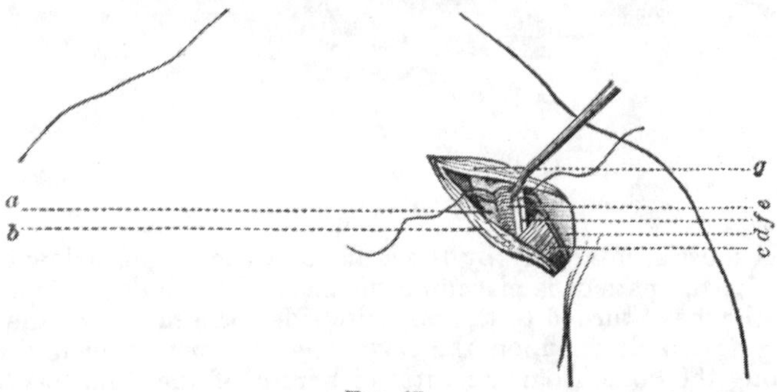

Fig. 67

over the deltoid and pectoral muscles, meeting the first nearly in the centre; the cellular membrane and fat are removed; the clavicular portion of the pectoralis major, *g*, *b*, is detached and the cellular tissue overlying the subclavian vessels removed; the artery now appears and its pulsations are detected; the pectoralis minor, *c*, and the margin of the deltoid, *d*, are brought to view, and the artery, *e*, is isolated from the vein, *a*, lying in front, and the brachial plexus behind.

Subclavian Artery.—The subclavian artery arises from the innominata on the right side, and from the arch of the aorta on the left; it extends in a curved direction from its origin to the lower border of the first rib. It may be ligated in three places.

I. **Outside of the Scaleni Muscles.**—(Fig. 66.) This portion of the artery, *g*, passes downwards and outwards, lying in a groove on the first rib; it first passes through the supra-clavicular triangle, and is then covered only by the deep fascia, the platysma, and skin; lower in its course it is covered by the clavicle and subclavian muscle; the subclavian vein, *h*, lies lower and in front of the artery, separated from it by the insertion of the scalenus anticus muscle, *c*; the external jugular vein crosses in front of the artery; the brachial plexus of nerves lies above and behind the artery. The artery may generally be compressed on the first rib.

Operation.—(Fig. 68.) The artery is sought for in the supra-clavicular triangle, which is bounded externally by the omo-

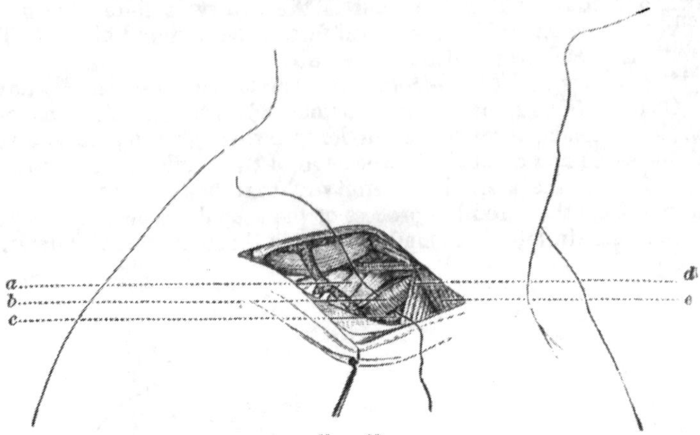

FIG. 68.

hyoid muscle, internally by the scalenus anticus, and below by the first rib, the patient is placed on his back, the shoulders depressed, and the head turned to the opposite side; the skin over the parts being drawn down upon the clavicle, an incision is made through it along the bone, from the anterior border of the trapezius to the posterior border of the sterno-mastoid, *e;* the platysma and superficial fascia are divided, care being taken to draw the external jugular outward, or, if cut, to tie the ends; with the director and finger the cellular and fatty tissue are separated, and the omo-hyoid muscle made out and held aside; the deep fascia is now divided and the border of the scalenus, *d*, defined; the finger is now passed along its margin down to the first rib; the tubercle for the attachment of that muscle is recognised, just external to which the artery, *b*, will be felt pulsating. The attachments of the artery are separated with the finger nail, and the aneurism needle (the American, Fig. 52, being the best) is gently insinuated beneath it, from before backwards, avoiding the vein, *c*, and slightly from within outwards; the point of the needle is guided by the end of the finger, and prevented, when it emerges upon the opposite side, from engaging any branch of the brachial plexus, *a*.

Variations.—Roux made an incision perpendicular to the clavicle; Lisfranc divided the external attachments of the sterno-mastoid; Physick made a V incision; Ramsden and Liston give the horizontal incision, with a second running along the outer margin of the sterno-mastoid; Blizard made an incision parallel with the external jugular.

Complications.—The sterno-mastoid may have an unusually extended insertion upon the clavicle, as also the trapezius, in which case the incision must involve the clavicular attachments of the former; the external jugular may run so near to the sterno-mastoid as to be involved in the incision, unless it is carefully isolated and drawn to the outer side; the transverse cervical and supra-scapular arteries may be met with in this dissection, and if wounded should be immediately ligated; the tubercle of the rib is sometimes not well defined, in which case the attachment of the scalenus to the rib is the guide to the artery, which is found just posterior to its insertion.

III. Between the Scaleni.—The artery at this point is very short, and passes between the two scaleni muscles; it is covered by the integuments, platysma, sterno-mastoid, and the scalenus anticus, upon which lies the phrenic nerve; below is the pleura and above the brachial plexus. The ligature has seldom been applied at this point.

Operation.—The incision is made as before, and the tubercle of the rib being recognised, and the insertion of the muscle into it, the director is passed behind it and between the muscle and the artery, and with a bistoury the muscle is divided; its retraction exposes the artery, which is readily ligated. The needle is passed from without inwards.

Modifications.—Dr. Mott advises to divide the muscle internally; Malgaigne directs to divide the muscle from without inwards, commencing some distance from the rib.

Complications.—The phrenic nerve is divided, unless the proceeding of Mott or Malgaigne is adopted; the internal mammary artery is outside the nerve, and is liable to be wounded if the incision is too near the rib.

III. Within the Scaleni.—On the right side the artery passes upwards and outwards from its origin from the innominata across the neck to the internal border of the scalenus anticus muscle; it is very deeply situated, and lies upon the pleura; its anatomical relations are, in front, the skin, fasciæ, platysma, origin of sterno-mastoid, sterno-hyoid, and thyroid muscles; it is also crossed by the pneumogastric, cardiac, and phrenic nerves, and by the internal jugular and vertebral veins; behind, it is in relation with the recurrent laryngeal and sympathetic nerves.

On the left side the artery extends from the left portion of the arch of the aorta to the scalenus anticus, situated very deeply, and passing upwards, almost vertically; in addition to the anatomical relations of the right, the left has in front the pleura, the lung, and the carotid, and internally, the œsophagus, trachea. and thoracic duct.

Operation on the Right Subclavian.—The patient is placed on his back, the shoulders raised, and the head turned to the opposite side; two incisions are made, one parallel with the inner part of the clavicle, and the other along the inner border of the sterno-mastoid;

a director is passed behind the sternal attachment of the sterno-mastoid, which is divided; the cellular tissue is divided with the handle of the scalpel, and finger; small arteries and veins in this part, and especially the anterior jugular, are avoided; the sterno-hyoid and thyroid muscles are divided on a director; the deep fascia now divided with the finger-nail, or end of the director, exposes the internal jugulars, which being pressed aside, the needle is passed around the artery from below upwards to avoid the pleura.

Operation on the Left Subclavian.—The following is the operation as performed by Dr. Rodgers, of this city:—The patient being placed in the position above described, an incision three inches and a half long was made on the inner edge of the sterno-mastoid, terminating at the sternum, through the skin and platysma; this was met by another incision along the sternal extremity of the clavicle, two and a half inches; the flap was dissected, and the sternal and half the clavicular origin of the sterno-mastoid divided on a director, and the flap raised; the deep fascia was then divided by the handle of the scalpel and the fingers, the dissection continued along the outer side of the deep jugular vein to the inner edge of the scalenus anticus muscle, half an inch above the rib, to avoid the thoracic duct; the phrenic nerve was detected and avoided, and the fingers pressed to the bottom of the wound, discovered the rib, and then the artery; the needle was passed from below upwards.

Internal Mammary Artery.—This artery arises from the subclavian, and descends behind the clavicle to the inner surface of the costal cartilages near the sternum; the internal jugular and subclavian veins and the phrenic nerve cross its upper part; in the chest it at first lies on the costal cartilages and intercostal muscles, covered by the pleura behind; but lower it is covered also by the triangularis sterni muscle; it may be tied in the second, third, or fourth intercostal spaces.

Operation.—An incision is made from the upper edge of the rib, commencing at the sternum, in either space, and carried slightly upwards, and outwards, an inch and a half in length; the skin, cellular tissue, pectoralis major muscle, fascia, and intercostal muscle are successively divided; a thin layer of cellular tissue opened, when the artery is exposed, and the needle cautiously passed from within outwards.

Vertebral Artery.—The vertebral artery arises from the subclavian artery in the first part of its course, and passes directly along the spinal column, entering the foramen in the transverse process of the sixth cervical vertebra; it passes along the foramen in each of the vertebræ to the brain. It may be tied at the following points:—

I. Before entering the Vertebral Canal.—The artery passes to the vertebral canal, behind the internal jugular vein and inferior thyroid artery, to the spine, where it lies between the scalenus anticus and the longus colli, and in a line drawn from the posterior part of the mastoid process, to the junction of the internal fourth with the external three-fourths of the clavicle.

Operation.—The patient is placed on the back, the shoulder depressed, and the head turned to the opposite side; an incision is made, three inches in length, along the inner border of the sterno-mastoid muscle, between it and the sterno-hyoid, and terminating at the middle of the upper extremity of the sternum; the skin, cellular tissue, and the aponeurosis, uniting the sterno-mastoid muscle and sterno-hyoid, are divided, bringing into view the common sheath of the carotid, the internal jugular, and the pneumogastric nerve; the cellular connexion of the sheath with the sterno-thyroid muscle, and finally, with the longus colli, is separated with the finger; the head is now raised, though still turned to the opposite side, and the sides of the wound forcibly separated; the cellular tissue at the bottom is divided, and exposing an aponeurosis which passes from the scalenus anticus to the longus colli, the anterior part of the transverse process of the sixth cervical vertebra, the "carotid tubercle" of Chassaignac, is recognised; the aponeurosis is opened an inch below this point, at the external border of the longus colli muscle; the artery lies very deeply, and should be isolated with the American needle.

Modifications.—Chassaignac makes an incision, three inches in length, in the course of the line above given, as marking the course of the artery. Ippolito makes his incision in the triangular space formed by the external jugular vein, the posterior edge of the sterno-mastoid, and the clavicle, and seeks for the inner margin of the scalenus anticus.

II. Between the Atlas and Axis.—The artery lies in a triangular space formed by the rectus posticus minor, and superior and inferior oblique muscles, and is covered by the rectus posticus major, and complexus.

Operation.—The head is turned to the opposite side, and inclined forwards; an incision two inches long is made on the posterior edge of the sterno-mastoid, commencing half an inch above the mastoid process; a second incision is made, an inch in length, from the upper fourth of the first incision backwards and obliquely downwards; the skin and cellular tissue are divided; then the splenius muscle with its fibrous expansion; a fibrous layer now appears, which must be cautiously divided to arrive at the small arteries which lie beneath it; the edges of the wound being separated, a layer of fat appears, which is cautiously opened with the finger or handle of the scalpel, and the artery is found within; the two branches of the occipital artery are to be drawn aside, as also branches of the second cervical nerve; the artery is isolated, and the needle passed from without inwards to avoid the internal carotid artery.

III. Between the Atlas and Occiput.—The anatomical relations are as given above.

Operation.—The incisions are the same as in the last operation, except that the first cut commences one-fourth of an inch above the mastoid process; the skin, fascia, and splenius muscle, are divided, the occipital artery appears at the upper angle of the first wound and is held aside; the underlying aponeurosis, with the cellular tissue, is divided; the edges of the wound are separated, and in a triangle formed by the muscles of the part, the cellular tissue, loaded with fat, covers the artery; this is divided and the artery exposed; the needle is passed from below upwards.

Inferior Thyroid Artery.—This artery is a branch of the thyroid axis; it ascends the neck obliquely, passing behind the internal jugular, the pneumogastric nerve, the carotid artery, and omohyoid muscle, to the thyroid body.

Operation.—The inferior thyroid may be ligated through the same incision as is made for the ligature of the common carotid (Fig. 70).

Innominata.—The innominata, arising from the right superior portion of the arch of the aorta, in front of the left carotid, passes in an oblique direction, upwards, outwards, and backwards, to the superior margin of the sternal articulation of the clavicle, when it divides into the right subclavian and right common carotid, being from one and a half to two inches in length. It is in relation on the right with the pleura, right vena innominata, and right pneumogastric nerve; behind, with the trachea; in front, above, with the sternum, and the origin of the sterno-hyoid, and thyroid; below, with the inferior thyroid vein, and left vena innominata; and on the left, with the left carotid.

Operation.—The following are the steps of Dr. Mott's operation:—The patient being placed on the back, the shoulders slightly raised, and face turned to the opposite side, an incision three inches in length was made just above the clavicle, and terminating over the trachea; another incision, of the same length, extended from this point along the inner border of the sterno-mastoid; the integuments were dissected off, the platysma divided; the sternal and part of the clavicular portion of the sterno-mastoid were then divided on the director at the first incision, and turned outwards; the sterno-hyoid and thyroid were divided and drawn inwards, exposing the sheath of the carotid, par vagum, and internal jugular vein; the par vagum was now separated from the carotid, and with the vein, drawn to the outside, while the artery was drawn towards the trachea, enabling the operator to expose the subclavian; the innominata was now reached by separating the cellular tissue, and the needle passed from below upwards and inwards.

The following method by Manec represents many of the modifications of this operation:—The patient is placed on the back, the head thrown backwards, in order to bring upwards the artery, the face turned slightly to the left shoulder; an incision is made, three inches in length, extending from a point midway between the two sterno-mastoid muscles, towards the right shoulder, half an inch above the clavicle (Fig. 69); the skin and platysma are incised; then, on a director, the sterno-mastoid, *e*, and sterno-hyoid and

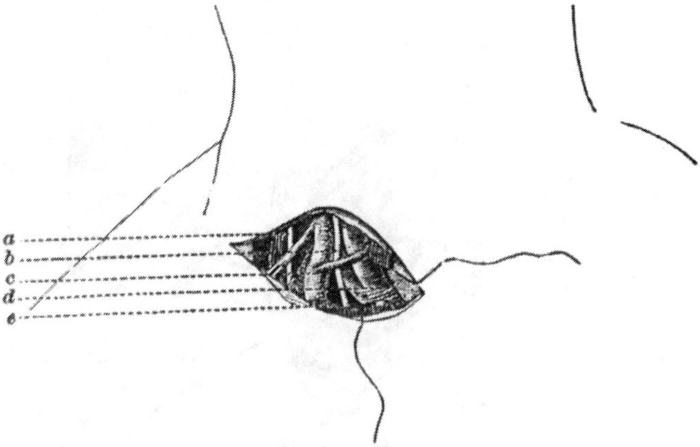

FIG. 69.

thyroid are successively divided; with the handle of the knife the artery, *d*, is isolated, care being taken to avoid the pneumogastric nerve, *b*, the internal jugular vein, *c*, and the phrenic nerve, *a*.

ARTERIES OF THE NECK AND HEAD.

Subclavian and Common Carotid Arteries.—(Fig. 70.) These two vessels may be ligated, according to Sédillot, by the following operation:—The patient being placed in the position for ligature of the innominata, an incision three inches in length is made through the integuments, along the space separating the clavicular and sternal attachments of the sterno-cleido-mastoid muscle; this interval is marked by a depression above the clavicle, at the articulation of the clavicle and sternum; the head is now slightly flexed, and the internal portion of the muscle, *a*, is separated from the external, *b*, the sterno-hyoid and thyroid are divided on the canula; the operator now readily exposes the innominata, *h*; the common carotid, *e*; the pneumogastric, *d*, and its branch, the recurrent laryngeal; the origin of the subclavian, *g*, and its branches, the vertebral, *c*, and inferior thyroid.

Common Carotid Artery.—This artery extends on the right side from the innominata, and on the left from the highest point of the arch of the aorta, to the upper border of the thyroid cartilage; their direction is obliquely from before backwards, and from within outwards, along the external side of the trachea and larynx, in a line drawn from the sternal end of the clavicle, below, to a point

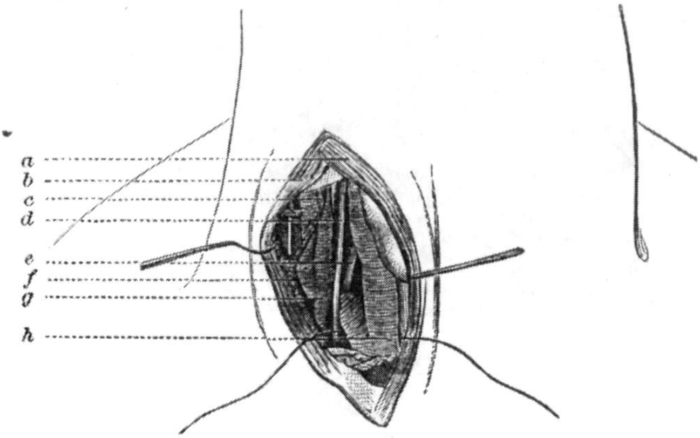

FIG. 70.

midway between the mastoid process and angle of the jaw above. Its sheath is derived from the deep fascia, and contains the internal jugular and the pneumogastric nerve, the vein being external, and the nerve between. The vessel may be ligated at two points:—

I. AT THE BASE OF THE NECK.—The artery is here deeply seated, having in front the platysma, superficial and deep fasciæ, the sterno-mastoid, sterno-hyoid, and sterno-thyroid muscles; externally it is in relation with the pneumogastric nerve and internal jugular vein; internally with the trachea; posteriorly with the longus colli and rectus anticus major muscle; the internal jugular of the right side recedes from the artery, but on the left approaches and often overlaps it.

Chassaignac lays great stress on what he calls the "carotid tubercle," as a guide to the position of the artery; this tubercle is the anterior projection of the transverse process of the sixth cervical vertebra, which is two inches above the clavicle, and is a precise guide to the artery when the neck is straight; it corresponds in front and a little inside to the artery.

Operation.—(Fig. 71.) The following operation is proposed by Sédillot:—The patient is placed on the back, the head extended and inclined to the opposite side; the interval between the two attachments of the sterno-mastoid muscle is recognised, and an incision is made from the clavicle, two and a half inches, obliquely, along this interspace; the skin, platysma, and deep fascia are divided; the internal portion of the muscle, *c*, is drawn inwards, and the external, *a*, outwards, by means of spatulas; this exposes the internal jugular vein, *b*, and the pneumogastric nerve, *e*, lying between the vein, *b*, and the artery, *f*, and the omo-hyoid muscle, *d*, crossing the upper part of the wound; the common vascular

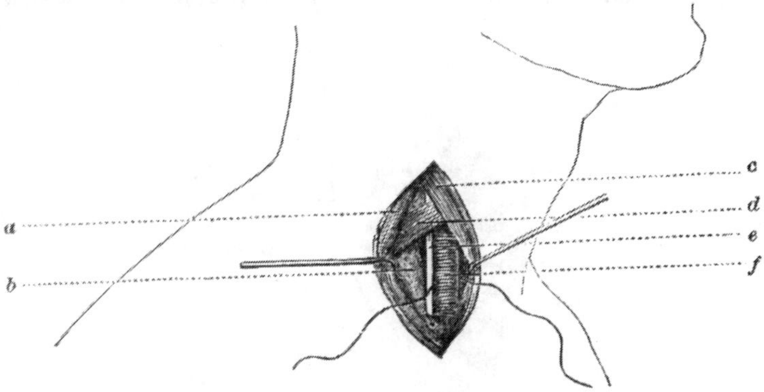

Fig. 71.

sheath is opened and the needle passed from without inwards, carefully avoiding the internal jugular vein and par vagum; a finger pressed upon the vein at the upper part of the wound will cause it to collapse.

Modifications.—Malgaigne rejects this operation, and proposes (*Bernard* and *Huette*) the following:—1st. Make an incision from two and a half to three inches in length, extending from a point one-third of an inch above the sterno-clavicular articulation, upwards in the direction of a line which, if produced, would meet the symphysis of the chin; 2d. The skin, cellular tissue, and deep cervical fascia being divided, the sternal insertion of the sterno-mastoid muscle is laid bare; 3d. Divide this in the direction of the external incision, and beneath it will be found the sterno-hyoid and sterno-thyroid muscles, which are to be pushed inwards towards the trachea; 4th. The sheath containing the vessels is now in view, and it should be opened, in the usual manner, as near to the trachea as possible, in order to avoid the vein.

II. Below the Omo-Hyoid.—The artery at this point is covered by the integument, the platysma, the superficial and deep fasciæ, the sternal part of the sterno-mastoid, the sterno-hyoid, and thyroid muscles; it is crossed obliquely, from within outwards, by the sterno-mastoid artery, also by the superior and middle thyroid veins, and lower down by the anterior jugular; on the outer side are the pneumogastric nerve and internal jugular vein, and on the inside are the inferior thyroid artery and recurrent laryngeal nerve, which separates it from the trachea and thyroid gland; the descendens noni nerve lies on the sheath of the artery.

Operation.—(Fig. 72.) The patient is placed on the back, with the head thrown back, an incision three inches in length is made along the inner border of the sterno-mastoid muscle, in the line above given; commencing on a level with the cricoid cartilage, the skin, superficial fascia, platysma, and deep fascia, are successively divided, and the inner border of the sterno-mastoid, *e*,

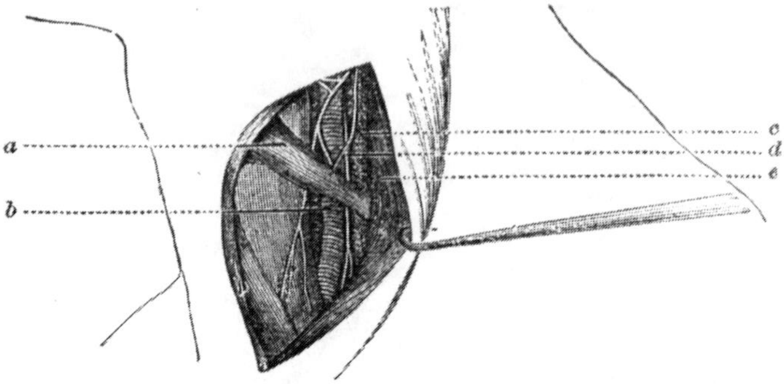

FIG. 72.

exposed; the sterno-mastoid artery and middle thyroid vein are here carefully avoided; the head is now thrown forward and the sterno-mastoid muscle is drawn outward, and the sterno-hyoid and thyroid muscles inwards, exposing the anterior belly of the omo-hyoid muscle, *a*, which should be drawn upwards; the deep fascia being divided, the sheath of the vessel is exposed; this is opened directly over the artery, avoiding carefully the descendens noni, which runs along the tracheal side; the pneumogastric nerve, *d*, and internal jugular vein, *c*, are pressed outwardly, and the needle passed from without inwards, carefully isolating the vessel from the inferior thyroid artery, and recurrent laryngeal nerve, which lies behind it.

Complications.—The thyroid body may be so large as to mislead as to the margin of the muscle, and then requires careful dissection; if the omo-hyoid muscle interferes with the operation it may be turned aside, or even divided by dissection.

III. ABOVE THE OMO-HYOID.—The artery is more superficial in this part of its course, being covered only by the skin, the two fasciæ, platysma, and the border of the sterno-mastoid; it is in relation internally with the larynx and pharynx, and externally with the pneumogastric nerve, and internal jugular vein.

Operation.—The patient is placed on the back, the shoulders raised, and the head turned to the opposite side; an incision is made from a little below the angle of the jaw, in the line given, along the internal border of the sterno-mastoid, three inches in length; the integuments, superficial fascia, and platysma, are divided, and the deep fascia raised carefully on a director, to avoid the small underlying veins, and incised; the head is now flexed to relax the muscles, the wound drawn apart by spatulas; the descendens noni nerve and superior thyroid arteries are avoided, and the sheath opened over the artery; if the internal jugular vein swell up into the wound, it should be compressed in the upper and lower part of the wound, and drawn outwards; the ligature is passed from without inwards, the point being kept close upon the artery to avoid wounding the vein, or including the pneumogastric nerve.

External Carotid Artery.—The external carotid ascends from its origin at the upper margin of the thyroid cartilage, at first, slightly forwards, then backwards, to the space between the condyle of the lower jaw and the meatus auditorius; it may be ligated as follows:—

I. BELOW THE DIGASTRIC.—At its origin the external carotid is more superficial and nearer the median line than the internal carotid; it occupies the triangle formed by the sterno-mastoid behind, the omo-hyoid below, and the posterior belly of the digastric and stylo-hyoid above; it has two veins, and is crossed by the hypoglossal nerve, and by the lingual and facial veins.

Operation.—An incision is made along the inner margin of the sterno-mastoid, three inches in length, from the angle of the jaw to the cricoid cartilage, through the skin, platysma, superficial and deep fascia; the internal margin of the sterno-mastoid now appears, the cellular tissue is cautiously separated, and the wound being drawn apart, the artery is exposed, the digastric muscle and hypoglossal nerve are separated from the sheath and drawn upwards, the internal carotid artery and internal jugular outwards, and the needle passed from without inwards.

II. ABOVE THE DIGASTRIC.—The artery here lies more deeply and is crossed by the stylo-hyoid muscle.

Operation.—The incision should extend from the lobe of the ear to the great corner of the hyoid bone, along the inner margin of the sterno-mastoid; the skin, platysma, and fascia being divided, the posterior belly of the digastric and stylo-hyoid are separated from the parotid gland, and depressed, exposing the artery, which is to be ligated as above described.

Superior Thyroid Artery.—This artery arises from the external carotid, just below the greater cornu of the hyoid bone, and passes inwards to the thyroid gland in a tortuous course; it is at first superficial, lying in the triangle formed by the sterno-mastoid, digastric, and omo-hyoid muscles.

Operation.—The head being placed in an extended position, an incision of an inch and a half is made along the internal border of the sterno-mastoid, the centre of which corresponds to the great cornu of the thyroid cartilage; the skin and platysma being incised, the sterno-mastoid is drawn outwards, exposing the omo-hyoid muscle, internal jugular vein, and primitive carotid artery; the artery lies between these vessels and the lobe of the thyroid body, and is readily ligated.

Lingual Artery.—The lingual artery is the second branch of the external carotid; it arises just above the superior thyroid, ascends to the great cornu of the hyoid bone, runs parallel with the greater cornu, and passes directly to the base of the tongue.

Operation.—(Fig. 73.) The head is turned to the opposite side, an oblique incision is made, an inch and a half in length, a little

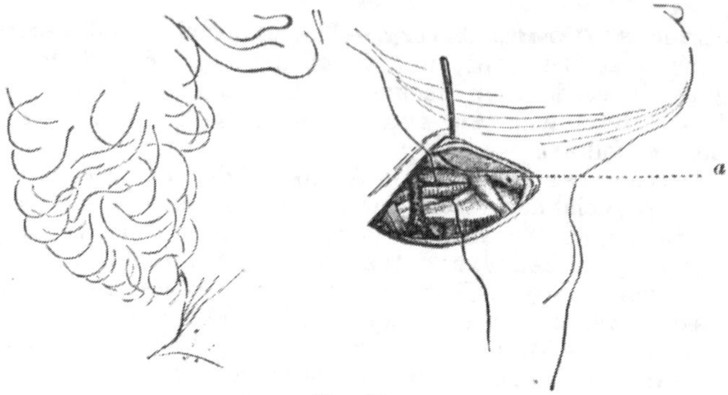

FIG. 73.

above the body of the hyoid bone, and parallel with it, near the median line, and curved backwards, outwards, and downwards, parallel with the superior border of the great cornu of the thyroid cartilage; the superficial parts being divided, the finger carried into the wound recognises the direction of the great cornu and divides upon it the aponeurosis which covers the deep parts; this exposes the digastric muscle, the submaxillary gland, hypoglossal nerve, and stylo-hyoid muscle, *a;* the great cornu of the hyoid bone is now isolated, and the fibres of the hyo-glossus muscle, which are attached at this point, come into view; this muscle is divided at the superior border of the great cornu, is drawn upwards and backwards, and the artery, is found behind it; the needle should pass from below upwards.

Malgaigne's method (*Bernard* and *Huette*):—1st. Having recognised the position of one of the greater cornua of the hyoid bone, make an incision about an inch in length, parallel with, and about two lines above it, through the skin, cellular tissue, and platysma; 2d. This incision will expose the lower border of the submaxillary gland, on lifting which slightly, the shining tendon of the digastric will be recognised; 3d. Less than a line below this lies the great hypoglossal nerve, and at the distance of a line below the nerve, a transverse incision through the fibres of the genio-hyo-glossus muscle, will certainly expose the artery, which, in this situation, is accompanied by neither vein nor nerves.

Facial Artery.—(Fig. 74.) This artery passes over the lower jaw, at the anterior border of the masseter muscle, *a;* it lies on the periosteum, and in a groove which is recognised at the junction of the posterior third with the anterior two-thirds of the body of the bone; the facial vein lies on the outer side.

Operation.—The pulsation of the artery being recognised, make an incision an inch in length, along the course of the vessel as

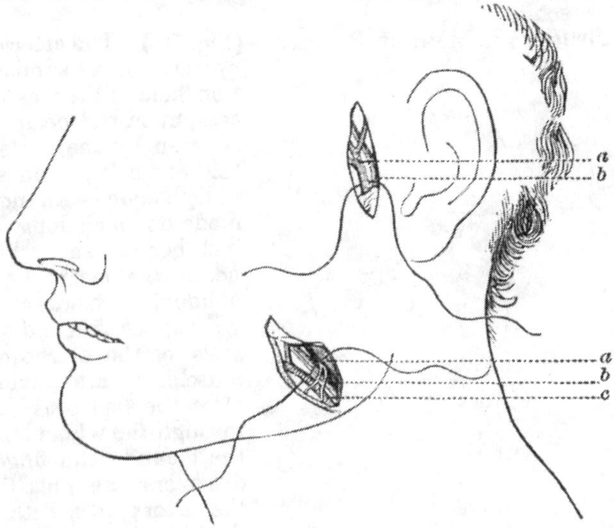

FIG. 74.

already given, through the skin, fascia, and platysma; the wound being separated, and the fibrous tissue divided, the artery, *c*, is exposed, and the vein, *b*, and masseter muscle, *a*, are drawn outwards, and the needle passed.

Temporal Artery.—(Fig. 74, upper part.) The temporal artery runs upwards towards the temporal region from its origin at the condyle of the jaw, in front of the concha; two inches above the zygoma it divides into the anterior and posterior branches.

Operation.—Recognising the position of the artery by its pulsation, at a point a little above the zygomatic arch, and in front of the ear, an incision is made through the skin, an inch in length, the dense cellular tissue is divided on a director, the artery, *a*, exposed, and the needle passed from without inwards, to avoid the temporal vein, *b*, and the auriculo-temporal nerve.

Occipital Artery.—The occipital arises from the external carotid, opposite the facial, ascends to the space between the transverse process of the atlas and the mastoid process, and passes up upon the occiput; it may be ligated—

I. At its Origin.—The artery is here covered by the stylo-hyoid and digastric muscles, and the hypoglossal nerve winds around it from behind forwards.

Operation.—An incision is made along the inner border of the sterno-mastoid muscle, two inches in length, at the angle formed by this muscle and the digastric; the deep fascia being carefully divided, the artery is exposed and isolated, the nerve being carefully protected.

II. Behind the Mastoid Process.—(Fig. 75.) The artery passes upwards, in a tortuous direction, behind the mastoid process, upon the occiput; it is covered by the sterno-mastoid and splenius muscles.

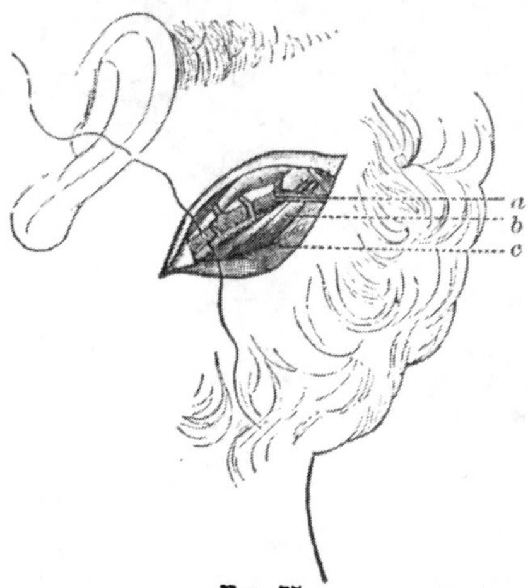

Fig. 75.

Operation.—An incision is made one inch long, half an inch behind, and a little beneath the mastoid process, obliquely upwards and backwards; the skin and aponeurosis of the sterno-mastoid muscle, *c*, are divided, as also the splenius muscle, through the whole length of the wound; the finger now discovers the pulsations of the artery, *a*, a little above the oblique muscle, *b*, and it is isolated from its veins.

ARTERIES OF THE LOWER EXTREMITIES.

Dorsalis Pedis Artery.—This artery terminates the anterior tibial, and runs in a line drawn from the middle of the intermalleolar space, measured from the extremities of the malleoli, to the space between the first metatarsal bones; it is covered by the integuments, fascia, and innermost tendon of the extensor brevis digitorum; on its inner side is the extensor proprius pollicis, and externally, the inner tendon of the extensor longus digitorum; it has two veins, and on its external aspect is the anterior tibial nerve.

Operation.—(Fig. 76.) An incision is made two inches in length on the line indicated, being parallel to the external border of the tendon of the extensor proprius pollicis muscle, *c;* the skin and deep fascia are divided on a director, and the internal division of the extensor brevis digitorum, *a*, is drawn outwards, exposing the artery, *d*, and its accompanying veins, *b;* the nerve is to the outside; the needle is passed from within outwards.

Anterior Tibial Artery.—The anterior tibial artery emerges upon the anterior part of the leg, at its upper part, through the interosseous membrane, and passes down to the ankle, in a line drawn from the inner side of the fibula to a point midway between the two malleoli; it may be ligated at any point in its course.

I. In its Lower Third.—The artery is covered by the teguments and fascia, and is crossed by the extensor proprius pollicis; it lies at first between the tibialis anticus muscle and the extensor proprius pollicis, the latter muscle crossing to the inner side; the artery lies between the tendon of this muscle, and that of the extensor longus digitorum; it is accompanied by venæ comites, and the anterior tibial nerve, which here lies to the outer side.

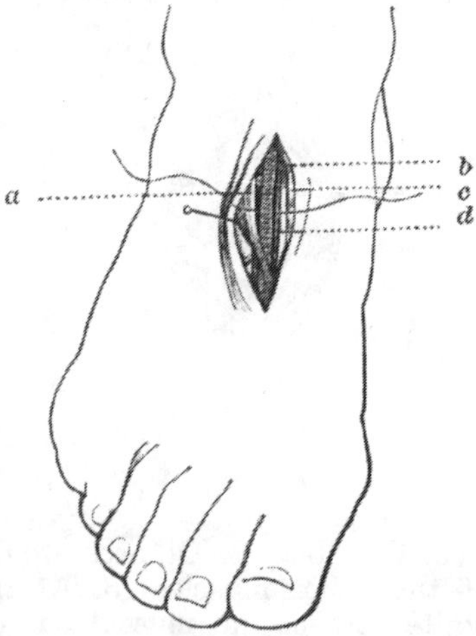

Fig. 76.

Operation.—The leg being placed in a horizontal position the foot is extended, and the tibialis anticus muscle recognised; an incision is made along the external border of that muscle, on the line already indicated, three inches in length, but not extending to the annular ligament; the deep fascia is carefully incised on a director, the space between the tibialis anticus and extensor proprius pollicis is found, and the two muscles separated with the index finger; the foot is now flexed, and the artery exposed, resting on the tibia, with the nerve superficial to it; it is isolated from the two veins, and the needle passed from within outwards, the nerve being drawn inwards. If the incision falls between the extensor proprius pollicis muscle, and the extensor communis digitorum, the ligature may still be applied.

II. In its Middle Third.—The artery is covered by the skin, superficial and deep fascia; on the inner side it has the tibialis anticus muscle, and on the external the extensor longus digitorum and extensor proprius pollicis.

Operation.—(Fig. 77.) The limb being placed as in the former position, an incision is made three inches or more in length, in the course of the artery, through the integument; the septum in the deep fascia uniting the two muscles is recognised by a white line; this is divided longitudinally, and also by a crucial incision; the foot is flexed to relax the muscles, and the wound being separated by drawing the tibialis anticus, *b*, internally, and the extensor longus digitorum and extensor proprius pollicis, externally, the nerve is met with more superficially than the artery, *d*, with its veins, *c*; the needle is passed from within outwards.

III. In its Upper Third.—The artery lies deeply between the tibialis anticus and extensor longus digitorum; those muscles having their origin in part from the deep fascia, the intermuscular septum is not easily recognised, nor are the muscles readily separated.

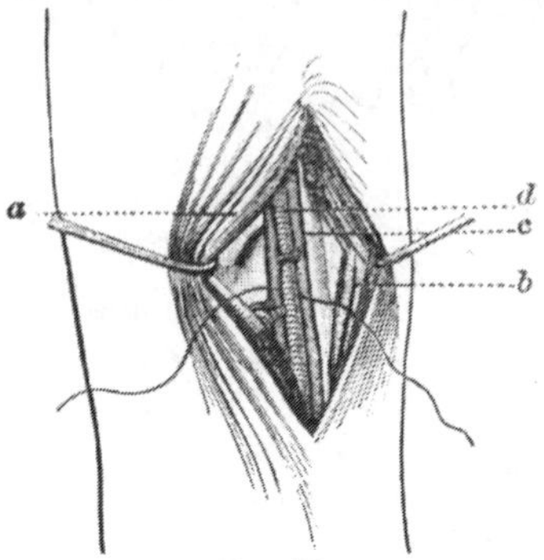

Fig. 77.

Operation.—The limb being turned inwards, the foot extended, take as a guide the line already given, or a point ten lines to the outer side of the spine of the tibia, and make an incision about four inches in length through the integument; the deep fascia is divided with a crucial incision to allow of its complete separation; the intermuscular septum is now sought for, and may be recognised, 1. As the first intermuscular space from the tibia; 2. On pressure from within outwards the resistance of the other muscles; 3. At the lower part of the wound the white line of the muscular interspace is more marked; the foot being flexed, the muscles are separated with the index finger, and the wound held apart, the artery is exposed with its two veins and nerve, the latter being outside; the needle is passed from without inwards.

Modifications.—Chassaignac makes an incision commencing three fingers' breadth below the head of the fibula, four fingers' breadth in length, in a line running from the anterior border of the head of the fibula to the anterior border of the internal malleolus; Lisfranc extends the incision from the external side of the crest of the tibia upwards and outwards, terminating an inch from the crest of the tibia superiorly.

Posterior Tibial Artery.—The posterior tibial, a branch of the popliteal artery, extends from the lower border of the popliteus muscle, in an oblique direction, from without inwards, to the annular ligament; its course is in a line commencing in the centre of the popliteal space and terminating behind the internal malleolus; it may be ligated—

I. In its Lower Third.—The artery passes down behind the internal malleolus, running at first parallel with the tendo-achillis, and then midway between the internal malleolus and the tuberosity of the os calcis; it is very superficial, and is in relation anteriorly with the tendons of the tibialis posticus and flexor longus digitorum, and posteriorly with the posterior tibial nerve; it has venæ comites.

Operation.—(Fig. 78.) The leg being placed on its external aspect, the foot flexed, an incision is made two inches in length, a finger's breadth posterior to the inner edge of the tibia, and parallel with it; the integuments are divided, the deep fascia, *a*, raised on a director, and a small mass of fat opened, which will expose the artery, *d*, and the venæ comites, *c*, and the posterior tibial nerve, *b;* the sheaths of tendons should be carefully avoided; it should be noticed that the artery sometimes lies anterior to the incision here given.

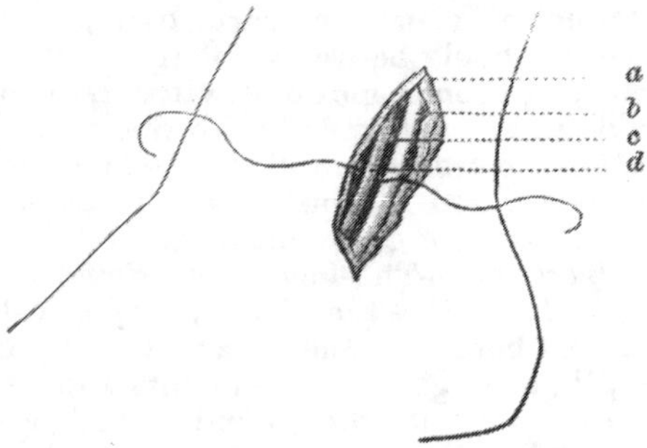

FIG. 78.

The artery may be ligated a little lower by making a curved incision one-third of an inch behind the posterior border of the external malleolus.

Complications.—At this part of the leg the anastomosis of large branches of the internal saphena vein are numerous, and generally run transversely; these may be brought out by compressing the trunk of the vein above, and thus be avoided, at least in part.

II. IN ITS MIDDLE THIRD.—The artery lies superficial, running parallel with the inner border of the tibia, from which it is separated by the flexor longus digitorum; it is covered by the internal border of the soleus; it has venæ comites, and the posterior tibial nerve is on its inner side.

Operation.—(Fig. 79.) The limb is placed as in the last position, and an incision made three inches in length, three-fourths of an inch posterior to the internal border of the tibia; the integument and deep fascia being divided, the fore border of the gastrocnemius, *d*, is seen and drawn backwards, exposing the soleus; the fibres of this muscle should be divided on a director; the artery is now felt pulsating about an inch from the margin of the tibia; the pearl-colored deep aponeurosis which overlies it is divided, and then the muscles relaxed by the position of the limb; the artery, *c*, is isolated from its veins, *b*, the nerve being pressed to the outside; the needle is passed from without inwards.

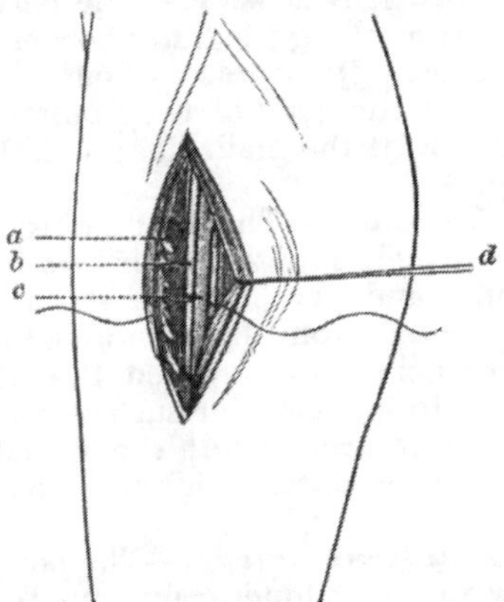

FIG. 79.

Modifications.—Lisfranc makes an oblique incision, from the border of the tendo-achillis, to the inner border of the tibia.

Complications.—The tendinous fibres of the soleus are liable to be mistaken for the deep aponeurosis; if there is doubt as to the anatomical relation of parts, owing to the size of the muscles, the incision should be freely enlarged; anomalies in the origin of the artery are sometimes met with; large branches of the soleus are liable to be confounded with the posterior tibial.

III. AT ITS UPPER THIRD.—The artery here lies very deep, being covered by the tibialis posticus, the deep aponeurosis, the soleus, and the gastrocnemius.

Operation.—The following (*Bernard* and *Huette*) is Malgaigne's method:—1st. At a distance of two-thirds of an inch from the internal border of the tibia make an incision at least four inches in length, through the integuments and deep fascia; 2d. Carrying the index finger into the wound, detach and push outwards the internal head of the gastrocnemius, and divide also the attachments of the soleus, thus exposed, from the posterior surface of the tibia; 3d. Whilst an assistant keeps this muscle held backwards and outwards with a blunt hook, divide the deep layer of aponeurosis upon a director, and search for the vessel immediately beneath; 4th. Detach the artery, and pass the ligature beneath it with the artery needle.

Modifications.—Manec directs the division of the soleus muscle through its entire thickness, at least one inch from the internal edge of the tibia, the wound is gently separated, the anterior aponeurosis of the muscle, a thick, pearly layer, is recognised, and incised the length of the wound; Guthrie advises to make an incision of six or seven inches in length perpendicularly through the calf.

Peroneal Artery.—The peroneal arises from the posterior tibial and runs along the inner border of the fibula to the outer side of the os calcis; its course is marked by a line drawn from the posterior part of the head of the fibula to the external border of the tendo-achillis, at the malleolus; it is ligated just below the middle of the leg.

Operation.—The foot being extended, make an incision, two or three inches long, one or two lines behind the external edge of the fibula and parallel with it; if the soleus is met with, it must be separated from the fibula and drawn inwards; the edge of the bone being now exposed, the attachments of the flexor pollicis proprius to its posterior surface are separated, and the artery is found at its internal side; the muscle has a strong aponeurosis on its anterior surface, which must be divided, as the artery lies under it.

Popliteal Artery.—The popliteal artery extends from the opening in the adductor magnus to the lower border of the popliteus muscle, in an oblique direction, downwards and outwards. The anatomical relations of parts in the popliteal space are as follows:—The external saphenous vein runs perpendicularly in the median line, and in the middle of the popliteal space perforates the deep fascia; then ascends, winds around the popliteal nerve, and empties into the popliteal vein. It is accompanied by the external saphenous nerve, from which it is separated by a process of the deep fascia; the popliteal nerve passes down the middle of the popliteal space, beneath the deep fascia, superficial to, and on the outside of the popliteal vessels, from which it is separated by adipose tissue; it gives off the external saphenous and the peroneal nerves; the popliteal artery is covered in its whole course, and crossed at the middle of the popliteal space, by the popliteal vein, the direction of which is vertical; the artery always beneath the vein, is somewhat internal to it above, and external to it below; the vessels are covered superiorly by the belly of the semi-membranosus; below they pass between the two heads of the gastrocnemius. They are connected together, throughout their course, by dense cellular tissue, which renders their separation difficult. It may be ligated in the following places:—

I. Below the Internal Condyle.—(Fig. 80.) The following is Marchal's method:—The patient is placed on his back, the limb flexed and lying on the outer side; the surgeon, standing on the outside, feels for the internal side of the muscular mass bounding the popliteal space internally and below, makes an incision, *b*, two and a half inches in length, from above downwards, from without inwards, and from behind forwards, along the edge of the internal head of the gastrocnemius, *a*, to within half an inch of the internal border of the tibia; care is taken to avoid the internal saphenous vein, *f*; the aponeurosis is divided a little further back than the skin; the finger is introduced to break down the intermuscular septum, the leg being flexed on the thigh to relax the muscles; at the bottom of the wound is seen the nerve, *e*, to the inside, the artery, *d*, and the accompanying vein, *c*, drawn outwards.

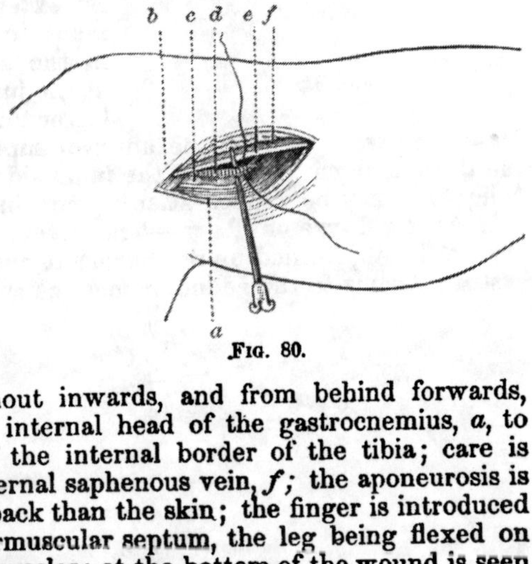

Fig. 80.

II. In its Lower Portion.—(Fig. 81.) The patient is laid on his face, the leg extended, and an incision made through the integument, three inches long, slightly on the outside of the median line; the external saphenous vein, *f*, which lies under the skin, is carefully avoided; the fascia, *a*, is divided, and the cellular substance in the space between the two heads of the gastrocnemius is separated with the finger, exposing the popliteal nerve, *c*, the vein, *b*, and most external, the artery, *d;* the nerve and vein are drawn inwards, and the needle is passed from within outwards.

III. In its Upper Part.—The patient is placed in the same position as last given; an incision is made three inches in length, commencing at the inferior third of the thigh, and passing along the posterior margin of the semi-membranosus muscle; the skin and fascia being divided, the cellular tissue is separated with the director and finger; the leg is now flexed, and the nerve first appears, then the vein to its inside, and lastly the artery; the needle is passed from within outwards.

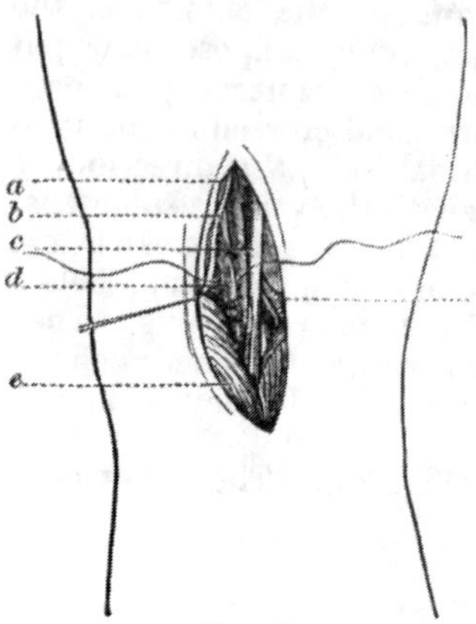

Fig. 81.

Femoral Artery.—The femoral extends from Poupart's ligament to the tendinous opening in the adductor magnus muscle, at the junction of the middle and lower third of the thigh, in a line drawn midway between the anterior superior spine of the ilium, and the symphysis pubis, and the inner side of the internal condyle. A ligature may be applied at any point, but it is generally tied—

I. At its Inferior Part.—The artery at this point enters a fibrous sheath, formed by the fibrous bands which extend from the vastus internus to the adductor magnus and longus, having over it the sartorius muscle, fasciæ, and integuments.

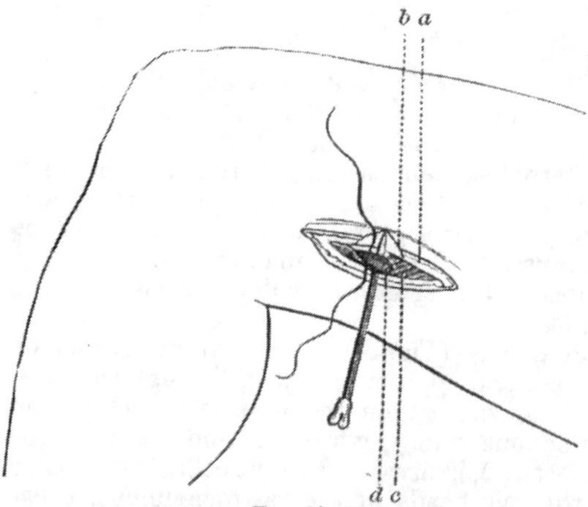

Fig. 82.

Operation.--(Fig. 82.) The thigh is flexed on the pelvis, and the leg on the thigh, and the limb rests on its external surface; an incision is made three inches long on the outer margin of the sartorius muscle, if recognised, or on the line above given; the skin being divided, the sartorius, *c*, recognised, and the fascia, *a*, divided on a director, two lines within its external border; the muscle is drawn backwards and the posterior part of its sheath divided; the space between the vastus internus and adductor magnus is now recognised, which contains the canal of the artery; this canal, *b*, is laid open on a director, and the artery, *d*, exposed, with the vein on its inside, and the saphenous nerve on the outside; the vessels are united by very dense cellular tissue, and great care is necessary to isolate the artery; the needle is passed from without inwards.

II. At its Middle Portion.—The artery is covered by the skin, superficial and deep fasciæ, and sartorius, and is contained in a fibrous canal; the femoral vein lies on the outer and posterior part of the artery, and the long saphenous nerve more externally.

Operation.—The limb is placed in the position above described, and an incision three or four inches in length is made at the middle of the thigh, on the line given, or on the inner border of the sartorius muscle, its upper extremity being six lines, and the lower two lines from the internal border of that muscle; care being taken to avoid the internal saphenous vein, the course of which is made apparent by compression above; the sartorius is exposed by dividing the fascia lata, and drawn outwards, and the fibrous connexion between the vastus and adductor muscles is exposed and divided; the sheath of the vessel now appears and is opened, and the needle passed from within outwards, avoiding the vein and long saphenous nerve.

III. At its Upper Portion.—The artery lies in a triangle formed by Poupart's ligament above as its base, the sartorius externally, and the adductor brevis internally, and known as Scarpa's space; the artery is very superficial, being covered by integument, the superficial and deep fasciæ, and lymphatic glands; the vein is on the inner and slightly posterior part.

Operation.—(Fig. 83.) The artery is tied near the apex of the triangle; the thigh is slightly flexed on the body and abducted, and placed on its external aspect; an incision is made commencing about four inches below Poupart's Ligament, along the inner margin of the sartorius muscle, three inches in length; the saphena vein, first made prominent by pressure above, is left to the inner side; the fascia lata, *a*, is divided, the sartorius, *b*, exposed and drawn outwards, and the sheath of the vessels becomes apparent; the position of the artery

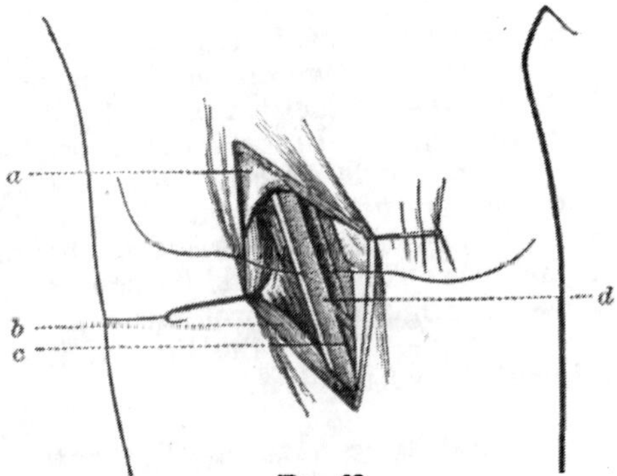

Fig. 83.

is recognised by its pulsations; the sheath is opened to a sufficient extent to pass the needle, which is cautiously done from within outwards to avoid the vein, *c*; the point of the needle should be kept close to the artery, *d*, as the vein lies closely on its inner and posterior aspect.

Complications.—If the saphena vein is wounded, compression is sufficient for its treatment; if the incision falls upon the sartorius, this must be drawn aside.

IV. Beneath Poupart's Ligament.—The artery is superficial, being covered by the skin, superficial and deep fasciæ, and lymphatic glands; the vein lies on its inner side, and the anterior crural nerve half an inch to its outer side; the vessels lie in a canal formed by the parting of the two layers of the fascia lata, and are separated by this septum.

Operation.—The pulsations of the artery being recognised, midway between the anterior superior spine of the ilium and the pubes, an incision is made two inches in length, over the artery, commencing at the crural arch; the skin and cellular tissue are divided, the fascia, *a*, raised on a director, and the sheath exposed; this is opened, the vein, *c*, drawn inwards, and the needle passed around the artery, *b*, from within outwards, ligating it above the profunda femoris. Porter makes the incision parallel with Poupart's ligament.

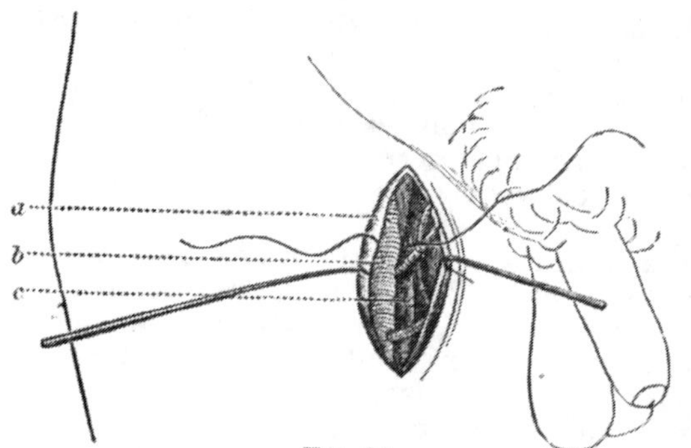

Fig. 84.

Complications.—In persons of ordinary flesh, the fold of the groin corresponds exactly with Poupart's ligament, but in those who are very fleshy the fold is somewhat below Poupart's ligament; and should this be taken as the guide to the commencement of the incision there would be danger of applying the ligature just below the origin of the profunda. It is advisable to bring the ligament into view before the ligature is applied, and pass the needle a finger's breadth below.

External Iliac Artery.—The external iliac, about four inches in length, passes obliquely downwards and outwards, from the sacro-iliac symphysis to Poupart's ligament, in a line drawn from the left side of the umbilicus to a point midway between the anterior superior spine of the ilium and the symphysis pubis; it may be ligated in any part of its course, except near its upper and lower extremities. Its anatomical relations are (Fig. 86):—In its upper portion it has in front the peritoneum and intestines, and near Poupart's ligament the spermatic vessels, genito-crural nerve, circumflex iliac vein, lymphatic vessels and glands; externally, the psoas magnus, M, from which it is separated by the iliac fascia; internally, the external iliac vein; below, and curving along its side, the vas deferens; behind, it rests above upon the external iliac vein, which gradually passes to its internal side.

Operation.—(Fig. 85.) The patient being placed in a recumbent position, the abdominal muscles relaxed, an incision is made three or four inches in length, commencing about an inch and a half within the anterior superior spine of the ilium and on a level with this process, and extending in a curved direction downwards and inwards, nearly parallel with Poupart's ligament, and terminating an inch and a half above it, just outside of the external abdominal ring; on the left side it will be found convenient to commence the incision internally, at the external ring and carry it upwards and outwards to the point indicated within its anterior superior spine; the integuments and fascia are incised and the superficial epigastric artery, if divided, tied; the aponeurosis, *c*, of the external oblique muscle is now exposed and divided on a director; in the same manner the fibres of the internal oblique and transversalis muscles, *a*, are divided until the transversalis fascia, recognised by its white, opaque appearance, is exposed; this membrane is cautiously opened and incised on the director; the peritoneum, *d*, is now exposed and carefully detached from the iliac fossa, and pushed towards the pelvis; the artery, *b*, is readily felt pulsating at the bottom of the wound, along the inner border of the psoas muscle, the vein being on the inner aspect, the genito-crural nerve external; the sheath is opened and the needle insinuated beneath it, from within outwards, to avoid the vein.

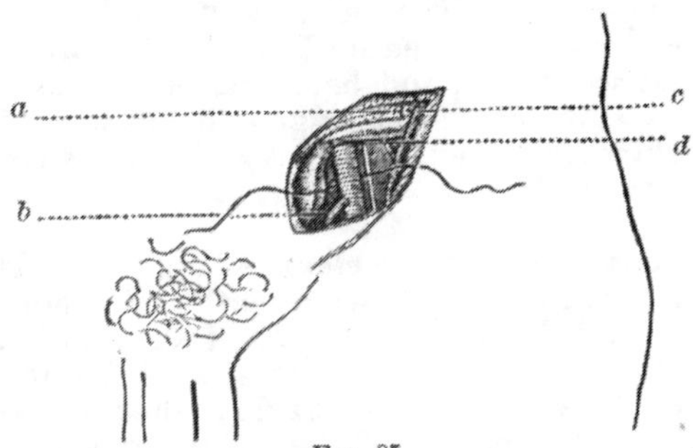

FIG. 85.

Modifications.—Abernethy made an incision in the course of the artery (Fig. 86, A), three inches in length; Cooper made a curved incision (Fig. 86, C), commencing a little above the spine of the ileum, and terminating a little above the internal edge of the inguinal ring; Bogros made an incision (Fig. 86, B), in the centre of the space between the anterior superior spine, and the symphysis pubis.

the finger may be passed into the internal ring along the spermatic vessels, and the iliac fascia raised in this manner.

Epigastric Artery.—This artery (Fig. 86, G), arises from the fore part of the external iliac above Poupart's ligament; it at first descends, then passes obliquely upwards and inwards between the peritoneum and the transversalis fascia, in a line drawn from the middle of Poupart's ligament to the umbilicus; it lies behind the inguinal canal, and to the inner side of the internal abdominal ring; it has two veins nearly to its origin.

Operation.—The incisions in the last operation, but not so long, are equally adapted for ligating this artery; the spermatic cord is first sought for, and being raised, the inner border of the internal ring is exposed; the ring is dilated with the end of the finger, and behind the layer of transversalis fascia constituting its border, the artery is felt.

Common Iliac Artery.—(Fig. 86.) The common iliac, D, two inches in length, passes from the bifurcation of the abdominal aorta, on the left side of the body of the fourth lumbar vertebra, a point corresponding with the left side of the umbilicus, on a level with a line drawn from one crista ilii to the other, downwards and outwards along the margin of the pelvis to the sacro-iliac synchondrosis. The artery upon the right side is longer than that upon the left, and has in front, the peritoneum, and at its point of division, the ureter: behind, the accompanying vein, J, is partly external above, but below it lies behind and slightly internal; on the outer side, the common iliac vein above, and the psoas muscle, M, below. The left common iliac has the rectum and superior hæmorrhoidal artery in front, the left common iliac vein internal and partly beneath, and the psoas magnus external.

Operation.—(Fig. 86.) The patient being placed on the back, inclining to the opposite side, an incision, R, is made commencing just anterior to the extremity of the eleventh rib, and carried downwards, one and a half inches within the anterior superior spine, and terminating just above the internal ring by a sharp curve upwards and inwards of an inch; the entire length being about seven inches; the integuments and superficial fascia are divided; then the three abdominal muscles are incised and divided; the fascia transversalis, cautiously raised from the peritoneum, first at the upper part of the wound where the union is slightest, the peritoneum is now gently elevated and pressed inwards from the iliac fossa towards the pelvis; the pulsations of the external iliac, F, are first recognised, and the finger carried upwards along this vessel reaches the common trunk; the ureter, H, in front is carefully pushed aside, and the needle passed from within outwards.

Complications.—There is great danger of lacerating the peritoneum, both in the act of separating it from the transversalis fascia, and in raising it from the iliac fossa; to avoid the first accident the transversalis fascia should be first raised high up in the wound, where the attachments are the slightest; to avoid the second, the peritoneum, with the inclosed bowels, o, should be raised on the palms of an assistant standing upon the opposite side of the

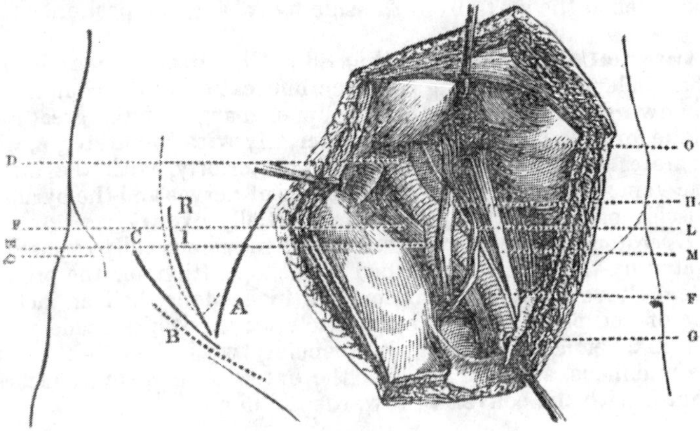

FIG. 86.

patient, while the surgeon gently separates with his fingers its attachments; if the operator work too deeply into the iliac fossa, he may get behind the psoas, instead of in front.

Modifications.—Mott carried his inoision five inches, commencing above the external ring, passing in a curved direction, half an inch above Poupart's ligament, upwards, a little above the spine of the ilium; Crampton made an incision several inches long from the seventh rib, downwards and forwards, curved outwards, to the front of the spine of the ilium; Dumricher makes an incision from just above the anterior superior spine towards the umbilicus, nearly to the sheath of the rectus; other modifications are immaterial.

Abdominal Aorta.—This artery lies in front, and a little to the left side of the bodies of the vertebræ, having the vena cava on its right side, the sympathetic nerve on its left, and behind, the left lumbar veins; it may be ligated about one inch above its bifurcation.

Operation.—The abdominal aorta can be exposed and successfully ligated by the operation above described for the common iliac; the artery being separated from the vein with the finger or a director, the needle passed from left to right. Cooper made an incision along the linea alba, three inches in length, the middle of it on a level with the umbilicus, but a little to the left; the peritoneum was opened, the intestines pushed aside, the artery detected by its pulsations, the peritoneal covering was torn by the finger nail on the left side; the finger carried under the vessel, and the needle passed from left to right. Murray made an incision from the extremity of the tenth rib downwards six inches, curving backwards to within an inch of the anterior spine of the ilium, Q, and reached the aorta from the side by raising the peritoneum.

Internal Iliac Artery.—(Fig. 86.) This artery, E, is an inch and a half in length, extending from the bifurcation of the common iliac downwards and forwards to the upper margin of the great sacro-sciatic foramen; it is in relation anteriorly with the ureter, H, which separates it from the peritoneum; posteriorly, with the internal iliac vein; it rests on the sacral plexus of nerves and the pyriformis muscle; on the left the rectum lies partially over it.

Operation.—The internal iliac artery may be readily exposed and ligated by the method described in the operation on the primitive iliac. Stevens made an incision five inches long, half an inch outside of and parallel to the epigastric artery. White made an incision in a semicircular form, commencing two inches to the left of the umbilicus, and ending near the external ring, seven inches in length, with the convexity towards the ilium.

Gluteal Artery.—This artery emerges from the pelvis, at the upper part of the great ischiatic notch, above the upper border of the pyriformis muscles; it is covered by the gluteus maximus muscles, and is accompanied by two veins; a line drawn from the posterior superior spine of the ilium to the top of the great trochanter marks the course of the artery.

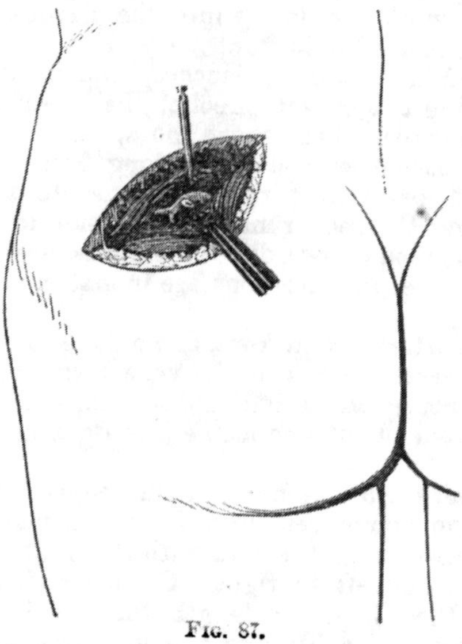

Fig. 87.

Operation.—(Fig. 87.) The patient placed upon his belly, the thigh extended, an incision is made on the line above indicated, four or five inches long; the cut is parallel with the fibres of the gluteus maximus, which should be separated, and the finger introduced to detect the pulsations of the artery; the pyriformis and gluteus medius muscles, the borders of which cover the vessel, are separated, and the artery isolated from its veins and the needle passed.

Sciatic Artery.—The sciatic artery escapes from the pelvis between the pyriformis and coccygeus muscles, and descends in the interval between the trochanter major and tuberosity of the ischium; it is covered by the gluteus maximus, and is accompanied by the sciatic nerve, and the vein which lies to its posterior and inner side; the centre of a line drawn from the posterior superior spinous process of the ilium to the tuberosity of the ischium, marks the point of exit of the artery from the pelvic cavity.

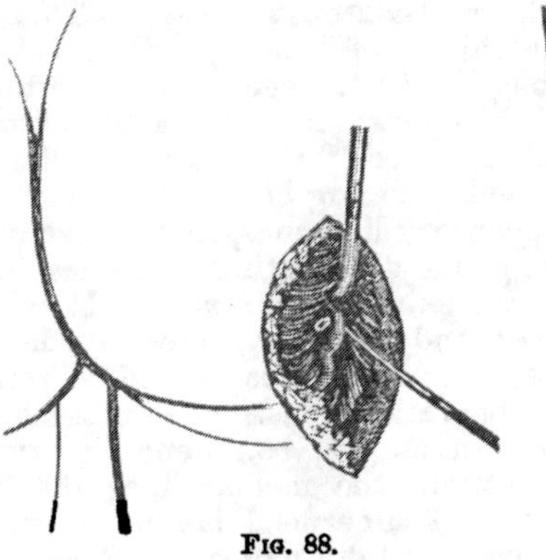

FIG. 88.

Operation.—(Fig. 88.) The patient being placed upon the belly, make a vertical incision, two inches in length, the centre of which falls upon the point of emergence of the artery, as given above; divide the skin, cellular tissue, and the fibres of the gluteus maximus; the artery is found to the inside of the nerve, and must be carefully isolated from the vein.

Internal Pudic Artery.—This artery, the smaller of the two terminal branches of the internal iliac, passes out of the pelvis through the great sacro-sciatic foramen, internal to the sciatic artery; it again enters the pelvis through the lesser sacro-sciatic foramen; it runs along the ramus of the ischium and pubes, and divides into the arteries of the penis; it may be ligated at two points:—

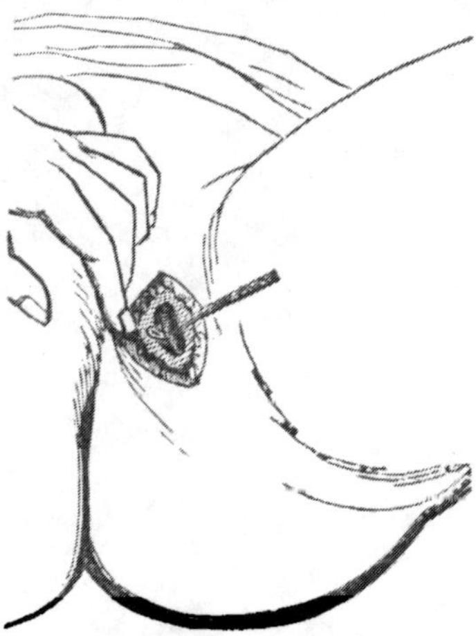

FIG. 89.

I. AT THE GREATER SACRO-SCIATIC FORAMEN.—In this operation the same incision is made as in the ligature of the sciatic artery; the pudic is found a little internal, accompanied by its veins and the pudic nerve.

II. IN THE PERINEUM.—(Fig. 89.) The artery may be ligated in the perineum as it ascends the ramus of the ischium; a line drawn from the middle of the pubes to the internal border of the tuber ischii, marks the course of the artery. The patient being placed in the position for lithotomy, an incision two inches in length is made along the ramus of the pubes, near the arch; by careful dissection the vessel is found along the inner border of the ramus, where it may be isolated and the ligature applied; care should be taken not to incise the corpus cavernosum.

Dorsalis Penis Artery.—This artery has been ligated by Dr. Hutchison, of Brooklyn, N. Y., Prof. of Operative Surgery in the Long Island College Hospital, who gives the following description of the operation:—The arteria dorsalis penis is one of the terminal branches of the internal pudic. It reaches the dorsum of the penis by passing between the crura, and runs forward, through the suspensory ligament, in the groove of the corpus cavernosum, to the glans, distributing branches in its course to the body of the organ, skin, and *prepuce*. It is enveloped in the subcutaneous layer, and is accompanied by the dorsalis penis nerve and vein—the latter structures should be remembered in ligating the artery. My operation consisted in making an incision three-fourths of an inch in length, commencing two inches in front of the pubes directly in the median line; the incision was carried through the skin and superficial lamina of the subcutaneous layer, when the artery was fully exposed. A small artery needle, carrying a ligature, was then passed around the artery, carefully avoiding the nerve, and tied.

CHAPTER III.

ON THE VEINS.

WOUNDS.

VEINS may be wounded in the same manner as arteries, but there is less liability to sudden and severe hæmorrhage; the largest veins, as the vena cava and subclavian, have been lacerated to the extent of an inch, and life has still been prolonged for several hours. They have, however, but feeble power of contraction, and hæmorrhage is more apt to continue in a passive manner than when arteries are wounded. Wounds of veins heal very readily and with but slight scar, though they are lacerated; the calibres of veins are much more seldom obliterated after wounds than arteries, owing to the sluggish and even current of blood of the former, and the rapidity with which the tissue of veins heals.

Venous hæmorrhage is readily suppressed by pressure, and unless the vessel is large a compress and bandage will prove sufficient to permanently arrest the bleeding. When large veins are partially divided the edges of the wound may be raised and inclosed in a ligature, applied upon its outside; union has frequently followed such treatment, and the calibre of the vessel has been preserved. If a large vein is completely divided, and firm pressure cannot be maintained, ligatures should be applied, as in similar wounds of arteries.

Wounds of large veins made during an operation are liable to be followed by the entrance of air, and sudden syncope. The finger should be instantly and firmly pressed upon the patulous vein to prevent a further admission of air, and efforts at resuscitation at once undertaken. The patient should be placed in a recumbent position, with the head low, and feet high, to favor cerebral circulation; the limbs chafed towards the heart; stimulants administered, and artificial respiration induced.

VARICOSE VEINS.

The treatment to be adopted for the cure of varicose veins depends upon the part of the body where found. It is our purpose to speak here only of varicose veins of the legs. All radical treatment aims at the obliteration of the larger trunks, and to effect this object the following methods have been adopted:—

With Pins and Needles.—Davat passed one needle underneath

the vein, and a second perpendicularly through the vein under the first needle, and upwards through the vein again to the skin; a thread was then passed around their extremities as in the hare-lip suture; Velpeau passes the pin transversely under the vein without wounding its parietes, and secures it by the twisted suture; Fricke transfixes the vein with the needle and allows it to act as a seton; Erichsen lays a piece of wax bougie upon the vein before applying the ligature; Lee, after three or four days, withdraws the pins and divides the veins subcutaneously; Wood uses the needles of the size of the ordinary hare-lip pin, one of which is first inserted subcutaneously over, the second, under the vein, both entering and emerging at the same opening, and when inserted the extremities are twisted upon each other, producing constriction of the vein.

Incision.—The largest knot is laid open by an incision of one or two inches in length, the cavity filled with lint, and a compress and bandage applied; the resulting inflammation extends sufficiently to obliterate the other varices; if varices exist above and below the knee, incision should be made at both points.

Section.—Velpeau directs that the vein be raised with the skin, by the surgeon and his assistant, a straight bistoury passed under it, and complete section be made, the wound filled with lint and pressure applied; Brodie makes subcutaneous section by passing a small slightly curved bistoury under the vein and dividing the vessel on its withdrawal; the hæmorrhage is restrained by compression; when several ligatures are applied to veins the vessel may be divided between them; Chassaignac employs the écraseur, and alleges that both hæmorrhage and suppurative phlebitis are thereby averted.

Excision.—This ancient operation consists in laying bare the vein and dissecting out a portion.

Ligature.—Home and Beclard applied the ligature directly to the vein, by raising a fold of skin transversely and incising it, and then dividing the vein above; Regnaud passed the ligature under the vein with a needle, and placing a roll of diachylon upon the vessel tied the ligature firmly; Gagnolès proposed to pass the ligature

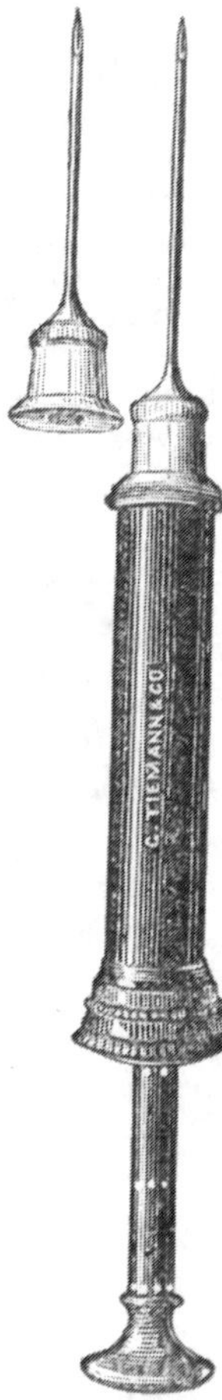

Fig. 90.

subcutaneously through a single puncture of the skin; Vidal applied a metallic ligature; Levis very ingeniously passed the metallic ligature *under* the vein and out on the opposite side, then re-entering the needle through the same opening, he passed it *above* the vein and out at the opening where it first entered, thus making a subcutaneous ligature; Ricord passed two silk ligatures, one above and the other below the vein, but both entering and emerging by the same opening, and the ends are then tied so firmly on each side as to strangulate the vessel.

Cauterisation.—The caustics generally selected are caustic potass, and Vienna paste, a mixture of caustic potass and powdered lime, made into a paste by adding spirits of wine. Several pieces of adhesive plaster, having small openings, varying in size from a split pea to a three cent piece, are placed over the most prominent parts of the vessel; the caustic is applied and covered with another strip of plaster and allowed to remain from twenty minutes to half an hour; the dressings should be poultices to hasten the separation of the slough; if the first application is not sufficient to obliterate the vein, a second should be made.

Compression.—Various instruments have been invented to make compression, but none have proved very effectual.

Injections.—Immediate coagulation of the blood has been produced by powerful astringents, as the perchloride and the persulphate of iron, diluted with water; the fluid is thrown into the vein with Pravaz's syringe, or the hypodermic syringe (Fig. 90), now in general use. The iron being diluted with two or three parts of water, a ligature is applied above the knee to distend the veins below, or the patient stands erect a few minutes, three or four drops of the preparation are drawn into the syringe, the amount being determined by the dots on the piston rod, an assistant compresses the trunk of the vein above the point of injection, the point of the syringe is then inserted into the enlarged vein, and the contents injected; to avoid all risks of the escape of coagula into the circulation, a compress should be firmly bound upon the main trunk of the vein; the injection should be made in a number of places.

CHAPTER IV.

ON AMPUTATIONS.

AMPUTATIONS IN GENERAL.

AMPUTATIONS are performed through the shafts of bones, or through the joints; the former are said to be *in the continuity*, and the latter, *in the contiguity*.

Amputations in the Continuity.—There are several methods of shaping the external parts to cover the stump in this operation:—

Circular Method.—There are three principal steps in this operation, viz.:—1. Incision of the skin; 2. Incision of the muscles; 3. Section of the bone. To incise the skin easily and neatly, the operator should stand upon the right side of the limb, the left foot thrown forward and placed firmly upon the floor, the right knee bending sufficiently to give freedom of motion to the body; the left hand grasps the limb above the point of operation, and the handle of the knife is taken between the thumb and forefinger of the right hand, being lightly supported by the other fingers; stooping sufficiently to allow the right arm to encircle the limb readily, he carries the knife around until the blade is nearly perpendicular to the long axis of the limb on the side next to him with the point downwards, and the hand of the operator above the limb; he now commences the incision with the heel of the knife, giving slightly sawing motions, and brings the hand under the limb, and then directly upwards upon the side next to the operator, until the heel touches the point of commencement; the handle of the knife held thus delicately will change its relative positions as it passes around the limb without the slightest embarrassment to the operator; if the handle is firmly grasped in the whole hand, the incision cannot be completed without the aid of the other hand, or an awkward movement of the hand holding the knife; the ease with which the incision is completed will depend much upon whether it commences well down upon the side of the limb next to the operator. The skin is raised from the first layer of muscles by dissection, and drawn upwards, two or three inches, according to the diameter of the limb, like the cuff of a coat. 2. The first layer of muscles is divided at the margin of the retracted integument, in the same manner as the incision of the skin is executed (Fig. 91); this layer is raised with the knife, and drawn still further upwards; and the last layer of muscles is divided down to the bone (Fig. 92) by the same sweep of the knife as before given. 3. The bone is then sawn at the apex of the cone.

Modifications.—The chief modifications are:—Louis divided the skin and superficial layer of muscles at one incision, drew them up

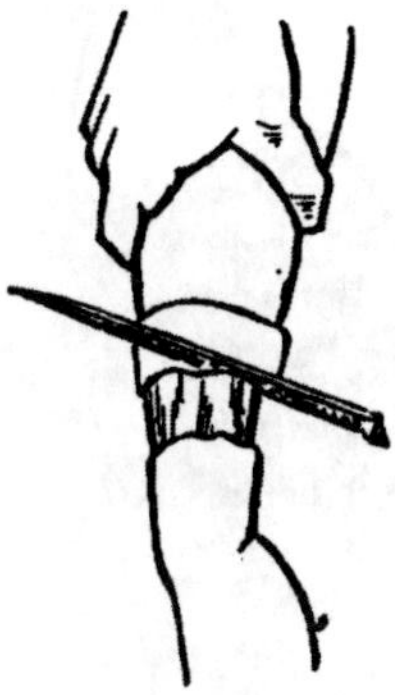

FIG. 91.

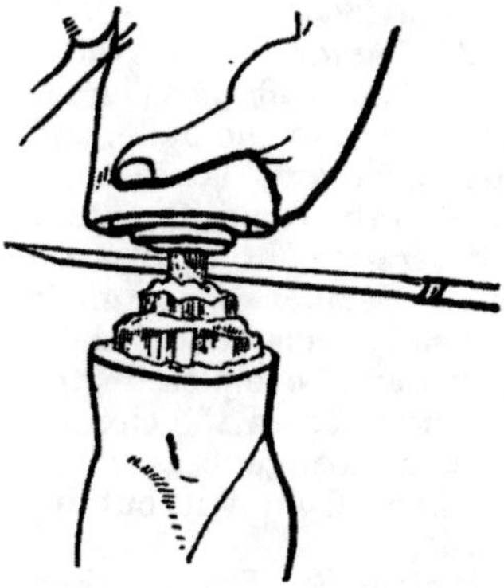

FIG. 92.

and divided the remainder; Petit incised the skin, drew it up an inch, and then divided the muscles directly to the bone; Alanson dissected up the skin and then cut the muscles completely to the bone; Bell followed Alanson, but concluded by detaching the muscles from the bone, an inch or more, with the point of a knife.

FLAPS.—Flaps may be anterior, posterior, or lateral; they may be made from without inwards, or from within outwards.

Single Flaps.—The operator grasps the tissues on the anterior part of the limb, with the left hand above the point of operation, and placing the heel of the knife at the point of the fingers on the opposite side of the limb, with a slight downward curve, he brings it over to the point of the thumb on the opposite side, with one stroke dividing the tissues to the bone; he now withdraws the knife until the point rests in the angle of the wound, when he thrusts it under the bone, taking care that the point emerges at the angle of the wound on the opposite side where the incision commenced; he now makes a flap from the posterior part of the limb of sufficient length to cover the stump; the muscles are dissected from the bone with the amputating knife or a scalpel; the operation is very rapid, the knife not being raised from the limb.

Double Flaps.—(Fig. 93.) The operator grasps the tissues on the upper part of the limb with the left hand, the thumb and fingers resting at the middle of the limb on opposite sides; the knife, *a*, is then entered at the thumb and thrust through above the bone, emerging on the opposite side at the point where the fingers rest, and passed downwards and outwards, *c*, making an anterior flap, *b*, of the required length; it is again re-entered at the same point, and passing beneath the bone emerges from the same point on the opposite side, and a flap is made from the posterior part of the limb; both flaps are forcibly retracted, the muscles dissected from the bone, and the bone divided.

Modifications.—Ravaton divided the soft parts circularly down to the bone, and then made two lateral incisions to the requisite extent and raised quadrilateral flaps; Sédillot first made two small flaps, turned them back, and completed the operation as in the circular method; Langenbeck made the flaps from without inwards.

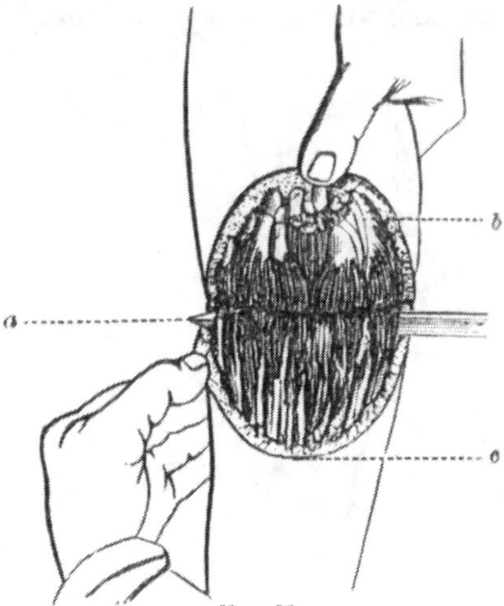

FIG. 93.

Rectangular Flaps.—(Fig. 94.) Mr. Teale recommends the following operation:—First mark on the limb with ink two flaps; the size of the long flap is determined by the circumference of the limb at the place of amputation, its length and its width being each equal to half the circumference. The long flap is therefore a perfect square, and is long enough to pull easily over the end of the bone. In selecting the structures for its formation, such parts must be taken as do not contain the larger blood-vessels and nerves. The flap so formed will be for the most part anterior in position as far as regards the general aspect of the body, but superior when the patient is in the recumbent posture, as during the after treatment. The short flap, containing the chief vessels and veins, is in length one-fourth of the other. The flaps being formed, the bone sawn, and the arteries tied, the long flap is folded over the end of the bone; each of its free angles is then fixed by suture to the corresponding free angles of the short flap. One or two more sutures complete the transverse line of union of the flaps. At each side the short flap is united to the corresponding portion of the long one by a point of suture, and one suture more unites the reflected portion of the long flap to its unreflected (Fig. 95) portion. Thus the transverse line of union is bounded at each end by a short lateral line at right angles to it.

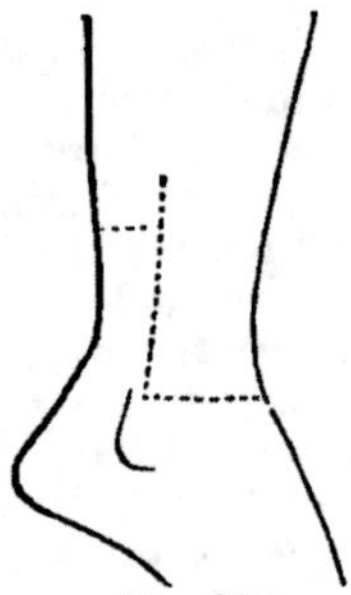
FIG. 94.

Oval Method.—In this operation the incision may be made like an inverted V, the apex being a little below the point where the

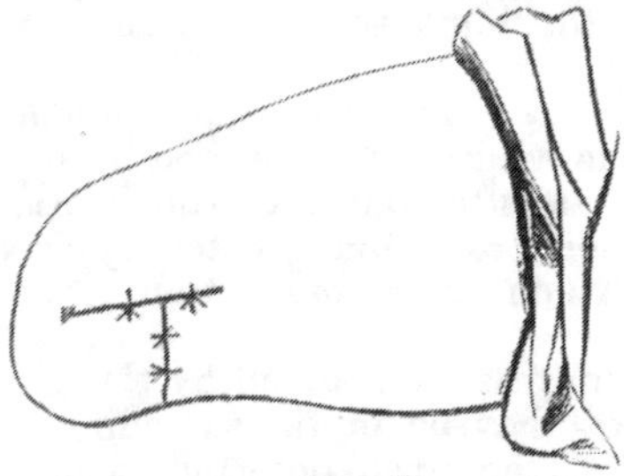

FIG. 95.

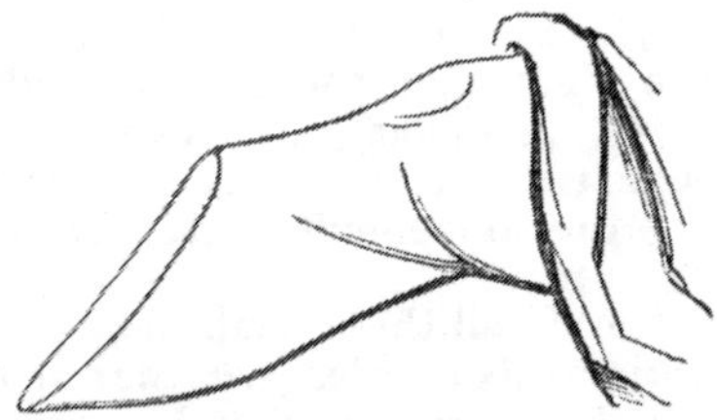

FIG. 96.

bone is to be sawn; the incision being extended quite down to the bone before the lower portion of the flap containing the large vessels is divided; or a perfect oval (Fig. 96) may be marked out by the first incision, and the operation completed as in the former case. The oval method is seldom adopted except in amputation at the joints.

Amputations in the Contiguity.—The methods of amputation already described may be employed in the disarticulation of limbs. The instruments required are a single knife, having a narrow blade, to enable it to move more readily over the irregularities of the joint, with a thick back to give it firmness, and an artery forceps. The chief points to be well considered by the operator are thus concisely stated by Malgaigne (*Operative Surgery*, *Am. Edition*):—

"The operator has here three special objects in view: 1. To well recognise the articulation before commencing. 2. The flesh being divided, to traverse the articulation without hesitation, destroying all its means of attachment. 3. To preserve flesh and integument enough. Whence the following rules:—

"*To Recognise the Articulation.*—The surgeon should have the disposition of the articulation so fixed in his mind, that he could, without having it under his eyes, trace it out exactly. In this way, recognising one part of the articulation, he is sure of the others, neither the blood nor the soft parts causing the knife to deviate. He must also know the direction of the ligaments, to attack them more surely; their length, to cut them between their attachments; their breadth, to divide them completely.

"1. The surest guides in finding the joints are the osseous projections. It is with them you must first occupy yourself. To find them, you may place the limb in a position that causes them to project; seek them on the side where they are most prominent; put aside by careful pressure the soft parts, fat, or œdema that mask their projections; and, lastly, seek them by starting from a known point: for example, passing the finger along the shank of a long bone till you reach its extremity.

"2. The second indication consists in the folds of the skin, sometimes placed immediately above the joint, sometimes some way from it.

"3. You may, as a third resource, cause to be prominent to the sight and touch the tendons which are inserted near the joint. To effect this, cause the muscles to contract; this is usually sufficient: or you may render their projection greater by opposing the movement of the limb which their contraction tends to execute.

"4. If all these trials fail, you may assist yourself by the neighboring tuberosities, whether or not they be in the same line, provided their distance and connexions are well determined beforehand. It is objected that the relations, and especially the distance, vary in different subjects; consequently, they can only give us a tolerably close indication: but certainly there is never more than some lines difference; and it is better to have such approximation than none at all.

"5. If these means do not suffice, seize the limb with the right hand, and seek the joint with the left, moving the limb slightly, and thus try to mark out the two diameters of the joint, or, in other terms, the point of entrance and exit of the knife.

"6. Lastly, supposing that all these indications do not afford a certain result, incise the skin in the most suitable direction, and, after having raised it, assure yourself by the touch of the articular line. If the touch does not point it out, place the knife in the angle of the wound nearest yourself, its heel perpendicular to the horizon, and the edge perpendicular to the bone, and thus move it along the bone with a sawing sidelong movement, without taking it off, and the pressure will cause the knife to enter the joint when it reaches it.

"*To Traverse the Articulation.*—1. The articulation recognised, or at all events presumed to be so, as we have directed, the index finger and thumb should rest applied on the two extremities of the articular diameter until the knife replaces them. If this search has been made with the right hand, substitute the left hand for it before seizing the knife. In this way you mark the point of entrance and exit of the knife.

"2. If you attack the joint by its dorsal surface, semiflex the limb, to extend the parts and enlarge the articular line. Without this precaution, you often fall on the neighboring joint, as happens on the foot and hand.

"3. The knife should not generally be carried into the joint without having first cut its principal means of connexion, which should be divided from without inwards.

"4. In joints with several projections and interlockings, commence by the internal or external side. As the knife opens one part, do not push it in there, but go on dividing and opening further. In this way, the ligaments are not put out of the reach of the knife, or shielded by bony projections.

"5. An important fact. An articulation, that offers to the anatomist a surface equal to one inch, presents to the operator at least four. So long as the ligaments are divided between their attachments, it is of slight importance whether during their division the knife fall on the articular line or at the side of it.

"6. The dorsal and lateral ligaments being cut, we can generally engage all the blade of the knife between the articular surfaces; but if there are interosseous ligaments, they must be first divided. Carry the point of the knife directly on them: as they are divided, the joint opens.

"7. To destroy these ligaments, you must know the interstices between the bones through which they may best be attacked. In general, on the hand and foot, the bones, very compact on their dorsal surface, leave between them on their palmar and plantar surfaces intervals which lodge these ligaments. Carry the knife under these intervals, inclining the handle towards yourself, and making it form an angle of forty-five degrees anteriorly; then raise it up to a right angle. The ligaments divided by this movement allow the articulation to be opened sufficiently for the knife to enter it.

"8. It is useless to luxate: it strains the parts very painfully; and if you separate the parts very much on one side, you apply those of the other together. If in cases of difficulty you have recourse to this means, luxate downwards as far as half the dorso-palmar diameter, and then *vice versâ*. But it is better to separate the parts by slight traction parallel to the axis of the stump: this ordinarily suffices. The heel and point of the knife should always move in the same line. If, in bringing the knife out of the joint, you dread jagging the integuments, push them gently aside with your left forefinger and thumb.

"*To Preserve Sufficient Flap.*—1. The proceedings vary according to the method, and often even in each method.

"2. In the circular, you can generally count only on the skin to cover the surface of the wound. Make the incision at a sufficient distance from the joint, and dissect back the skin as a cuff. If there are muscles under it, you may cut them obliquely on the plan of Alanson, or divide them perpendicularly on a level with the joint.

"3. The oval method is ordinarily performed by tracing on the dorsal surface a V incision reversed, the ends of which are joined by a semicircular incision round the palmar surface. When there are any large vessels, leave them in the portion to be divided last, as in the method by flaps, so as to be able to compress the artery before dividing it beyond the part compressed.

"4. In most of the oval proceedings, the second incision is made to join the first at its point of commencement. A loss of substance is the consequence; or, if the V terminates on a level with the articulation, there is considerable difficulty in getting the knife to act in disarticulating. I lay down here as a general rule, *expose the joint to be destroyed by a longitudinal incision passing half an inch, at least, above, and one inch below it.* The two branches of the V, which fall on the inferior part of this incision, leave, as it were, two small flaps at the upper part, which do not hinder immediate and linear union, and which perfectly cover the osseous prominences left by the disarticulation.

"5. The methods by one or two flaps are executed in two ways. Sometimes the flaps are made first, before touching the joint; but most usually a simple incision is made first, or the least important flap, and the second is not begun till after the disarticulation.

"6. The knife having traversed all the joint, when the bones are large and uneven, as in the foot and hand, the instrument must be withdrawn, and its point placed horizontally in the extremity of the joint next the hand operating, and its way cut by pressing from right to left.

"7. To avoid terminating the flap by a point, the knife must be held horizontally close to the bones, and kept so to the required extent, cutting freely.

"8. It is well, before you terminate your flap, to apply it to the part to be covered, to see if it is long enough.

"9. If there remain any tendons beyond the bleeding edge, cut them off with a scissors.

"10. If you fear too much retraction of the skin, do not divide it until the muscles have retracted.

"11. You may cut your flap from engorged tissues, so long as the engorgement is not malignant.

"12. You may operate when there is not enough skin to make a flap; a cicatrix will be formed on the articular surfaces."

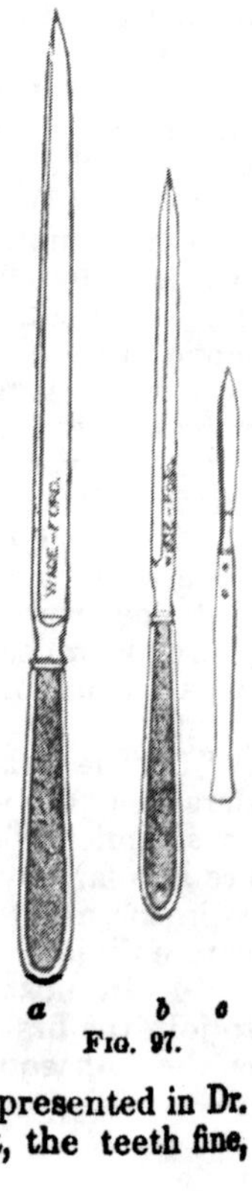

a b c

FIG. 97.

Instruments.—The following instruments are required to form a complete amputating case:—A long and short knife, catling, metacarpal saw, scalpel, tenaculum, saw, bone forceps, artery forceps, needles, and tourniquet.

Knife, Catling, and Scalpel.—The knife, *a*, selected for each operation should be of about twice the length of the diameter of the limb; the catling, *b*, is a double-edged knife, the two edges being parallel until they converge to form the point; the scalpel, *c*, is large and strong, having a firm handle.

The Saw.—The form of saw generally used is represented in Dr. Wood's case, Fig. 2; the edge should be straight, the teeth fine, and so *set* as never to allow the saw to *bend* in its passage through the bone; a saw having fine teeth is but little liable to lacerate the periosteum, and produces a comparatively small amount of comminution of the osseous tissue.

Bone Forceps.—The forceps in common use is that of Liston, and is represented in Dr. Wood's case, Fig. 2.

The remaining instruments have already been described. In

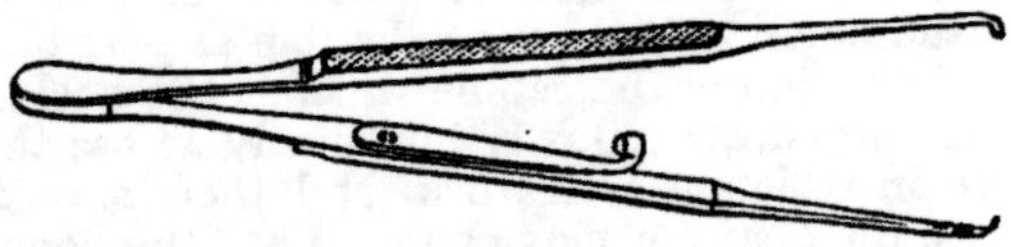

FIG. 98.

addition to the common artery forceps a pair of small forceps (Fig. 98) will sometimes be found useful in dissecting out vessels.

Arrangements.—The retractor is a piece of muslin, half a yard long, and half an inch wide, split in the centre, half its length; it is used by passing the tails on either side of the bone, and the extremities being seized by an assistant, the flaps are forcibly drawn upwards. The sponges should be fine, and in large number. These preliminaries being arranged, the patient is placed in a recumbent position, on a table of such height as to enable the operator to manipulate with his instruments about the limb with perfect freedom; if it is an amputation by the circular method the limb should be much more elevated than if the flap operation is performed. The anæsthetic is administered by an assistant, and when the patient is under its influence a second assistant applies the tourniquet as directed, page 26, but as far as possible from the point of operation; previously to its being tightened, if it is desirable to save to the system the largest possible amount of blood, the limb is elevated and rubbed towards the heart to force the blood in the superficial veins beyond the point of amputation; compression of the artery by the fingers of an assistant should never be relied on when a tourniquet can be used. A third assistant should hold and steady the extremity of the limb, and a fourth is in waiting to retract the flaps, either with his hands or with the retractor, and to apply ligatures; a fifth uses the sponges. It is usual to have an assistant to hand the instruments to the operator, but it is much better and more convenient for the operator to place the instruments which he will require on a low bench by his side, in the order of the steps of the operation; an assistant frequently mistakes the instrument called for, and by his confusion often delays vexatiously an important step of the operation. The operator takes a position, in general, upon the right side of the limb. In amputations of the leg, however, the best position for sawing the bones is on the inside.

Operative Procedure.—An amputation in the continuity involves the following steps:—

Incision of Soft Parts.—The method being selected, the operator proceeds, according to the rules already given, to form the coverings of the bone from the soft parts; the bone having been exposed, an assistant, either with his hands or the retractor, draws the flaps firmly upwards and maintains them in that situation.

Incision of the Bone.—The periosteum having been divided completely around the bone, as high up in the flap as possible, the saw is employed, in imitation of the cabinet-maker, the heel being first applied, and the saw drawn slowly but firmly across the bone to make a groove in which it will work, and then moved with as much rapidity as the operator may choose, until the bone is nearly divided, when it is to be moved more slowly to avoid splintering the last connexions. With the bone forceps any sharp or projecting edges are clipped off, and the end of the bone bevelled smoothly. Where there is a single bone it will be found easier to apply the saw nearly perpendicularly on the side opposite to the operator; where there are two bones the saw should be first and last applied to the larger and firmer bone, the smaller bone being completely divided while the saw is engaged in the larger bone.

Ligating Arteries.—The arteries should be tied according to the rules given, page 31. If a vein bleeds freely, a ligature should be applied. Before the stump is dressed any dark clot on its face should be removed, and a bleeding vessel sought for underneath it.

Dressings.—The flaps should be brought accurately together, and maintained by silk or metallic ligatures; the sutures should be taken deeply in the lips of the wound, from a quarter to half an inch, and at sufficient intervals to support the parts in apposition, with the assistance of adhesive straps applied in the intervals. The external dressings should be light and cool; the limb is then placed in an elevated position, and protected from all pressure and irritation.

AMPUTATION OF THE UPPER EXTREMITIES.

General Principles.—"It is of the utmost moment that you should use your most anxious endeavor, and try every method to save portions of the hand, however small, and not cut away more than you can help. You cannot get an instrument maker to contrive anything half so good as even one finger, or the smallest portion of one. I have often saved one finger only, and you should leave even the little finger if you can do nothing else. The hand, perhaps, has been caught by machinery, and been thoroughly bruised. On examination you discover that many of the fingers are squeezed to a mere pulp, but one or two are not quite so bad as the rest; you remove the parts that are irreparably injured, and at all events try to save the rest; if you can leave the thumb and the stump of a finger to oppose it, it is wonderful what use a patient will make of them."—*Liston.*

"In all injuries of the hand, the value of a thumb and a finger, or of two fingers, or even of one, should be borne in mind, and no part should be removed that can be saved and appears likely to be of use. When cannon-shot, large splinters of shells, or grape-shot, have struck the hand, amputation will often be necessary; but the foregoing precept should never be forgotten."—*Guthrie.*

Amputation of the Fingers.—The fingers present as points for operation three phalanges, and three articulations (Fig. 99); the first phalanx, *b*, articulates with the metacarpal bone, *a*, above, and with the second phalanx below; the second phalanx, *d*, articulates with the first and third phalanges; the third phalanx articulates above with the second, and below presents the free extremity of the finger. The anatomical guides to the articulations are the osseous prominences (Fig. 99, *c*), and the transverse depressions (Fig. 100, *c*), in the skin on the palmar surface. Between the bony projections on the side of the finger, at the articulation of the second and third phalanges, a depression marks the position of the articulation; a prominence is readily detected on the dorsum of the second phalanx, just in front of its articulation with the distal extremity of the first phalanx; the articulation of the first phalanx with the metacarpal bone, is immediately behind the bony prominences of the proximal extremity of the first phalanx. The linear depressions in the skin, on the palmar aspect of each finger, are three in number, and have the following relation to the corresponding articulations, commencing with the extremities of the fingers, held in an extended position (Fig. 99). The first depression is situated about a line and a half above the articulation, *f*, between the third and second phalanges; the second depression is situated exactly over the articulation, *d*, between the second and first phalanges; the third depression, *c*, situated at the commissure of the fingers, is twelve or thirteen lines, or about an inch below the articulation, *b*, of the first phalangeal with the metacarpal bones. When the finger is placed in a state of extreme flexion (Fig. 101), it will be seen that the relations of the articulations change, and hence the point at which the articulation is sought will depend upon the position of the finger.

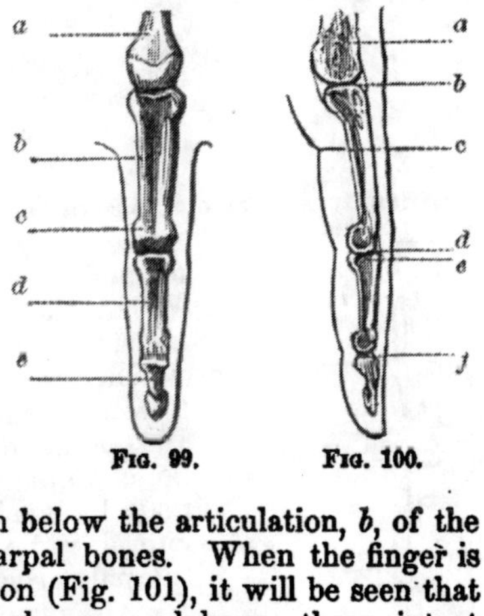

FIG. 99. FIG. 100.

The articulations of the phalanges with each other, are all ginglymoid; the anterior extremities of the first and second phalanges, *a, a* (Fig. 102), are smaller than the other, *b, b*, and terminate on each side in two lateral condyles, having a slight concave articular surface between them, which is prolonged on the palmar surface; the posterior extremities, *b*, present a corresponding prominence in the centre of their articulating surface, dividing it into two concave surfaces, and thus making a ginglymoid joint. They have strong lateral ligaments, and are in relation on the palmar aspect, with the tendons of the flexor muscles.

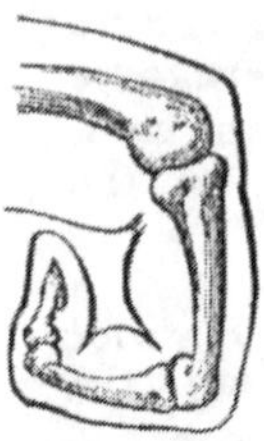
FIG. 101.

The articulations of the metacarpal bones, *a, a* (Fig. 103), with the first phalanges, *b, b*, are enarthrodial; the phalanx alone is movable, and when flexed at a right angle is carried below the extremity of the metacarpal bone, the articular surface of the latter alone presenting.

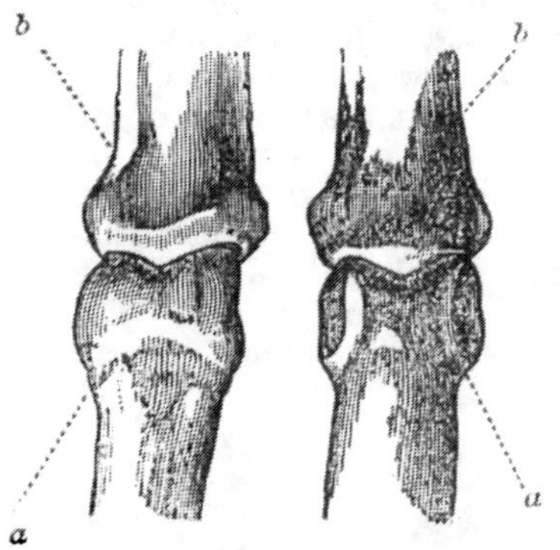

FIG. 102.

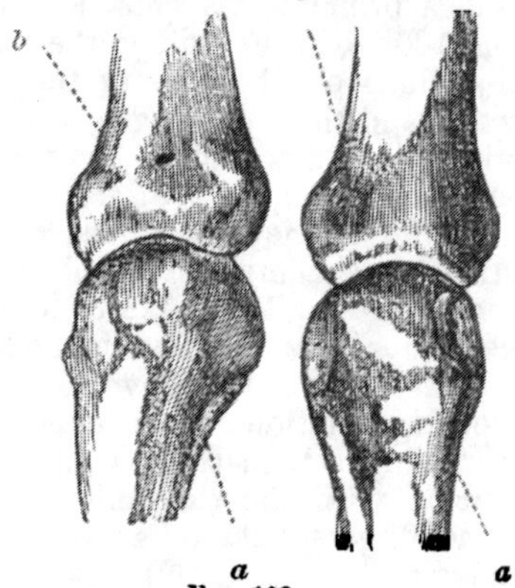

FIG. 103.

Amputation of the Fingers in the Continuity.—Amputation through the phalangeal bones may be performed by the circular or flap method. When the circular method is adopted an incision should be made through the skin, which is retracted three or four lines, the fibrous tissue incised, a retractor, *a* (Fig. 104), applied, and the bone divided with bone nippers, or a fine saw; a double flap may be made anterior and posterior, or lateral, and a single flap may be taken from the palmar surface.

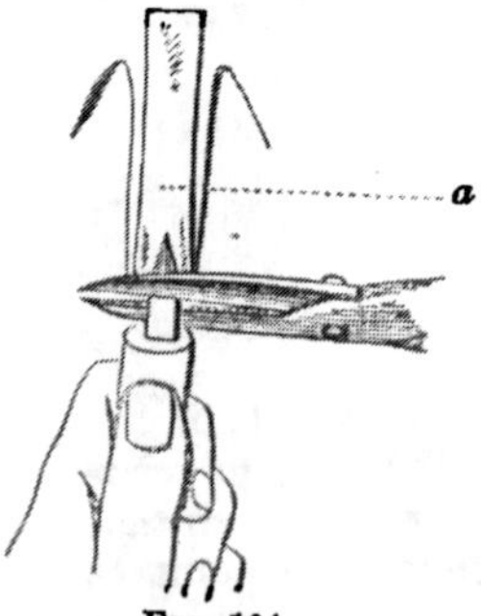

FIG. 104.

Disarticulation of the Phalanges.—Disarticulation at the joints of the fingers may be performed by the circular or flap operations:—

Circular Method.—The articulation being recognised, a circular incision is made three or four lines below, through the skin; this is dissected up to the joint, the lateral ligaments divided, and disarticulation completed.

Methods by Flap.—The following are Lisfranc's methods (*Malgaigne's Op. Cit.*), now generally followed:—

1. "*The Joint is opened on its Dorsal Surface.*—If you would remove the last phalanx, pronate the hand; an assistant holds away the sound fingers, and at the same time turns back the skin of the diseased finger, and retains it in position. The operator seizes the phalanx with the thumb and index finger of the left hand placed across it, on its palmar and dorsal surfaces, and bends it to an angle of forty-five degrees. There are three ways of recognising the line of the joint. 1. There is on its dorsal surface a well marked fold in the skin; the joint is half a line below it. 2. If you cannot find this, assure yourself of the dorsal projection formed by flexion, and cut half a line beyond it. 3. Seek the termination of the palmar fold; you will find the joint half a line below it. Then take a straight bistoury in the third position, and, applying its heel perpendicularly on the recognised extremity of the articular interline, cut from left to right a very small semicircular flap, which terminates at the other extremity. You should divide the capsular ligament in this cut: if you have not, seek it by the indications given. Then, without entering the joint, cut the lateral ligaments. For the ligament situated on the left of the surgeon, carry the bistoury on this side perpendicularly to the axis of the last phalanx; the handle nearer the operator than the point, and the edge also slightly turned towards the operator. In this way, the incision is perfectly suited to the articular surfaces, and the ligament is divided at the first cut. Bring back the bistoury to the other side, and attack the second lateral ligament in the same manner; only here the handle of the bistoury is turned downwards, and farther from the operator than the blade. When the surgeon is well practised, these three steps are comprised in one; and in the same cut, the skin, the left lateral ligament, the dorsal ligament, and the right lateral ligament are divided. In whatever way you attain this point, after having widely opened the joint, seize the phalanx by its sides, and by degrees extend it; while the bistoury, entering the articulation, divides the palmar ligament, passes round the head of the phalanx, slips parallelly under it, and at the same time cuts a semicircular flap, large enough to cover all the solution of continuity. If you would remove the last two phalanges, the proceeding is the same, only the dorsal incision should start on each side on a level with the termination of the palmar fold in the skin. In performing this proceeding, inexperienced operators are frequently misled. It has also another inconvenience in unpractised hands, viz. the base of the flap is cut and jagged in dividing the lateral ligaments; but a little practice gives all the necessary precision in this respect."

2. "*The Joint is opened on its Palmar Surface.*—Strongly supinate the hand, with all the fingers flexed but the one to be operated on, seize the phalanx by its dorsal and palmar surfaces with your left thumb and forefinger, taking care to have your own fingers parallel to the axis of the one to be operated on, or you may wound yourself. Moreover, the index finger should extend some way beyond the joint to be destroyed; the thumb, on the contrary, remains at some distance, to allow the bistoury to act freely in cutting the flap. Things being thus arranged, take a pointed straight bistoury in the third position, with the blade turned horizontally, and the edge towards yourself; place the point of it half a line in front of the palmar fold in the skin, if you amputate the third phalanx, and at the base of this fold if the second. Push it in this way right through, grazing the anterior and lateral surface of the bone (Fig. 105), and raising as much of the tissues as possible. For this purpose, it is recommended, when you put in the bistoury, to hold the handle not quite so much raised as the point. As it advances, again make it horizontal; and, when the point is almost through, raise the handle a little more than the blade. Push the instrument in up to its heel, and, in drawing it out, graze the anterior surface of the bone to the extent of half an inch; then turn up the edge to finish a semilunar flap, and, replacing the edge perpendicularly at the base of the flap, divide the ligament. In this proceeding, it is scarcely necessary to divide the lateral ligaments separately; generally, one cut divides them both at once, and allows the bistoury to pass through the joint. Finish by cutting the tissues on the dorsal surface without making any posterior flap."

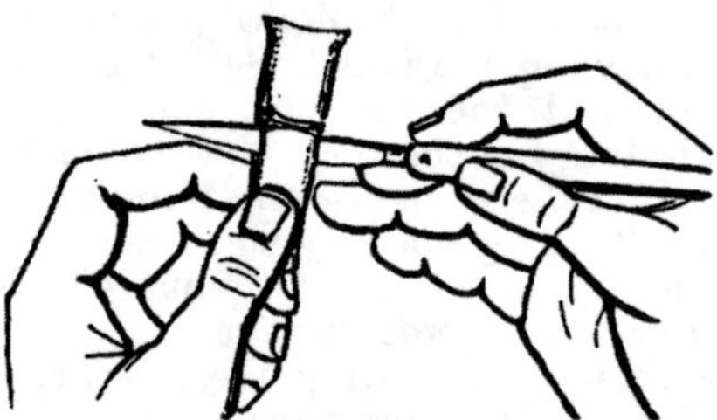
FIG. 105.

Modifications.—Guérin directs the operator to hold the condemned finger between the thumb and index finger of the left hand (Fig. 106), the extremities of which correspond to the margins of the articulation, while the flexed position of the hand upon the forearm places the body of the fingers so far posterior as not to be touched by the point of the bistoury. If there is any liability that the flap will not be sufficiently rounded, the operator should bring forward the heel of the knife, held in the position Fig. 106,

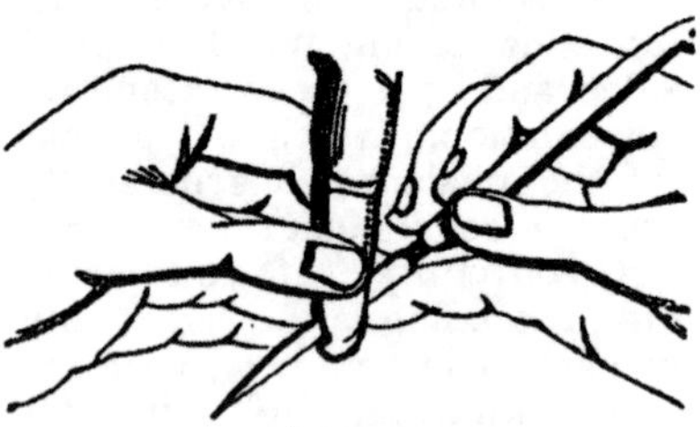
FIG. 106.

and cut the flap rounded upon the side of the finger nearest to his right hand; Ravaton made the circular incision, and two lateral incisions, thus raising two equal quadrilateral flaps; other operators have made lateral flaps, anterior and posterior flaps of different lengths, and also of equal lengths; Sédillot, reviewing these different operations, gives decided preference to the method of Ravaton, reserving, he says, the more brilliant processes of Lisfranc for the amphitheatre.

Disarticulation of a Finger.—The line of articulation may be detected an inch above the commissures of the fingers; or by making strong traction on the finger, the articular surfaces may be sufficiently separated to recognise it.

Oval Method.—(Fig. 107.) The finger in a prone position is grasped on its palmar and dorsal surfaces by the fingers of the operator's left hand, and flexed at an angle of forty-five degrees; an incision is commenced on the dorsal aspect of the joint, a quarter of an inch above, *a*, and carried down to the commissure, *c;* then across the palmar surface to the opposite side, *b*, in the fold of the skin, the finger being forcibly extended; thence the incision is continued upwards to *a*, the finger being again flexed; the borders of the wound are dissected from the head of the phalanx, the joint entered on the dorsal part, the extensor tendon and lateral ligaments divided, the flexion increased with an effort to luxate the joint which renders the division of the flexor tendons and soft parts easy of division. (*a, b, c, d*, Fig. 108.)

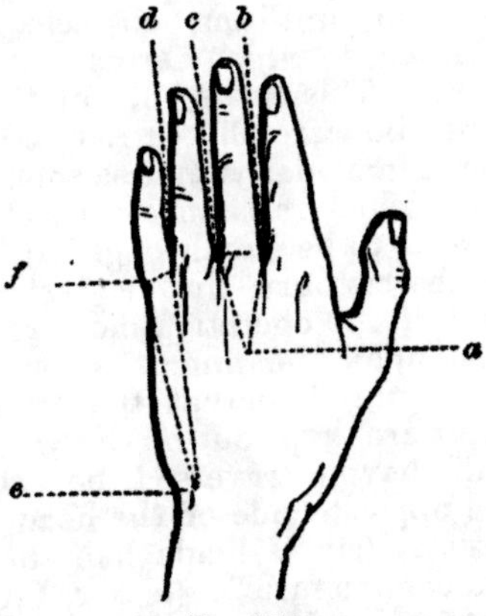

Fig. 107.

Double Flaps.—(Fig. 108.) Lisfranc's method (*Bernard* and *Huette*) is as follows:—"1. The first phalanx of the finger to be removed, is to be grasped by its dorsal and palmar surfaces, and flexed to an angle of forty-five degrees. With a straight bistoury, having a prominent heel to its blade, the surgeon commences an incision over the articulation above the head of the metacarpal bone, starting from the union of the internal two-thirds of the interarticular line with its external third, if he is operating upon the left hand, and *vice versâ* for the right hand, and carrying it down to the end of the commissure between the fingers. This incision, made by drawing the bistoury towards himself, and from heel to point, should divide at once all the soft parts down to the bone. Having attained the end of the web between the fingers, the blade of the bistoury should be brought to a perpendicular position, lying flatwise against the side of the phalanx, and then, at the same time that the hand of the patient is elevated so that the operator's eye shall precede the edge of the bistoury, he depresses its handle towards the palm of the patient's hand, whilst the heel of the knife is making an oblique incision on the palmar aspect of the joint similar to that on its dorsal surface. 2. By the process just described, a lateral semicircular flap has been circumscribed, which is to be detached from the phalanx. Then the bistoury, still held in the first position, is carried to the bottom of the wound, its blade lying flatwise against the phalanx, and by a gently sawing motion, upwards towards the articulation, until an obstacle is encountered which arrests its progress. This is the head of the phalanx; the blade of the bistoury must be carefully carried around it without allowing it to slip or move irregularly, and as soon as it arrives at the articulation, the diminished resistance will allow it to enter with facility. 3. The joint is to be cut through with the narrowest portion of the blade of the bistoury, that nearest its point, and in order to effect this part of the operation more readily, the surgeon should make traction upon the fingers, so as to separate the articular surfaces, at the same time that the integuments of the opposite side of the joint are kept out of the way of the edges of the bistoury. The knife having traversed the articulation, it is brought back hugging the opposite side of the head of the phalanx, and a second semicircular flap is made like the first, as it cuts its way out through the commissure." (*a*, *b*, *c*, Fig. 108.)

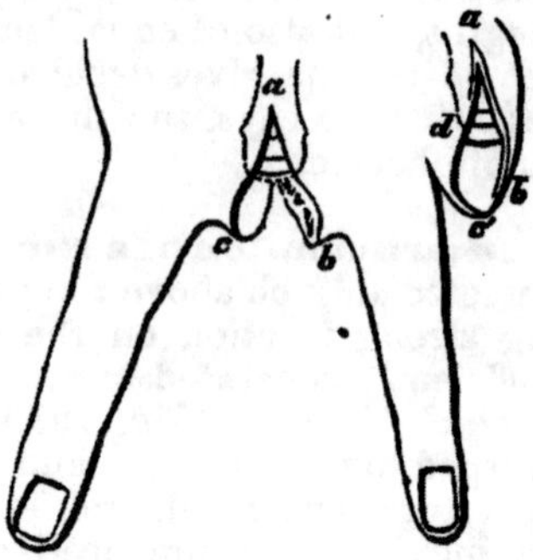

FIG. .08.

Circular Method.—The circular incision is made around the finger, on a line with the fold of the skin on the palmar surface; the integument is drawn back, and a second incision divides the tissues to the bone; the soft parts are retracted, the joint entered from the back, the lateral ligaments divided, and disarticulation completed.

Disarticulation of the Four Fingers.—The distal extremities of the four metacarpal bones are not all on the same straight line; those of the index and ring are nearly on a level, while that of the middle finger is about half a line lower, and that of the little finger is half a line higher.

Single Flap.—(Fig. 109.) Lisfranc's method (*Bernard* and *Huette*) is thus given:—"The hand being pronated, the surgeon grasps the four fingers in the palm of his left hand, whilst his thumb, placed on the dorsal aspect of the fingers, flexes them moderately; an assistant supports the hand, and retracts the skin as much as possible; then, with a straight narrow knife, the operator makes a curved incision, *a*, *b*, *c*, with its convexity looking downwards, from six to eight lines below the heads of the metacarpal bones, from the index towards the little finger if he is operating on the left hand, and in the opposite direction for the right. The extensor tendons being exposed by the retraction of the integuments, which the operator assists by a few strokes of the knife, each of the metacarpo-phalangeal articulations is then successively opened, the extensor tendon being first divided, then the lateral, and finally the palmar ligamentous attachments. It remains to carry the knife through the articulations to the palmar aspect of the phalanges, and cut out a flap, which is limited anteriorly by the folds in the skin at the base of the fingers on their palmar surface."

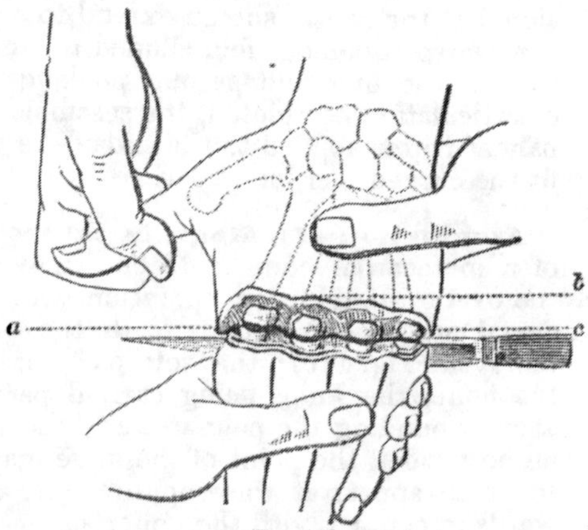

FIG. 109.

By the same method, two, or three fingers may be amputated, the sound fingers being held aside; the dorsal flap is then formed with the point of the knife; or the hand may be held in the supine position and the flap made first from the palmar surface. If the patient is under seventeen years of age, the probabilities are that the ossification of the articular portion of the metacarpal bones is not complete, and the knife may readily pass through them, thus enabling the operator to make longer flaps if desirable.

Circular Method.—The hand being supinated the operator grasps the fingers and makes a semicircular incision, following the depressions in the skin, at the commissure of the fingers, dividing the soft parts down to the joints; the hand is then pronated and an incision made on the dorsal aspect, on a line of the commissure of the fingers; the joints are laid open, and the ligaments divided.

Disarticulation of the Phalanges of the Thumb.—Removal of the second phalanx is effected in the same manner as disarticulation of the second phalanges of the fingers. The articulation of the first phalanx with the metacarpal bone requires larger flaps, owing to the greater size of the head of the metacarpal bone.

The circular or flap method may be adopted, but the operation best adapted to this articulation is, according to Malgaigne, performed as follows:—Make an incision on the dorsal aspect, convex upwards, the centre being a little above the joint, and the extremities terminating on each side at the commencement of the palmar transverse fold; the thumb is now extended and a second convex incision is made, uniting the extremities of the first incision, but the centre should extend to a point midway between the transverse cutaneous fold alluded to, and that making the articulation of the first and second phalanges; the joint is opened and disarticulation completed, the sesamoid bones being removed; the palmar flap is applied to the end of the bone, and should accurately fit the curved incision above.

Amputation of a Single Metacarpal Bone.—When a portion of a metacarpal bone is to be removed, an incision is made as in the oval or double flap operations; the extent of incision on the dorsal aspect corresponds with the portion of the bone to be removed (Fig. 110); the soft parts are cautiously separated from the bone, the knife being carried parallel with its long axis to avoid wounding the palmar arch; the incisions having been made on both sides, the point of the knife may be passed under the bone so as to appear at the opposite side, and then by carrying it forwards in contact with the under surface of the bone, the soft parts may be divided at one section; if the operation is on either the third or fourth metacarpal bone the section should be made with bone forceps; if the metacarpal bone of the thumb, it is sawn perpendicularly to its axis; if of the index finger, section is made obliquely, from without inwards, the hand being supine; if of the little finger, from within outwards (Fig. 110), *a*, the soft parts being withdrawn by the retractor, *b*.

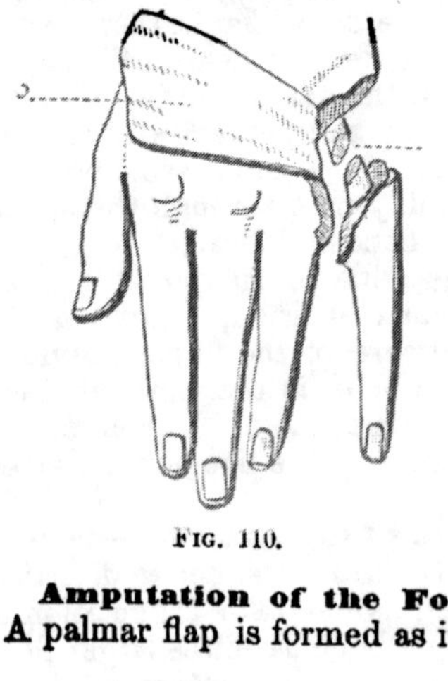

FIG. 110.

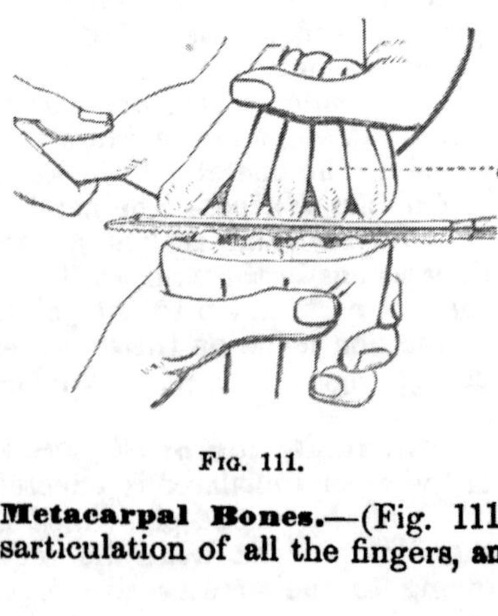

FIG. 111.

Amputation of the Four Metacarpal Bones.—(Fig. 111.) A palmar flap is formed as in disarticulation of all the fingers, and a similar incision is made upon the dorsum; the bistoury is then passed into the interosseous spaces, and the muscular attachments separated, and the periosteum divided; a retractor with five tails is applied, as in (Fig. 111) *a*, and the bone sawn through with a metacarpal saw. Malgaigne recommends the circular operation, and saws the bones separately, perpendicularly to their axes.

Disarticulation of the First Metacarpal Bone.—The metacarpal bone of the thumb, *a* (Fig. 112), articulates with the trape-

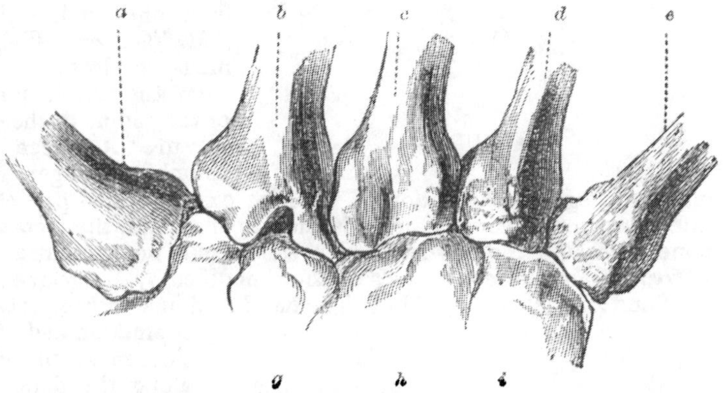

FIG. 112.

zium, *f*, which has a concave surface from within outwards; the joint is of a mixed character, between arthrodial and ginglymoid; on its dorsal surface it is almost subcutaneous, but on its palmar surface it is covered with thick muscles; the radial artery passes around its ulnar side; it has a loose capsule; the joint runs in an oblique direction, in a line drawn from its external side to the root of the little finger; it is easily determined by the projection of the enlargement of the head of the bone, on pressing the thumb into the palm; or, it lies an inch and a quarter below the styloid process of the radius.

Single Flap.—(Fig. 113.) An assistant holds the fingers away, and the operator abducts the thumb; an incision is made through the middle of the commissure between the thumb and fingers, the knife being held vertically, with the heel downwards, close to the bone, terminating at the articulation; the knife is inclined towards the joint, which is opened, the bone dislocated, and the external flap formed by carrying the knife close along the side of the bone, a few lines beyond the metacarpo-phalangeal joint.

Complications.—If the incision is carried too near the second metacarpal bone, the knife may become fastened; this is remedied by making the incision a line or more external; to avoid cutting the base of the external flap, open the joint with the point rather than the blade; if the line of the articulation is not found readily, seek it from before backwards, along the *end* of the metacarpal bone; if the knife is kept close to the first metacarpal bone at its upper extremity, the radial artery may be avoided; if cut, it must be at once tied.

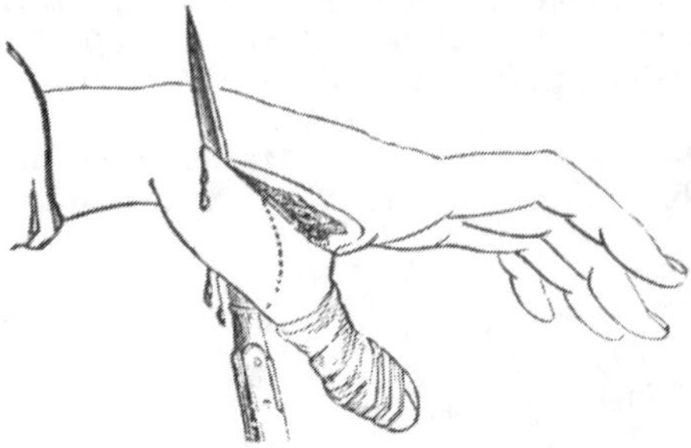

FIG. 113.

Modifications.—Velpeau made a dorsal incision from the styloid process of the radius to the commissure between the thumb and finger, dividing the integuments, tendon of the long extensor, and part of the interosseous muscle; the joint is then opened, and the metacarpal bone dislocated and dissected out; the palm is not wounded.

Oval Method.—Scoutetten's method modified by Malgaigne (*Bernard* and *Huette*):—(Fig. 114.) The hand held in a position between supination and pronation, make an incision along the dorsal surface of the metacarpal bone of the thumb, commencing six lines above its articulation, *a*, with the trapezium, and extending through all the tissues down to the bone, to the inner side of the head of the first phalanx of the thumb, on a level with the commissure, *b*, between the thumb and index finger. Then, carrying the hand into a state of pronation, continue the incision around the palmar surface of the phalanx to its outside, *c*, and thence to the dorsum of the metacarpal bone, to meet the first incision about at its middle. Detach the muscles and integuments from either side of the bone, and open the articulation from its dorsal aspect (Fig. 115, *a*); then, endeavoring to dislocate the bone outwards, complete the division of its remaining attachments.

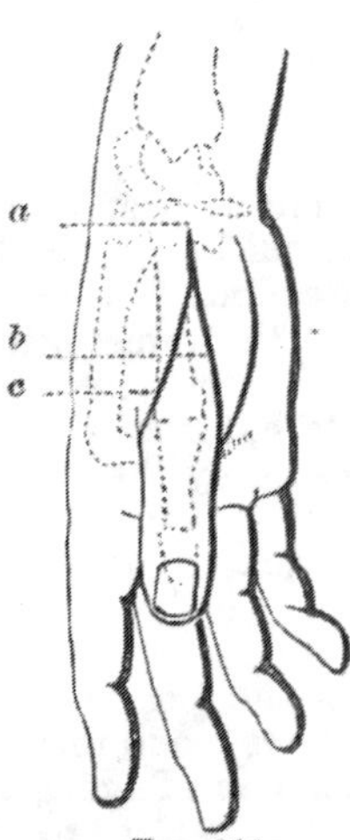

FIG. 114.

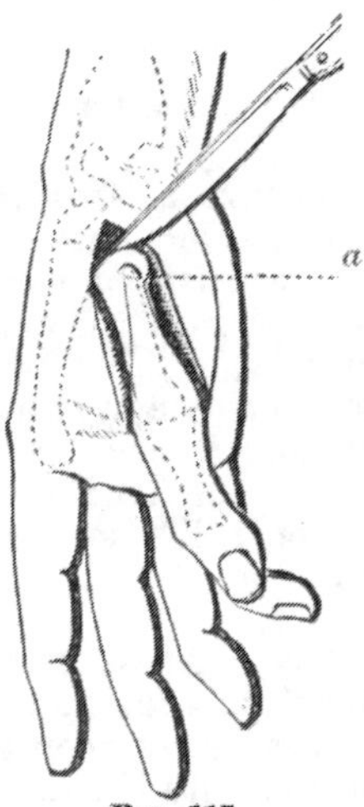

FIG. 115.

Disarticulation of the Second Metacarpal Bone.—The second metacarpal bone, *b* (Fig. 112), has four articular facets, corresponding with the following bones:—1. The trapezius, *f;* 2. The trapezoid, *g;* 3. The os magnum, *h;* 4. The third metacarpal bone, *c;* these bones are firmly united by strong ligaments. Disarticulation of the bone is rendered especially difficult on account of the prolongation of that part of the head that is in relation with the trapezoid, os magnum, and third metacarpal.

Oval Method.—The hand held in pronation, the thumb and fingers separated, an incision is made, commencing about half an inch in front of the styloid process of the radius, but on a line with the second metacarpal bone, *d* (Fig. 116), and is continued to the internal side of the base of the first phalanx, *a;* it is now carried around the dorsal surface in the cutaneous fold, represented on the dorsum by the line, *b; c;* the two points, *c*, and *d*, are now united by an incision; the soft parts are dissected by keeping the edge of the knife close to the bone, the wound being held apart; the knife is carried up along the internal side of the bone to the union of the two metacarpal bones, and turning its edge inwards the interosseous ligament is divided, and in the same manner the knife is made to enter the articulation of the metacarpal bone with the trapezius; the anterior and posterior ligaments are next divided, the bone dislocated, and the knife entered flatwise and horizontally under the upper part of the bone (*a* and *b*, Fig. 117), is carried downwards, completing the operation; care should be taken in dividing the ligaments not to penetrate any adjoining articular cavities.

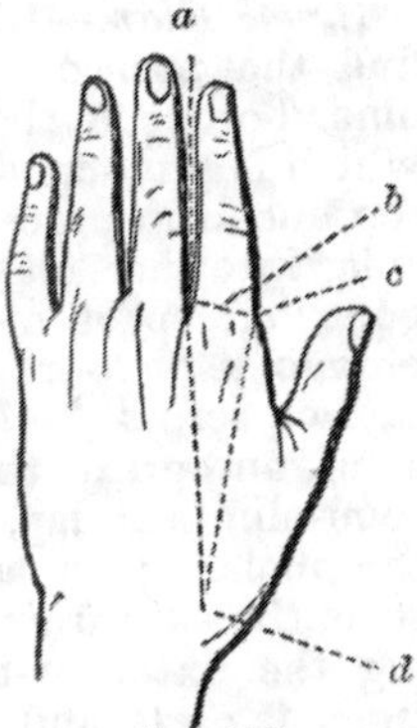

FIG. 116.

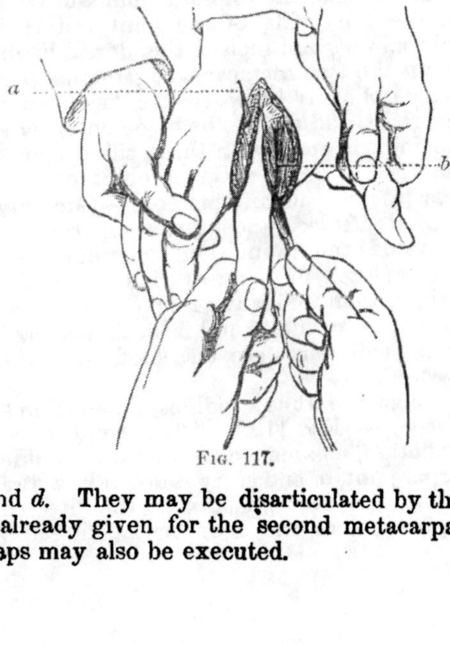

FIG. 117.

Disarticulation of the Third and Fourth Metacarpal Bones.—The articulations of these two bones are seen at (Fig. 112) *c* and *d.* They may be disarticulated by the same operation as that already given for the second metacarpal bone. The method by flaps may also be executed.

Disarticulation of the Fifth Metacarpal Bone.—This bone, *e* (Fig. 112), articulates with the os unciforme, *i*, forming an arthrodial joint; its articulation is continuous with that of the fourth metacarpal bone and the wrist; it has ligaments upon the palmar and dorsal face, and on the outside the interosseous ligament; the unciform bone receives the fifth metacarpal, upon a surface concave from behind forwards, and slightly from within outwards; the line of articulation, if prolonged, would fall upon the middle of the second metacarpal bone.

Single Flap.—Lisfranc directs thus:—The hand being pronated, find the position of the joint by carrying the finger along the ulnar border of the metacarpal bone, until it meets an eminence which is prolonged into a projection on the palmar surface; this is the unciform process; immediately below it is the joint; the articular interline may be seen on the dorsal surface by moving the bone; grasp as much flesh as possible with the left hand, and plunge a bistoury perpendicularly from the dorsal to the palmar surface across the skin and muscles opposite the ulnar side of the joint, and graze the bone with the edge of the knife, forming a semi-elliptical flap, which is finished a little beyond the head of the phalanx; an assistant holding away this flap, the surgeon dissects the skin from the dorsal surface of the bone, without including the extensor tendon; seizing at the same time this skin and the soft parts, and dragging them away, he plunges in his bistoury, still cutting from behind forwards, and a little from without inwards, so as to graze the bone without wounding the skin on either side; and freely divides, from above downwards, all that he meets with to the digital commissure. Lastly, he carries the edge on the ulnar side of the joint, enters it, following the direction pointed out, and incises the dorsal ligament with the point; then to cut the two metacarpal ligaments, plunges the point of the bistoury obliquely between the two bones, its edge turned towards the wrist, and makes the blade enter by elevating the handle; then the joint is opened on three sides, and you need only draw away the bone to finish with the point of the knife the section of the muscles and palmar ligaments.—(*Malgaigne, op. cit.*)

Oval Method.—Scoutetten operated as follows:—The hand is pronated, and an incision commenced one line above the articulation, *e* (Fig. 107), and carried along the dorsum to the commissure, *d*, then under the finger, along the fold of the integument to the opposite side, *f*, and from thence back to the point of departure, *e*; the soft parts are dissected from the bone, and disarticulation effected.

Malgaigne thus modifies Scoutetten's operation (*Bernard* and *Huette*):—(Fig. 119.) "The hand being held in a state of forced pronation, commence an incision six lines above the carpo-metacarpal joint, *a*, and carry it down in a straight line to the inner border of the first phalanx of the little finger, until it meets the depression at the base of the finger on its palmar surface, *b*;

then continue it around the base of the finger, following this depression exactly. Then the operator, lifting up the little finger, continues its incision around to its inside, *c* (Fig. 119), and upwards to join its first portion about opposite to the centre of the metacarpal bone. The integuments and muscles are then detached from the bone, and its articular connexions divided with the point of the bistoury in the manner already described." The wound after the operation is seen in Fig. 118.

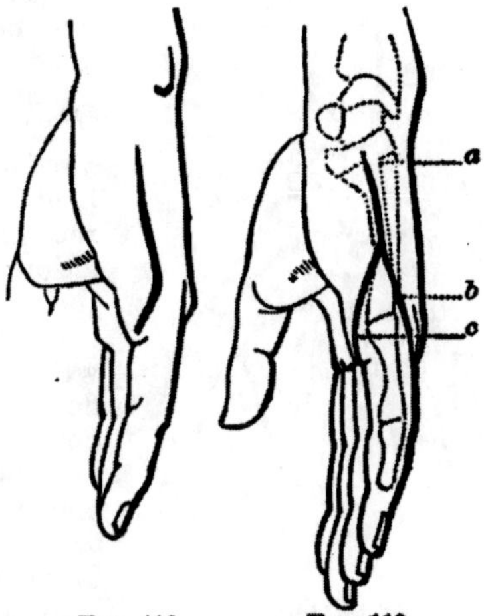

FIG. 118. FIG. 119.

Disarticulation of Two Metacarpal Bones at a Single Operation.—The second and third, the fourth and fifth, or any two or three metacarpal bones may be removed together. Velpeau advises, in removing the fourth and fifth, to make a transverse incision, a little in front of the articulations, another parallel to the axis of the metacarpal bones, upon the dorsum of that which supports the little finger, in order to cut upon that part a dorsal flap which is to cover the whole ulnar side of the wound after the operation; the disarticulation is then effected, and a small flap formed of one or two inches in length, which must be separated down to its base in the palm of the hand, in order to be able to raise it upon the transverse branch of the wound. The same process is adapted to any other two metacarpal bones.

Chelius says:—"If both middle metacarpal bones are to be exarticulated, the fore and little fingers being well adducted, one cut between the bones is to be made, close on the radial side of the middle finger, and another on the ulnar side of the ring finger to the carpus. These two long cuts are then to be connected on the volar and dorsal surfaces by transverse cuts, close down to the bone, the soft parts turned back, and the joint cut through."—(*System of Surgery.*)

Disarticulation of the Metacarpal Bones of all the Fingers.—To recognise the line of articulation fix the external and internal limits; externally it begins with the upper extremity of the first metacarpal bone, 1 (Fig. 120), with the trapezium, *g;* this point is made prominent by pressing the thumb into the palm; internally, it corresponds with the articulation of the fifth metacarpal with the unciform bone, *f;* being a line above the long process of the former, and just below the hook-like process of the latter the line of articulation between these points is irregular, but represents a slightly curved line, convex downwards (Figs. 112, 120); these articulations have only anterior and posterior ligaments, except the second and fifth, which have also lateral ligaments.

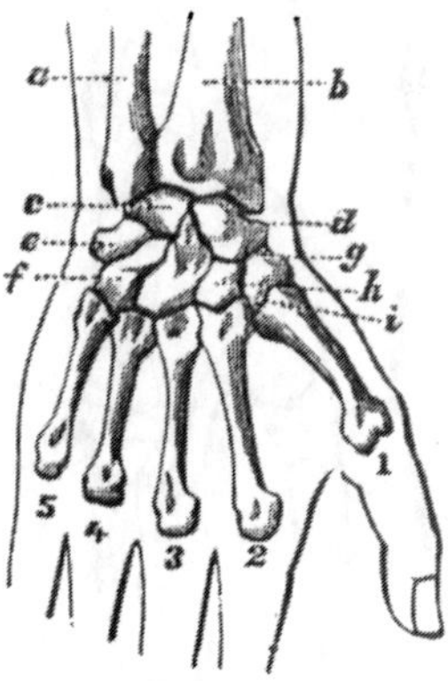

FIG. 120.

Single Flap.—Maingault's method (*Bernard* and *Huette*):—"1st. The hand being held in the position of forced supination, recognise at its outer border the articulation of the first metacarpal bone with the trapezium, and, at its internal side, the articulation of the unciform bone with the fifth metacarpal. 2d. Introduce a small straight knife between the bones and the soft parts, carrying it a little below the projections formed by the unciform and the trapezium, so as to bring out its point below the thumb. 3d. Carry the blade of the knife along the anterior surfaces of the metacarpal bones, and cut out a large flap of an elliptical outline, *a*, *b*, *c* (Fig. 121). 4th. Then turn the hand in the prone position, and make a semicircular incision across its back, two-thirds of an inch below the line of the articulations, and carrying the knife through the tissues connecting the thumb with

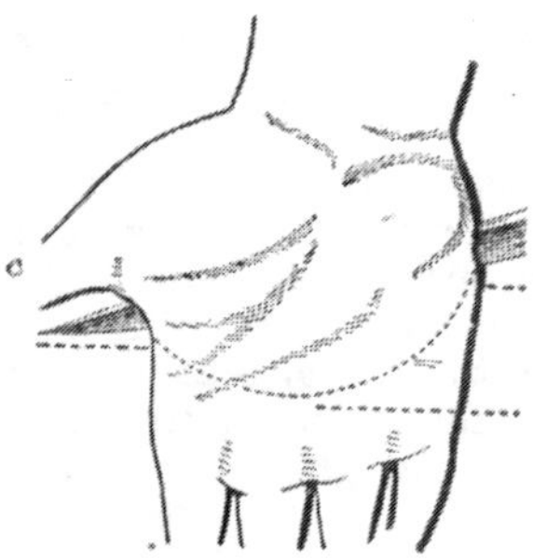

FIG. 121.

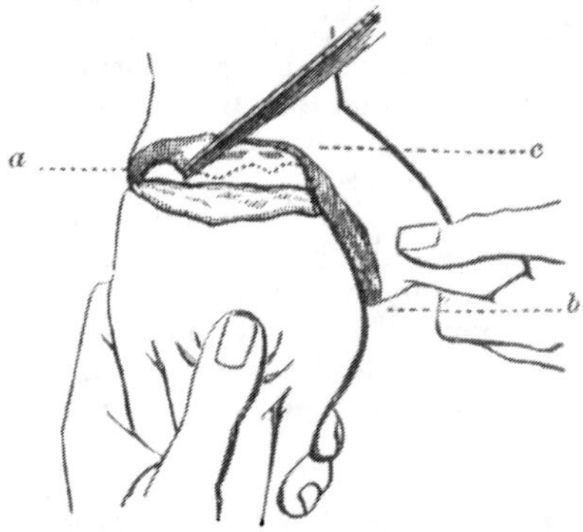

FIG. 122.

the index finger, *a*, *b*, *c* (Fig. 122), join the first incision. While an assistant is drawing the integuments upwards, the surgeon, holding the metacarpus in his left hand, proceeds with the disarticulation from the front of the hand, commencing with the metacarpal bone of the index or the little finger, according as he is operating upon the right or left hand."

Disarticulation of Metacarpal and Carpal Bones.—There are instances on record of the removal of the unciform, pisiform, and pyramidal bones, with the fourth and fifth metacarpal bones; of the os magnum with the three middle metacarpal bones; and finally, of the trapezium, trapezoides, and scaphoid, with the metacarpal bones of thumb and index finger. No rules need be given for these operations; the principal danger arises from the opening thus made into the cavities of the carpal articulations.

Disarticulation of the Radio-Carpal Articulation.—This articulation is composed of the radius and ulna above, and the scaphoid, semi-lunar, and cuneiform bones below (Fig. 120); the line of articulation is convex upwards, the three latter bones forming a convexity which is received into the concavity of the radius and ulna; the pisiform bone is in front and below the articulation; it has external, internal, anterior, and posterior ligaments.

Malgaigne (*op. cit.*) gives the following rules for determining the line of articulation:—"1. Strongly bend the hand backwards; the summit of the angle formed by it with the forearm indicates the radio-carpal articulation; 2. Feel in front the transverse projection of the radius; the joint is one line below it, and about half an inch above the crease in the skin that separates the palm of the hand from the forearm; 3. Determine the summit of the styloid processes, and draw a transverse line between them; the joint will be two lines and a half above this imaginary line; 4. Lastly, the styloid process of the radius being found, the styloid process of the ulna is two lines shorter, and the joint is a quarter of an inch above it."

Circular Method.—(Fig. 123.) The tourniquet being applied over the brachial artery, or compression being made, an assistant holds the forearm in a position between pronation and supination, and strongly retracts the skin at the wrist; a second holds the hand; the operator, standing upon the right side of the limb, makes a circular incision through the skin, about an inch below the styloid processes, grazing the thenar and hypo-thenar eminences; the skin is dissected and turned back as high as the joint; a second circular incision just above the pisiform and unciform bones, and over the joint, divides all the soft tissues; the joint is then entered on one side under the styloid process, and the knife, held perpendicularly, is carried along the curve of the carpal bones to the opposite side, completing the disarticulation at a single sweep; the radial and ulnar arteries are to be tied, the interosseous rarely; the styloid processes may or may not be removed, and the wound is closed by bringing together the parts antero-posteriorly.

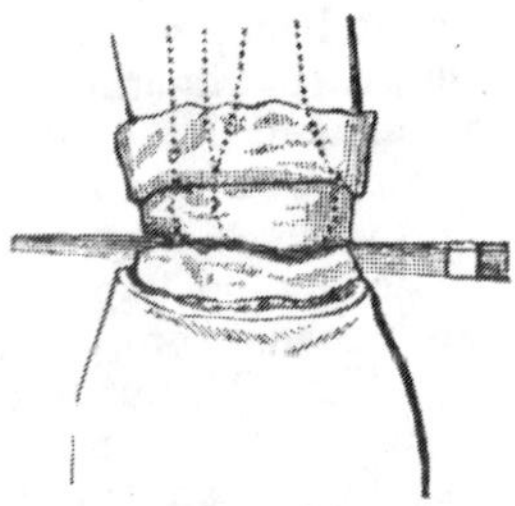

FIG. 123.

Modifications.—Velpeau directs the hand to be flexed when the incision is made on the back of the wrist, and to be extended when it is made in front; it has been advised also to direct the assistants to rotate the limb while the incision is made, rendering the movements of the knife more limited.

Flap Method.—Amputation at the wrist may be performed with single or double flaps, according to existing lesions. If a single flap is made, it may be taken from the dorsal or palmar aspect. If from the dorsum, the hand is held in a prone position, the integument strongly retracted by an assistant, the operator grasps the extremity in the palm of the left hand, placing the thumb and forefinger on the extremities of the styloid processes; a semicircular incision is then made on the dorsum, from just below the processes, having its concavity upwards (Fig. 124), the skin is dissected and

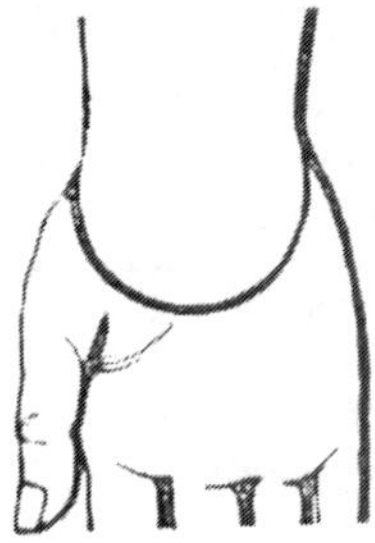

FIG. 124.

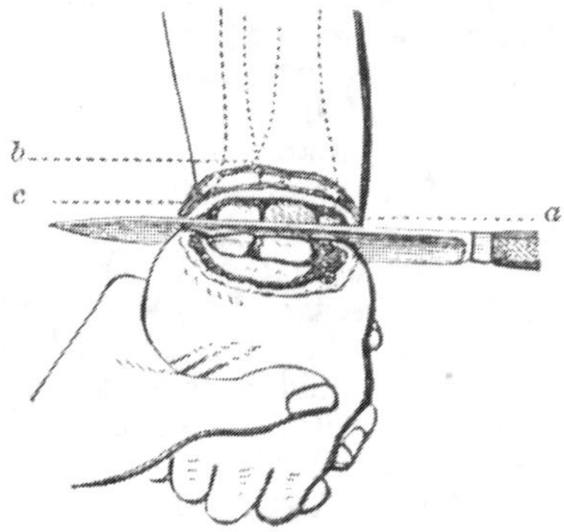

FIG. 125.

turned back, *a*, *b*, *c* (Fig. 125), and the joint, the tendons, and radio-carpal ligaments divided; the lateral ligaments are next cut, the articulation opened, and the knife passed through (Fig. 124), forming a palmar flap of two-thirds of an inch in length; the styloid processes may remain if desired.

The double flap is generally made as follows:—A semicircular flap is made from the extremity of one styloid process to another, as in Fig. 124, but not so low, first on the palmar, and then on the dorsum of the wrist; the ligaments being divided, the hand is forcibly flexed, and the knife carried through the joint from the dorsum (Fig. 125), or from the side, as in the circular amputation.

Amputation of the Forearm.—The forearm, in its upper portion, is covered by muscles, which in its lower part become tendons; its arteries are the radial, ulnar, and anterior and posterior interosseous; amputation may be performed in any part of its length, but the operator should save as much of the limb as possible. It must be remembered that there are two bones to be divided, of different diameters, at different parts of the limb, and the rule must be followed of applying the saw *first and last* to the larger and firmer bone. The following methods of operating have been practised:—

Circular Method.—The forearm is held in a position between pronation and supination; the surgeon standing upon the right side of the limb, makes a circular incision with a catling, dividing the skin and subcutaneous cellular tissue down to the aponeurosis; then turns up the skin like the cuff of a coat, if it should not easily retract; if the limb is large and conical, it may be necessary to make a lateral incision in the skin; next he divides circularly the muscles, with a sawing motion, at the border of the flap of skin which is turned up (Fig. 126); the deep muscles between the bones are divided by introducing the point of the knife, and carefully cutting all the soft parts in the interosseous space; the knife being entered on the dorsal aspect of the radius, and carried around and between the bones by a figure-of-eight incision; a retractor with three ends is introduced into the interosseous space, and the soft parts drawn up; at the point where the bones are denuded, the surgeon draws the saw slowly at first across the radius and ulna, taking care to saw through the radius first (Fig. 127), as the ulna, being more closely attached to the arm, serves as a support for the limb; the radial and ulnar, with the anterior and posterior interosseous arteries, are now tied.—(*Bernard* and *Huette.*)

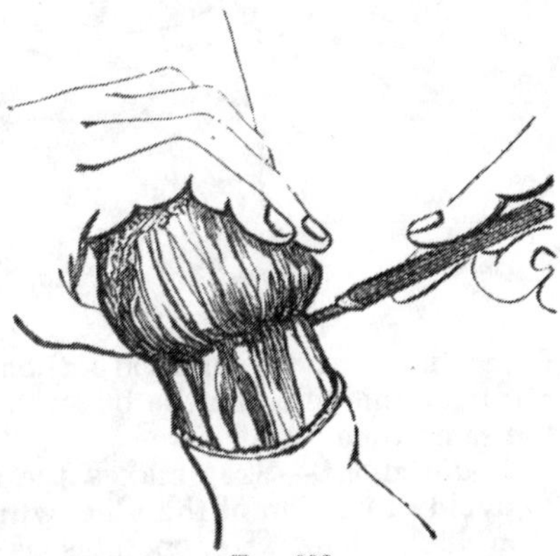

FIG. 126.

Single Flap.—The flap is made from the anterior part of the arm, and of sufficient length to cover the stump; the tissues on the posterior part are incised circularly.

Double Flap.—The flaps may be of equal or unequal length, according to the condition of the parts; if equal, the following rules by Mr. Guthrie may be followed:—"The arm being placed and held firmly in the intermediate position between pronation and supination, with the thumb uppermost, so that the radius and ulna are in one line, a sharp-pointed straight knife is to be entered close to the inner edge of the radius, and brought out below at the inner edge of the ulna. It is then to be carried forwards for half an inch, and made to cut its way out with a gentle inclination, so as to form a semicircular flap. Re-entered at the same point as before, a similar flap is to be made on the outside, the position of the bones being a little altered to admit of its easy execution.

The two flaps are to be turned back; the tendon of the supinator radii longus, and all other tendinous, muscular, or interosseous

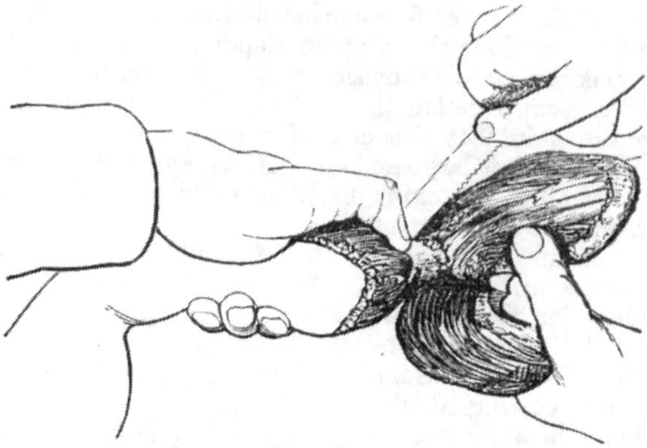

FIG. 127.

fibres, not cut through, are then to be divided, and the linen retractor run between the bones, which are to be sawn across at the same time."

Modifications.—Skey makes the double flaps of the integuments to avoid projection of the ulna, which is liable to occur in the common double flap. He operates as follows:—The flaps should be anterior and posterior; the point of division of the bones being determined on, an arched line in ink should be drawn in front from the central point of the radial to the ulnar aspect of the arm, and a corresponding one behind; commencing at the starting point, the lines formed for each should be run nearly longitudinally along the arm, to the extent of about an inch, and then curve almost suddenly inwards, and passing nearly transversely across the forearm; the depth of each flap should be about an inch, or something more; these two integumental flaps being separated up to the lines forming their base, and drawn upwards with some force, even beyond it, the muscles should be divided by the circular incision, as in the former kind of operation.

Mr. Teale's operation, with rectangular flaps (Fig. 94), is also recommended for the lower part of the forearm.

Disarticulation of the Elbow Joint.—The elbow is a true ginglymoid or hinge joint, formed by the lower extremity of the os brachii above, *a* (Fig. 128), and the upper extremities of the radius, *c*, and ulna, *d*, the former on the outside, and the latter on the inside; the ulna forms the principal part of the lower portion of the joint, having a large articular surface by the projection of the olecranon, *c* (Fig. 129), backwards, and the coronoid process, *b*

(Fig. 129), forwards, which embrace the irregular articulating surface of the os brachii; the radius is merely in contact with the os

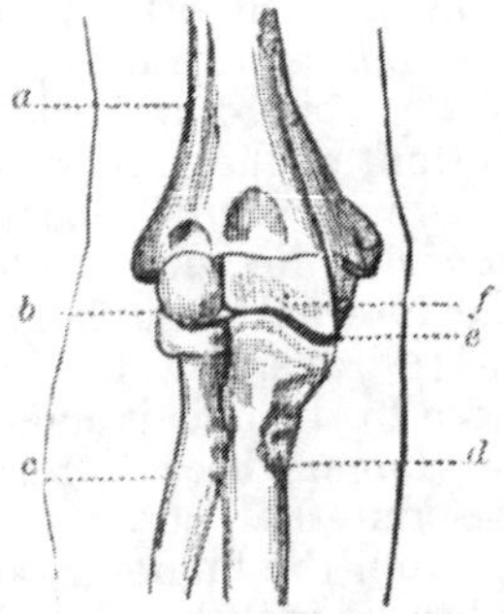

FIG. 128.

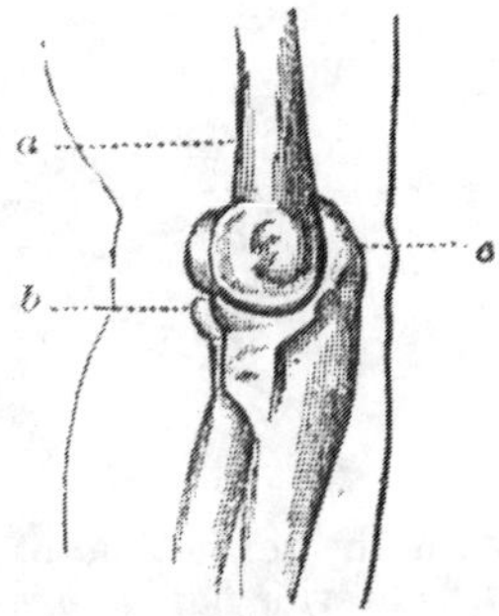

FIG. 129.

brachii; the articulation has anterior, posterior, and lateral ligaments. The exact position of the joint is determined only by careful attention to the anatomical relations of the following osseous prominences about the joint:—the epicondyles, or the most prominent points on the condyles of the os brachii (Fig. 128), are recognised, the internal more readily than the external, a line drawn through the lower points, is, on the outside, a quarter of an inch above the interarticular line, *b*, *f*, *e* (Fig. 128), and on the inside three-quarters of an inch; the articulation of the radius and humerus is transverse, that of the ulna irregular, and owing to its projections must be entered externally.

Malgaigne remarks of the position and direction of the interarticular line (*op. cit.*):—"Two facts result: first, that the articular interline is very oblique from without inwards, and from above downwards. Second, that it is very much below the tuberosities of the humerus. If, then, in cutting your anterior flap, you extend its base up to the level of these tuberosities, it will almost always be too short to cover the bone, which will project, especially on the inside and downwards: this often happened to Dupuytren, who put in his knife transversely at the internal and anterior part of the epitrochlea, to bring it out on the anterior border of the epicondyle. You should, on the contrary, plunge in the knife obliquely one inch below the middle projection of the epitrochlea, to bring it out half an inch below the projection of the epicondyle."

Circular Method.—The brachial artery being controlled, the arm is held in a supine position, and the operator standing on the outside of the limb makes a circular incision, through the skin only, around the arm, four fingers' breadth below the joint; the integuments are dissected up to the joint, and reflected backwards, *a*, *b* (Fig. 130); the muscles in front are then divided, the ligaments cut, and the joint entered, and disarticulation completed by dividing the triceps, or sawing off the olecranon; the brachial artery is divided before its bifurcation.

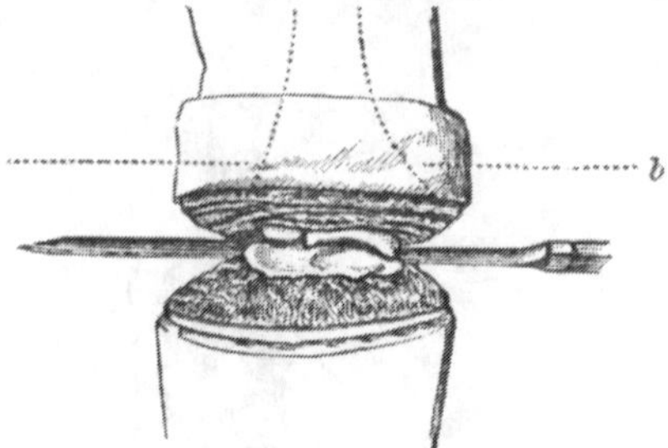

FIG. 130.

Single Flap.—The limb is placed in a supine position, but slightly flexed; the operator, raising the soft parts from the bone, in front of the joint, enters a straight knife about a finger's breadth below the internal condyle (Fig. 131); traversing the limb close to the ulna it appears two fingers' breadth below the external condyle, to allow for the retraction of muscles arising from the humerus, and cuts an anterior flap, *a*, *b*, *c* (Fig. 131), about three inches in length; this flap being retracted, *a* (Fig. 132), the knife is passed behind

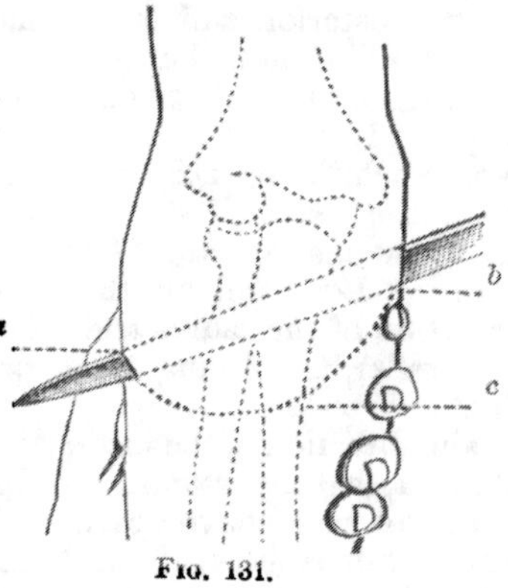

FIG. 131.

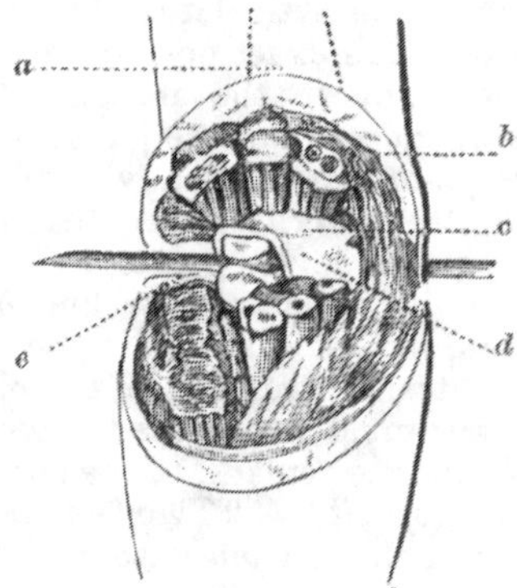

FIG. 132.

the limb, and the heel entered on the outside, between the articulation of the radius and os brachii, *e*, and continued across the back part of the joint, dividing all the tissues to the internal angle of the wound; the anterior ligament, *c*, *d*, and lateral ligaments are divided, the bones luxated forwards, the insertion of the triceps cut, and the operation completed.

Guérin recommends an external flap; this is made by transfixing the limb upon the outside, entering the point of the knife just within the head of the radius, *a* (Fig. 133), traversing its neck, *c*, and cutting out a large external flap, *b*; a second flap is made from the inside of the arm, by cutting from without inwards, and from below upwards, *d*; the soft tissues immediately covering the joint are divided, and disarticulation completed. A good covering is thus made for the condyles.

Oval Method.—Baudens performed the oval operation, commencing the incision over the border of the radius, five fingers' breadth below the fold of the joint, and passing around the limb, a finger's breadth higher, over the ulna; the dissection was then carried upwards to the joint, and disarticulation accomplished.

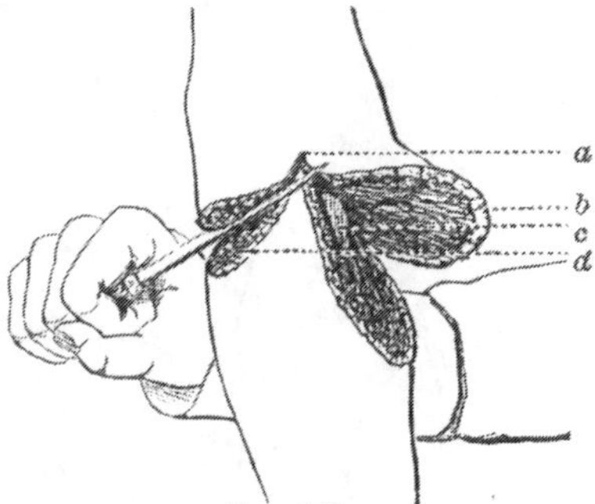

FIG. 133.

Amputation of the Arm.—The humerus is covered in its lower part by muscles, closely attached throughout its extent; but at the upper part large muscles are inserted into it which have their origin from the thorax, shoulder, and back, which, when divided, tend to leave the bone bare; the only artery always requiring the ligature is the brachial; the following methods are practised:—

Circular Method.—The patient placed in a recumbent position, the arm carried at right angles to the body, the operator standing on the right side of the limb, makes a circular incision through the integuments; these are loosened from the fascia with the point of the knife, and drawn up or rolled over by an assistant, an inch, an inch and a half, or two inches, according to the size of the limb; the second incision made at the margin of the retracted skin, divides the superficial muscles, which are also retracted; a third incision lays the bone bare (Fig. 92); this is sawn through; the brachial artery, lying on the inside, between the biceps and internal portion of the triceps muscles, is secured; the wound is generally brought together from before backwards; it may be closed from side to side, or even obliquely.

Single Flap.—Amputation may be performed with a single flap at any point presenting upon one surface a sufficient amount of tissues; Sabatier, in amputations on a level with the axilla, made a square flap of the deltoid, by uniting two lateral parallel incisions by a transverse, detaching the flap from the bone, incising circularly the remaining tissues, on a level with the base of the flap, and sawing the bone.

Double Flap.—The flaps are made of equal size (Fig. 134), and generally anterior and posterior; the arm being carried at right angles from the body, the operator grasps with his left hand the tissues on the anterior or lateral part of the arm, and passing the knife down to the bone, carries it over to the opposite side, cuts a flap of the requisite length, being two to three or more inches long, according to the size of the limb (Fig. 135); withdrawing the knife, it is re-entered and a second flap is made in a similar manner; the flaps are firmly retracted, the tissues covering the

*

bone divided, and the bone sawn at the highest point in the flap (Fig. 134).

Modifications.—The most rapid operation is that in which one flap is short, and is formed on the anterior surface by cutting from

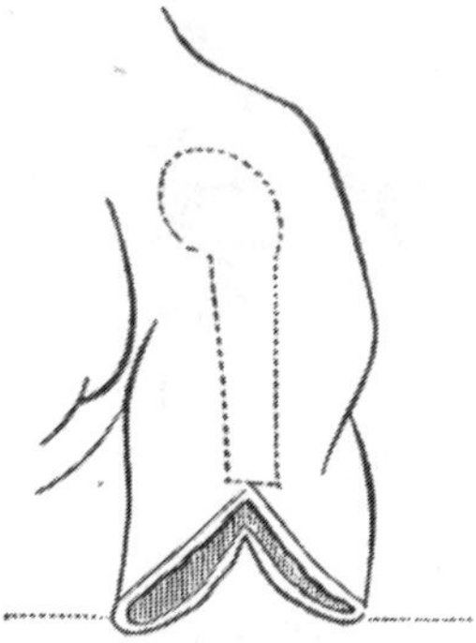

FIG. 134.

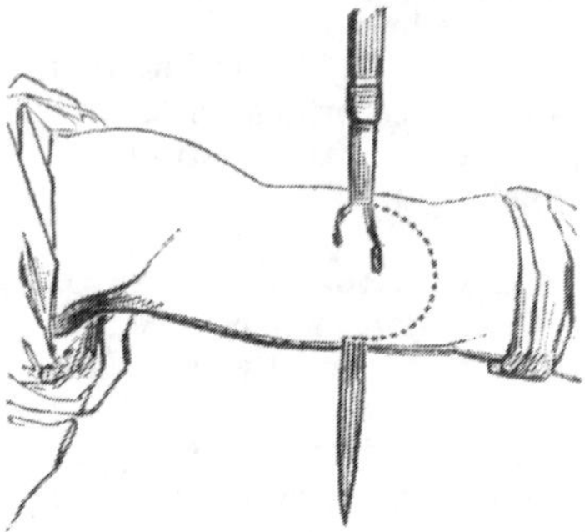

FIG. 135.

within outwards. Mr. Luke's amputation of the arm with two flaps is thus described by Mr. Guthrie:—"The first flap is made posteriorly to the bone, by transfixing the limb, for which purpose the knife is entered at the mid-point between the anterior and posterior surfaces, carried transversely across the limb, and made to cut towards the posterior surface, in an oblique direction, until all the soft structures are divided. It is necessary, in entering the knife, to bear in mind that the bone lies opposite to the mid-point, and that, in carrying the knife across the limb, it would strike against the surface of the bone, unless means were adopted for its prevention. This is easily done by grasping the structures which are to form the posterior flap between the fingers and thumb of the left hand, and by drawing them backwards during the time the knife is entering at the mid-point and being carried across the limb. Having formed the posterior flap, the anterior one is formed as in amputation of the thigh, by cutting inwards from the surface towards the bone with a sweep, which will make this flap equal in length to the posterior. The operation is completed by dividing the remaining soft parts by means of a cut carried circularly around the bone, and by sawing the bone in the line of division."

Rectangular Flap.—The method by a rectangular flap has also been adopted on the lower part of the arm, the line of incision being given in Fig. 136.

Oval Method.—Mr. Guthrie describes the following method of amputation of the arm immediately below the tuberosities of the humerus, which is similar to his amputation at the shoulder-joint, and is designed to supersede it:—"The arm being raised from the side, and an assistant having compressed, or being ready to compress, the subclavian artery, the surgeon commences his incision one or two fingers' breadth beneath the acromion process, and carries it to the inside of the arm, below the edge of the pectoral muscle, then under the arm to the outside, where it is to be met by another incision, begun at the same spot as the first, below the acromion process. The integuments, thus divided, are to be retracted, and the muscular parts cut through, until the bone is cleared as high as the tuberosities. The artery will be seen at the under part, and should be pulled out by a tenaculum or spring forceps, and secured as soon as divided. The bone is best sawn, the surgeon standing on the outside; the nerves should be cut short, and the flaps brought together by two or three silk or leaden sutures. There are few or no other vessels to tie, and the cure is completed in the usual time, while the rotundity of the shoulder is preserved."

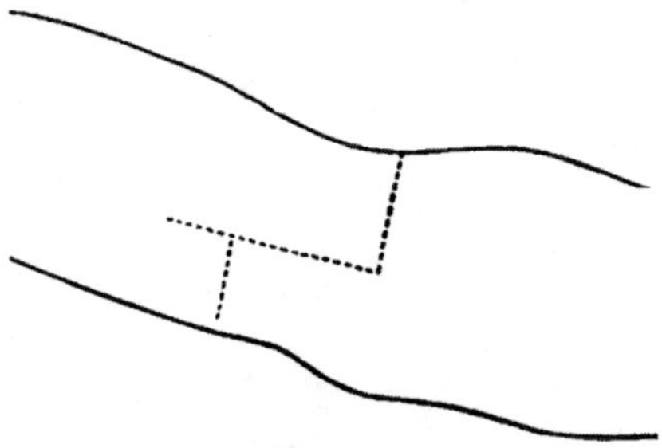

FIG. 136.

Disarticulation of the Shoulder-Joint.—The shoulder-joint is arthrodial; the articular head of the os brachii, *e*, is very broad, and articulates by scarcely one-third with the shallow glenoid cavity of the scapula; it is connected to it by a loose capsular ligament; the joint is strengthened by the long head of the biceps, and the muscles arising from the scapula, and inserted in the vicinity of the joint; the joint is protected above by the extremity of the clavicle, *b*, and the acromion, *c*; in amputations at the shoulder-joint, the artery must be compressed upon the first rib above the clavicle, with the thumb, or a padded key.

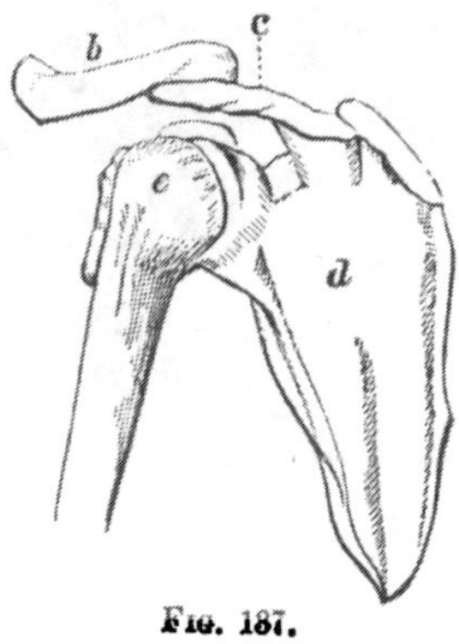

FIG. 137.

Oval Method.—The following is Larrey's operation (*Bernard* and *Huette*):—"Make a vertical incision on the outer surface of the shoulder through the skin and subjacent tissues down to the bone, and extending from the edge of the acromion process to a point one inch below the top of the humerus (Fig. 137); 2d. Make then two oblique incisions starting from the centre of the vertical one, one on the anterior, and the other on the posterior aspect of the joint, carrying them through the tissues composing the anterior and posterior walls of the axilla, to the lower border of each, and dividing their attachments to the humerus; 3d. Push the edges of the wound on either side to expose the joint, and open it, making traction on the bone to put its ligament on the

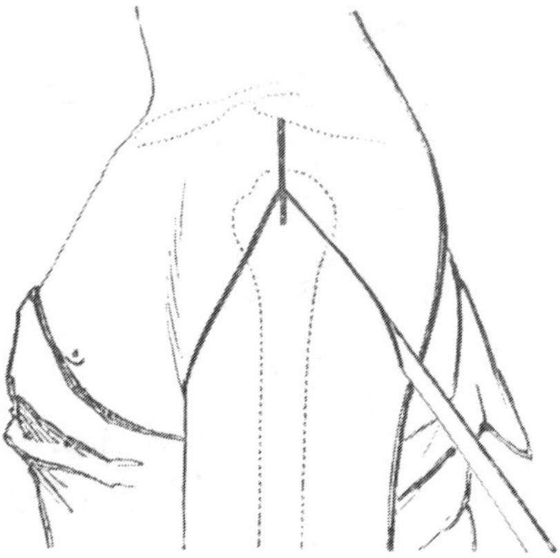

Fig. 138.

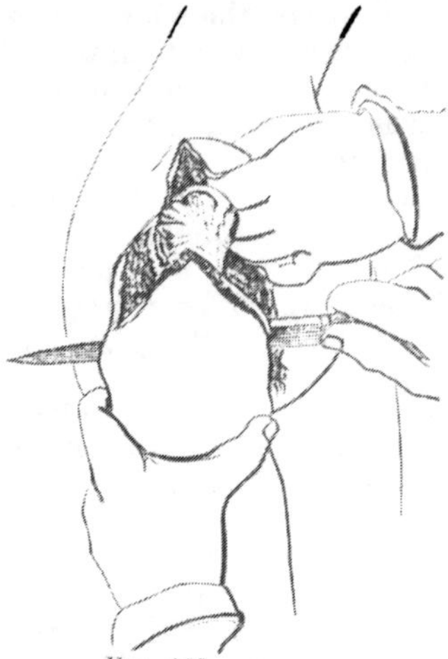

Fig. 139.

stretch; 4th. Luxate the bone, pass the knife behind it (Fig. 138), and finish the operation by cutting directly through the tissues in the axilla, which intervene between the extremities of the incisions already made, recollecting that the artery is contained in them, and requires to be compressed by an assistant. The wound which results from this operation is almost perfectly oval in shape."

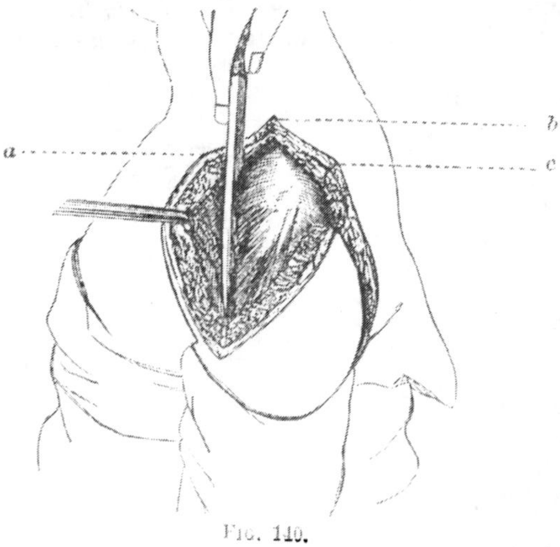

Fig. 140.

Modifications.—Guthrie commences his incision just below the acromion, but endangers the exposure of the glenoid cavity, by the subsequent contraction of the muscles and integuments; Guérin dissects the head of the bone from its cavity with the knife held vertically, first upon one side and then upon the other, *a*, *b*, *c* (Fig. 140), and completes it by dividing the axillary portion.

Single Flap.—Malgaigne (*op. cit.*) gives the following description of Dupuytren's operation with a single flap:—"The arm being held away from the trunk, grasp the deltoid in its entire length and thickness in the left hand; with the right pass a double-edged knife through its base, under the acromion, and grazing the surface of the humerus, cut an external and superior flap of sufficient extent; an assistant raises it; then, by approaching the arm to the body, expose the tendons of the muscles inserted into the head of the humerus. Cut them, commencing with those posterior, which are more easily divided on account of the greater interval between the acromion and the head of the humerus, than between the latter and the coracoid process, and finishing with the anterior tendons. To a practised hand, a semicircular incision on the anatomical neck of the humerus with the edge of the knife held perpendicularly suffices. The fibrous tissue that unites it to the acromion is also divided. Then the operator, grasping the diseased arm with his left hand, dislocates the head of the bone outwards; and, passing the knife behind it, detaches the flesh that covers it, in which the nerves and vessels are comprised. At this moment, the assistant compresses these soft parts, with his thumb on the bleeding surface, and his fingers placed in the axilla, so as to compress the artery; and the operator, assured against hæmorrhage, finishes dividing them, on a level with the inferior attachment of the great pectoral and latissimus dorsi to the humerus."

Modifications.—Guérin, instead of making the flap by transfixion, cuts from without inwards; commencing the incision (on the left side) near the anterior border of the deltoid, on a level with the articulation; it descends in a curved direction to within two-thirds of an inch of the insertion of the deltoid, and then ascending on the posterior part (Fig. 141) at the same level as it was commenced; the flap is dissected up, and the limb disarticulated.

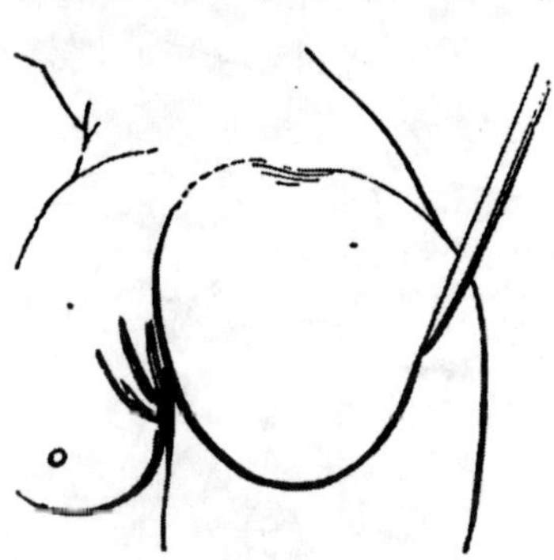

FIG. 141.

Double Flaps.—The method of Lisfranc, now generally adopted, is as follows (*Bernard* and *Huette*):—1st. The patient is supported in a convenient position upon a chair, and the arm kept close to the trunk, the head of the humerus at the same time being pushed upwards and outwards as much as possible. The surgeon then, being provided with a long straight knife cutting on both edges, assures himself of the exact position of the acromion and coracoid processes. If it is the left shoulder upon which he is about to operate, the point of the knife should be entered in a direction almost parallel with the humerus at the outer side of the posterior border of the axilla, in front of the tendons of the latissimus dorsi and teres major muscles, *c* (Fig. 142). As the knife passes in, the plane of its blade should form an angle of thirty-five degrees with the axis of the shoulder, and its point should graze the posterior and external surface of the humerus, until it reaches the under surface of the acromion; at this point the handle of the knife should be raised, and its point lowered, so that it is brought out below and in front of the clavicle, *a*, in the triangular space between the acromion and coracoid processes, which is bounded posteriorly by the clavicle. The knife should then be made to cut its way outwards around the head of the humerus, *b*, and as soon as it becomes disengaged from beneath the acromion, the arm is carried a little distance away from the trunk, and the surgeon grasps with his left hand the deltoid muscle, raising it as much as possible from the bone, and carries the knife directly downwards, grazing the bone, and cutting out a posterior semicircular flap about three inches in length. In making this flap the upper part of the capsule of the joint should be divided, as well as the tendons of latissimus dorsi, the teres major and minor, and a part of the deltoid; 2d. The head of the humerus being readily separated from the glenoid cavity after the division of the parts just mentioned, the operator passes the blade of the knife behind it, and carries it downwards and forwards, grazing the humerus, to cut out the internal flap, and at this moment the artery contained in the substance of this flap should be compressed

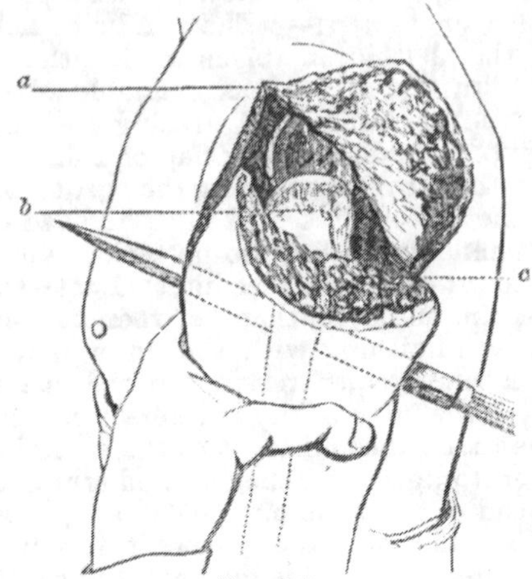

FIG. 142.

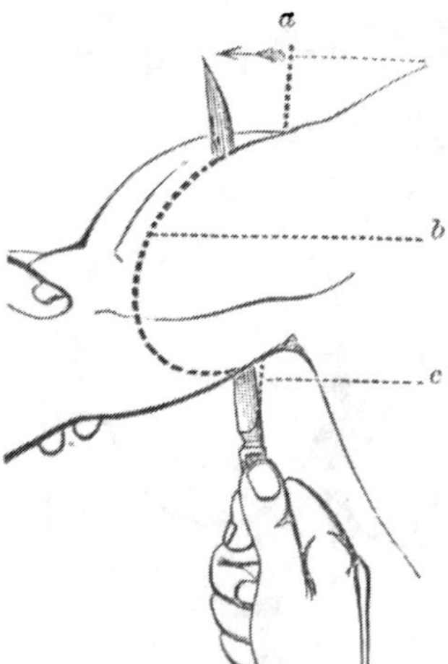

FIG. 143.

by an assistant. In operating upon the shoulder of the right side the same rules are followed, except that the knife should be entered in the infra-clavicular triangle described above, to be brought out at the posterior border of the axilla, thus reversing the direction of the knife in transfixing the articulation to cut out the posterior flap."

The manner of cutting out the first flap by transfixing the parts above the joint, is illustrated in Fig. 143; *c*, point of entrance of the knife, *a*, of emergence, and *b*, the flap; the knife may, as here represented, have a single blade.

AMPUTATION OF THE LOWER EXTREMITIES.

General Principles.—"*Under all circumstances, except where poverty and advanced age, and confirmed dissolute habits, so combine in the individual, as to render it certain that mechanical appliances would be of little service, give the patient the stump best adapted to the most useful artificial limb.*"

"I. In all amputations of the lower extremity, the surgeon should be governed in the selection of the point of operation and the method to be adopted—1. By the mortality of the operations in question; 2. By the adaptability of the stump to the most serviceable artificial limbs.

"II. In all injuries of the foot, involving parts anterior to the medio-tarsal articulation, the surgeon should sacrifice as little as possible of the structures essential to progression. He should preserve, 1. Single phalanges, the importance of which increases from the small to the great toe; 2. The metatarsus, by amputation of the phalanges, or by the excision of individual metacarpal bones; 3. The tarsus, by amputation at the tarso-metatarsal articulation (Hey's or Lisfranc's method).

"III. Of the amputations through the tarsus or at the ankle-joint, preference should be given to Syme's operation as affording a minimum mortality, with a stump best adapted to an artificial limb.

"IV. In the after treatment of the amputations and resections above considered, it is good practice to leave the wounds open to heal by granulation."—*Report* of Drs. Valentine Mott, Gurdon Buck, John Watson, Alfred C. Post, Willard Parker, Ernst Krackowizer, W. H. Van Buren, and Stephen Smith, a committee of Associate Medical Members of the U. S. Sanitary Commission.

Bones of the Foot and Ankle-Joint.—(Fig. 144.) *a* and *b*, inferior extremity of the tibia and fibula; *c*, astragalus; *d*, os calcis; *e*, scaphoid; *f*, cuboid; *g*, internal cuneiform; *h*, middle cuneiform; *i*, external cuneiform; 1, 2, 3, 4, and 5, first, second, third, fourth, and fifth metatarsal bones; *k*, *k*, *k*, *k*, *k*, phalanges of the toes.

Amputation of the Toes.—Amputation in the continuity of individual toes is performed by the same rules as have been given for similar amputations of the fingers.

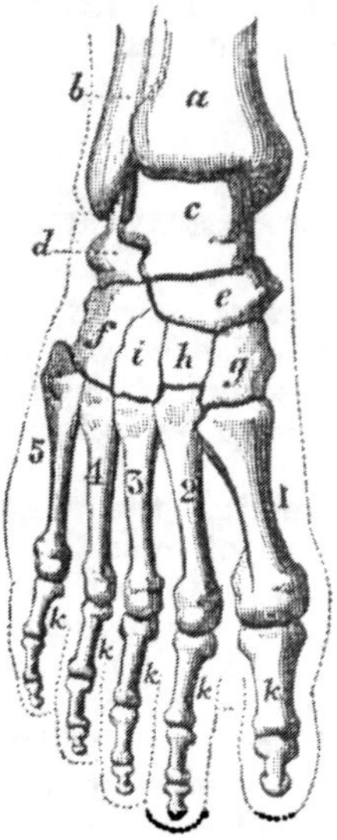

Fig. 144.

Disarticulation of the Second Phalanges.—Amputation through the phalangeal articulations may be performed by the same methods as are given for the fingers; a flap is generally formed from the palmar surface.

Disarticulation of Single Toes.—The metatarso- and metacarpo-phalangeal articulations present but slight differences. The following peculiarities are to be noticed:—The extremity of the first metatarsal bone, 1 (Fig. 144), is large, and requires a very liberal flap to cover it; on the plantar face of the articulation are two or three sesamoid bones; the inter-articular line is further from the inter-digital commissure than in the hand, but the second space is much nearer the joint than the others.

Oval Method.—Holding the toe with the finger and thumb of the left hand, commence an incision over the joint and carry it downwards and forwards, along the side of the toe to the commissure of the toes, around, under the toe, along the transverse linear depression to the opposite side, and thence back to the point of commencement; the extensor tendons and lateral ligaments are divided with the point of the knife, the joint opened, and the disarticulation completed by cutting the tissues upon the under part of the joint.

Single Flap.—A flap may be made from the dorsal or plantar surface, or, in amputation of the great and small toes, from the internal and external surface. If the flap is made upon the dorsum, make two lateral incisions, extending from the joint to the first phalangeal articulation, join their lower extremities by a transverse dorsal incision, dissect up the flap to the joint, dislocate by depressing the toe firmly, and divide the tissues on the lower surface. If the flap is palmar, make a transverse incision over the joint, and lateral incisions to divide the connexions of the joint, depress the toe, and pass the knife through the joint and along the under surface of the bone until a sufficient flap is formed. If the flap is upon the outer side of the great or small toe, enter the joint by cutting through the commissure, the knife being held vertically, and complete the operation by carrying the knife through the joint and along the outer side of the bone, forming a flap of the requisite size. (Fig. 145.)

Double Flap.—The operator holds the toe between the left

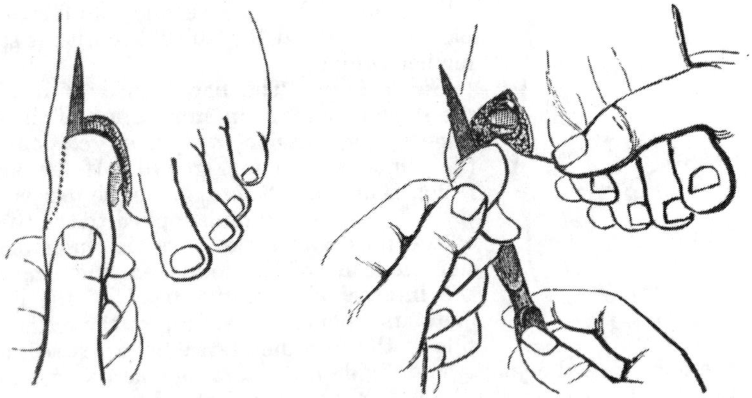

FIG. 145.

thumb and finger, and recognising the articulation, transfixes the soft parts by passing the knife from the palmar to the dorsal surface on one side, emerging over the middle of the joint, and cutting a flap from the side as far forwards as the edge of the commissure; the joint may now be opened on the side, the knife passed through, and a flap cut from the opposite side by passing the knife along the bone; or the parts may be transfixed, and the second flap cut out as the first, and disarticulation completed as the last step.

Skey describes (*Op. Surg.*) the following methods of forming flaps:—"A second mode of effecting this separation of the great toe is by a double flap. Bend the toe downwards, and make a dorsal flap, which is carried round across the middle of the phalanx, from the integumental fold, between that and the second toe, to the side of the ball of the first toe, and reflect it. A similar line below, uniting the ends of the first flap by a circular sweep of the knife, forms the lower flap. The bone is then disarticulated, and the lower flap completed by cutting out. A third mode of performing this amputation, which insures sufficient integument, consists in making a straight longitudinal incision along the inner side of the toe, commencing about half an inch behind the articulation, and carrying it onwards to the middle of the first phalanx. At this end of the line make a circular incision around the toe down to the bone, reflect back the integuments and soft parts from it, and open the joint from above. These operations on the toe often require a ligature or even two."

Disarticulation of all the Toes.—It will be seen (Fig. 144), that the metatarso-phalangeal articulation represents a curved line, having its convexity downwards, due to the following difference in the metatarsal bones: the second is half a line longer than the first, the third is half a line shorter than the second, the fourth is half a line behind the third, the fifth is still further behind.

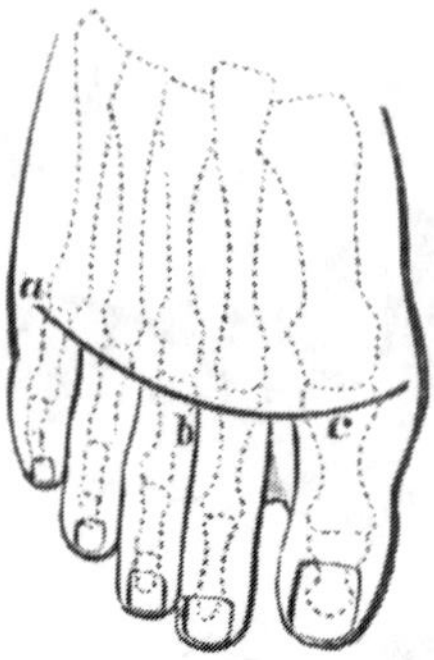

Fig. 146.

Single Flap.—The flap is made in nearly the same manner as in amputation of all the fingers; the incision, *a, b, c,* in relation to the joints is seen in Fig. 146. If the operation is on the left foot, grasp the toes with the left hand, the thumb applied to the back of the toes, and make a semicircular incision, in front of the joints, commencing at the internal side of the head of the first metatarsal bone, and ending at the external side of the fifth metatarsal bone; dissect up the flap, open the joints, and divide the lateral ligaments with the point of the knife; the knife is now passed behind the phalanges, and a flap cut from the palmar surface. The lower flap may be made, according to Guérin, by an incision on the palmar surface, commencing on one side, and passing in a curved direction along the cutaneous fold at the root of the phalanges (Fig. 147).

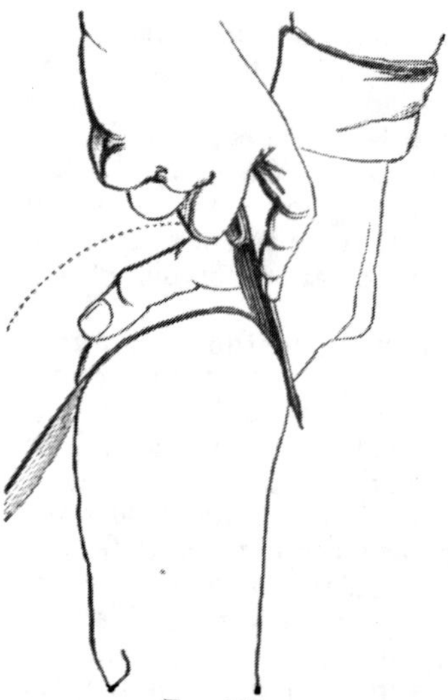

Fig. 147.

Circular Method.—The steps of this operation are the same as for circular amputation of the fingers, *en masse.*

Amputation through the Metatarsal Bones.—Amputation of all the metatarsal bones is performed with palmar and dorsal flaps, as on the metacarpus; an incision is made on the dorsum of the foot, convex downwards, the soft parts divided down to the bone; the knife should then transfix the palmar surface, grazing the bones, and make a flap nearly or quite to the commissure of the toes; the interosseous muscular substance is divided by the point of the knife, a six-tailed retractor applied and the soft parts retracted; the metacarpal saw is now used to divide the bones (Fig. 148).

Disarticulation of the First Metatarsal Bone.—The first metatarsal bone has a large, slightly concave, articular surface for the internal cuneiform; it has four ligaments, an internal, dorsal, plantar, and interosseous; the articulation is one or two lines behind the first projection discovered on the posterior part of the inner margin of the metatarsal bone, and an inch anterior to the prominence of the scaphoid, *e* (Fig. 144); the direction of the line of articulation is from within forwards and outwards; the dorsalis pedis artery passes to the sole of the foot on the outer side of the joint.

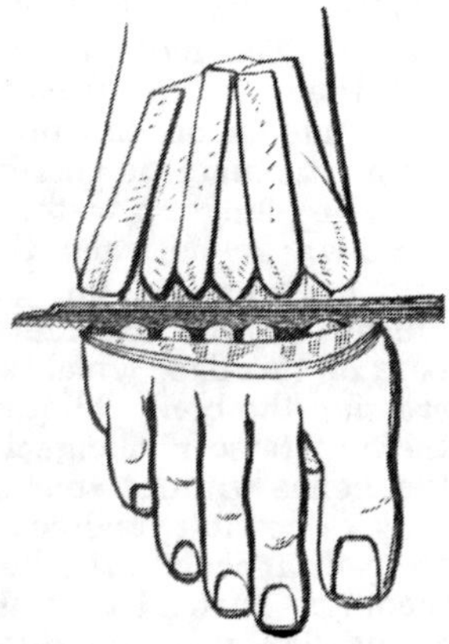

FIG. 148.

Oval Method.—Scoutetten operated as follows (*Malgaigne, op. cit.*):—"Commence two lines behind the joint, *a* (Fig. 149), an incision directed obliquely from within outwards, to the commissure of the toes, *c*, and passed round the base of the first phalanx, following the crease on its palmar surface; withdraw the bistoury and replace it on the internal side of the phalanx, *b*, in the inferior angle of the incision, ascend on the internal side of the metatarsal bone and phalanx, and by a line slightly oblique from within outwards, rejoin the point of commencment; the skin being cut, divide successively in the whole extent of the incision the extensor tendons of the toe, and the fibres of the dorsal interosseous muscle. Dissect the skin from the sole of the foot, leaving the sesamoid bones on the phalangeal articulation, and exposing all the internal surface of the bone. The operator then again seeks the joint, divides the internal ligament, holding the point of the instrument perpendicular to the horizon, and the edge slightly oblique from within outwards and from behind forwards to follow the directions of the joint. Next divide the superior ligament, and then direct the edge of the bistoury upwards, and push its point obliquely at an angle of forty-five degrees into the interosseous space, formed by the external surface of the first cuneiform and the extremity of the second metatarsal bone. When the point has penetrated to the plantar layer, raise the blade again to the perpendicular, and the interosseous ligament is divided. There remain only a few muscular and ligamentous

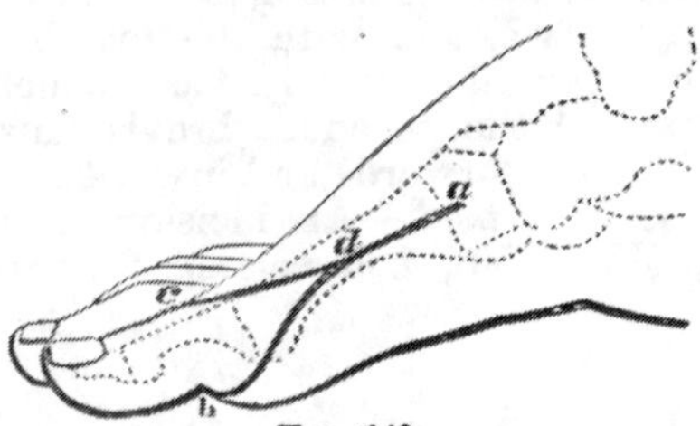

FIG. 149.

fibres, which are easily divided." The incision in Fig. 148 is not precisely that described above, but is preferable.

Single Flap.—Lisfranc's method is as follows (*Malgaigne, op. cit.*):—"The foot being placed on a table, and fixed by an assistant, the operator seizes with his fingers and thumb the muscles and integuments on the internal side of the bone, and draws them from it as much as possible, to obtain a flap of suitable thickness; then he plunges a bistoury, held in the third position, from above downwards, between the inside of the bone and the soft parts, two lines behind the joint; cuts a flap all along the bone, and finishes beyond the metatarso-phalangeal articulation. From the base of this flap, which an assistant draws back, make an incision, crossing the bone obliquely to the internal and superior surface of the metatarso-phalangeal joint. Then push the bistoury between the bones without touching the skin, as near the posterior extremity as possible, and cut directly down to the commissure of the toes; disarticulate the bone as we have shown in the former proceeding. Instead of making a second incision after the formation of the flap, you may dissect off the skin from the base of the flap to the metatarso-phalangeal articulation, and have it drawn outwards by an assistant. The essential point is to be able to introduce the knife between the bones without jagging or cutting the integuments."

Disarticulation of the Fifth Metatarsal Bone.—The fifth metatarsal bone articulates with the cuboid (Fig. 144) by a triangular surface, and with the fourth metacarpal; it has a tubercle on the external part of its base, which is easily felt, and into which is inserted the peroneus brevis muscle; the line of articulation is obliquely forwards and inwards.

Oval Method.—An incision is commenced just behind the joint, *a* (Fig. 150), and carried forwards towards the commissure, *b*, thence under the toe, along the transverse linear depression to the opposite side, *c*, and then along the external margin to *a*, the point of departure; the soft parts are dissected from the bone, the joint entered from the outside, behind the tubercle; divide the ligaments which unite it to the fourth metatarsal, and complete the operation by dividing the plantar ligaments.

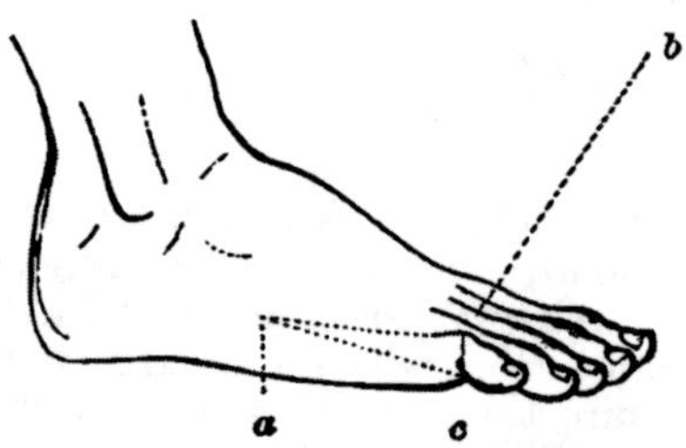

Fig. 150.

Single Flap.—Velpeau directs as follows:—"The knife being held perpendicularly, the point upwards, cut through the entire interosseous tissues between the fourth and fifth metatarsal bones, from before backwards to the cuboid bone; disarticulate the bone, detach it, pass the knife to the outside, and cut an external flap."

Lisfranc transfixes the tissues at the base of the metacarpal bone, and cuts forward, making an external flap; then he transfixes on the inner side and cuts out to the commissure, making an internal flap.

Disarticulation of Single Metatarsal Bones.—Any singl metatarsal bone may be removed by the oval method; the incisio commences just behind the joint, *a* (Fig. 151), is carried forwards to the commissure, *c*, then under the toe in the transverse line to the opposite side, *b*, and terminates at *a*, the point of beginning; the soft parts are dissected from the bone; the ligaments uniting it to the third and fifth metatarsal, and the cuboid, are cut, and the disarticulation is completed by dividing the plantar ligaments.

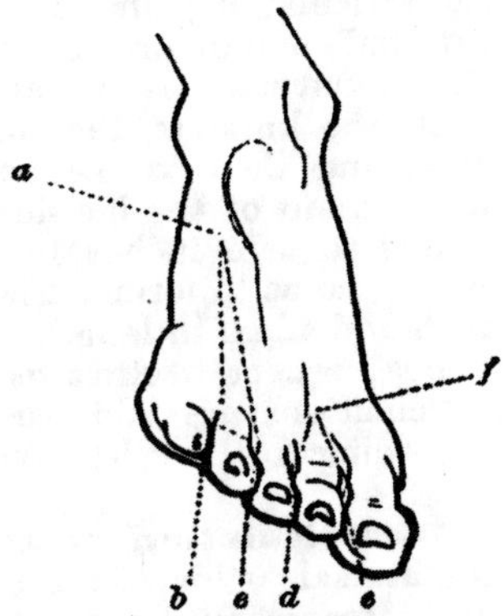

FIG. 151.

If it is desirable to amputate only the head of the metatarsal bone, the oval incision may be made, commencing on the dorsum, as at *f* (Fig. 151), passing downwards to the commissure, *e*, then along the under surface in the cutaneous fold to *d*, and terminating at the point of beginning, *f*.

Flap Method.—This operation may be performed in the same manner as the similar operation on the metacarpal bones.

Disarticulation of the Two Outer Metatarsal Bones.—The fourth and fifth metatarsal bones articulate with the cuboid, the fourth having a more transverse line of articulation than the fifth.

Oval Method.—An incision is commenced a finger's breadth behind the joint of the fifth metatarsal bone, in the middle, between the articulation of the two bones; it is carried forwards to the commissure, then along the under surface in the transverse line to the outer side of the little toe, and thence back to the beginning; the soft parts are dissected from the bones, the lateral ligament divided, and the joints disarticulated by entering them from the outside, and following the line above given (Fig. 152).

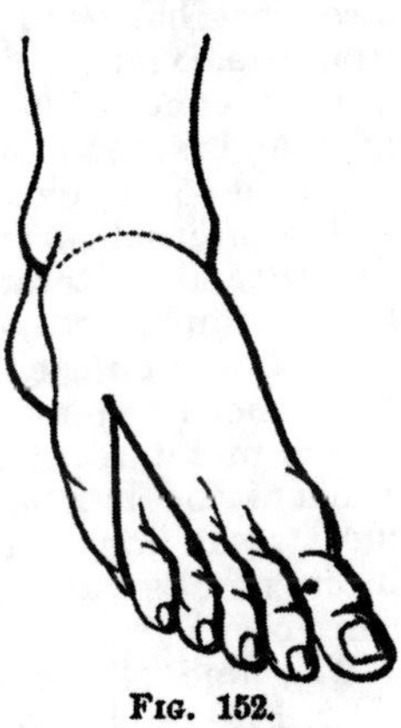
FIG. 152.

Disarticulation of the First Two Metarsal Bones.—It must be borne in mind that the articulation of the second metatarsal bone is on a line posterior to the first

(Fig. 144), and if the knife is carried along the posterior part of the first metatarsal bone, it strikes the second, and if it be then turned backwards, it will reach the articulation of the second metatarsal bone.

Oval Method.—Béclard operated as follows:—The point of the knife is carried on the first interosseous space of the dorsal surface of the foot, from six to seven lines in front of the cuneo-metatarsal articulation; incise obliquely the skin as far as the second internal commissure, around which the knife is carried, following the transverse groove at the root of the two toes, and bringing back the knife to the internal and dorsal surface of the first toe, returning then to the point of departure; at the point of commencement of the incision make two other incisions from one and a half to two inches in length, one inwards, and the other outwards, so as to form a triangular flap, the base of which, about one inch and a half in length, is a little behind the two first metatarsal bones; reflect backwards the flap, and the two tarso-metatarsal articulations are laid bare; the disarticulation is then completed according to the rules given.

Disarticulation of all the Metatarsal Bones.—The tarso-metatarsal articulations are arthrodial; they have dorsal, plantar, and interosseous ligaments, as follows: the first metatarsal is bound to the internal cuneiform by a single ligament, the second has three uniting it to the three cuneiform bones, the third one from the external cuneiform, and the fourth and fifth have one each from the cuboid; the plantar ligaments are irregular fibrous bands, uniting the metatarsal and tarsal bones; the interosseous ligaments, three in number, the most important to the operator, are thus described by Malgaigne (*op. cit.*):—"The first or internal, the strongest, has been justly called *the key of the articulation.* It starts from the external side of the first cuneiform, and from the inside of the second, to be inserted on the corresponding surfaces of the first and second metatarsal bones. The second or middle is attached to the external surface of the second cuneiform bone, and to the internal surface of the third, it goes to the external side of the second metatarsal, and on the inner side of the third. The last is implanted on one hand into the internal surface of the cuboid, and on the external surface of the third cuneiform; and on the other hand on the outside of the third, and the inside of the fourth metatarsal bone. According to this disposition, the lateral walls of the mortise are only immediately applied to the second metatarsal bone, at their dorsal surface; on their plantar exist intervals filled up by the interosseous ligaments, in which the knife can enter."

The line of the tarso-metatarsal articulation is very irregular (Fig. 144), and requires careful study. Malgaigne (*op. cit.*) gives the following as the relative positions and directions of the lines of individual tarso-metatarsal articulations:—

"1. The external side of the joint at the union of the fifth metatarsal bone with the cuboid, has a double obliquity; first, in the direction of a line which would pass from this point to the internal surface of the first joint of the great toe; second, in the direction of another line, passing from the same point to the middle of the first metatarsal bone.

"2. The joint of the fourth metatarsal bone is in the direction of a curved line, one inch long, beginning on the outside following the above-mentioned inflexions, and terminating on the inside, one-third of an inch in front of its external end.

"3. The articulation of the third is usually half a line in front of the fourth, and almost transverse.

"4. The second, more prolonged backwards, is lodged in a kind of mortise formed by the three cuneiform bones. The internal wall of this mortise is one-third of an inch deep, oblique backwards and outwards, and forms with the axis of the foot an angle of five or six degrees; the external wall, one-sixth of an inch deep, oblique behind and internally, makes with this axis an angle of seven or eight degrees; the posterior wall, half or three-quarters of an inch wide, is almost even and transverse. These relations are not subject to much variety.

"5. The articulation of the first is a quarter of an inch in front of the third; it is oblique in the direction of a line passing from its internal side to the middle of the fifth metatarsal bone."

The arteries of the leg, the posterior and anterior tibial, are compressed by an assistant during the operation.

The articulation is recognised on the inner side of the foot just posterior to the projection, *g* (Fig. 144), on the base of the first metatarsal bone, or one inch anterior to the prominence of the scaphoid, *e* (Fig. 144); on the outer margin of the foot the finger readily detects the prominence, *f* (Fig. 144), of the posterior part of the fifth metatarsal bone, immediately behind which is the articulation.

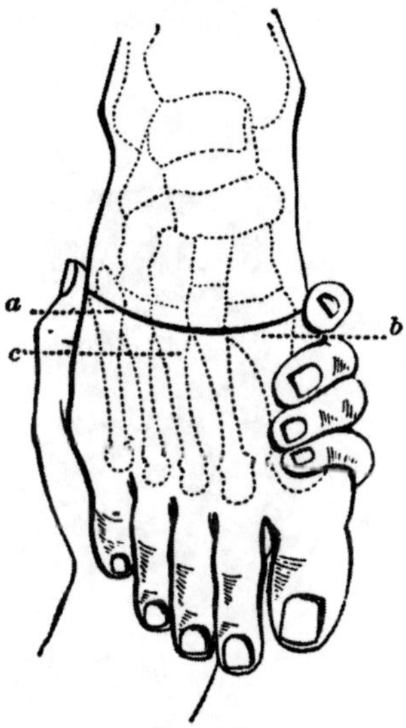

FIG. 158.

Flap Method.—Lisfranc's operation is as follows (*Bernard* and *Huette*):—"The patient is placed upon his back, and the foot rotated moderately inwards. The surgeon recognises the exact articulation by the rules already laid down, and then grasps, with the palm of his left hand, the sole of the foot, his thumb being placed on the outer side of the proximal end of the fifth metatarsal bone, *a* (Fig. 153), and the index finger at the internal extremity of the articulation, *b*. He then makes a semilunar incision with its convexity looking downwards, from without inwards, across the dorsum of the foot, passing about half an inch below the articulation, and extending from one of its extremities to the other down to the bones.

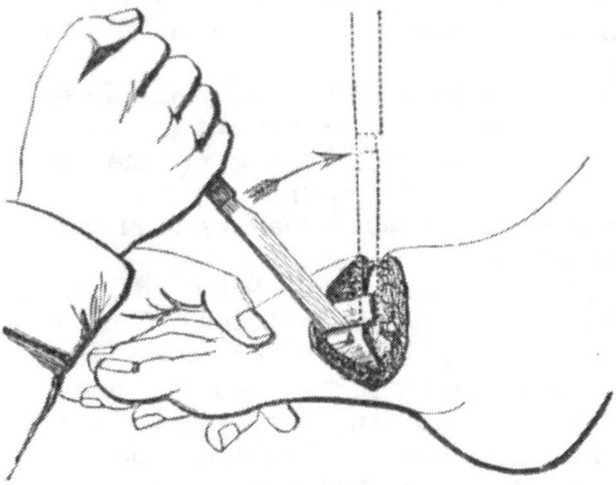

FIG. 154.

"2d. The surgeon divides, with the point of his knife, the dorsal ligaments, carrying it along the line of the articulation, from without inwards, as already indicated, and recollecting that the articulation of the second metatarsal lies a third of an inch posterior to the others.

"3d. The mortise in which the head of the second metatarsal is inclosed remains to be opened. This is effected by introducing the point of the knife between the internal cuneiform and the head of the first metatarsal bone, its edge being turned upwards, and making an angle of forty-five degrees with the axis of foot (Fig. 154). The knife is then carried up to a right angle, its point traversing the whole of the inner surface of the mortise, in order to insure the division of the interosseous ligament; it is then withdrawn, and applied to the external surface of the mortise.

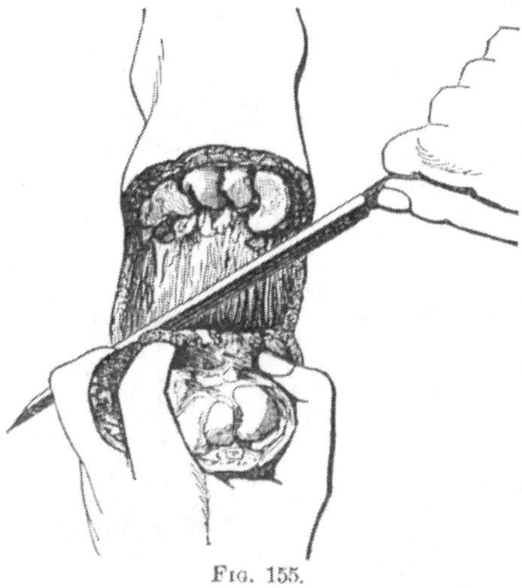

FIG. 155.

"4th. When this has been accomplished, pressure is made upon the metatarsus to separate the articular surfaces, and their remaining ligamentous attachments are successively divided, especially on the plantar aspect of the articulation, so that the knife may be carried readily beneath the heads of the metatarsal bones, and the operation is then finished by cutting out a flap from the sole of the foot, which should be somewhat larger at its internal than at its external part."

Care should be taken to make the plantar flap sufficiently large; the internal portion should extend nearly to the base of the great toe, the external may be of less extent (Fig. 155); the shape of the flap should be bevelled, and not transverse.

Modifications.—Hey, who first performed this operation, made a dorsal transverse incision from side to side, one inch in front of the articulation, and lateral incisions from the extremities of the first incision to the toes, disarticulated all the toes, and dissected back from the metatarsal bones the tissues forming the sole of the foot; he then separated the four external metatarsal bones from their articulation with the tarsal bones, and divided with a saw the projecting portion of the internal cuneiform bones, on which rests the great toe. Skey advises to divide the second metatarsal with forceps and allow the posterior extremity to remain in the mortise, disarticulating the remainder; Baudens directs the disarticulation of the first metatarsal bone, and the transverse division of the remainder with the saw, on a level with the internal cuneiform bone; Edwards makes a plantar flap by cutting from without inwards; Cloquet makes a transverse section of the bones; Guérin makes a plantar flap by a curved incision, commencing at the inner angle of the wound (Fig. 156), and passing to the sesamoid bones, then across the sole of the foot with a curve forward, but terminating at the junction of the anterior with the middle third of the fifth metatarsal bone; he then transfixes the base of the circumscribed part, and cuts the flap outward.

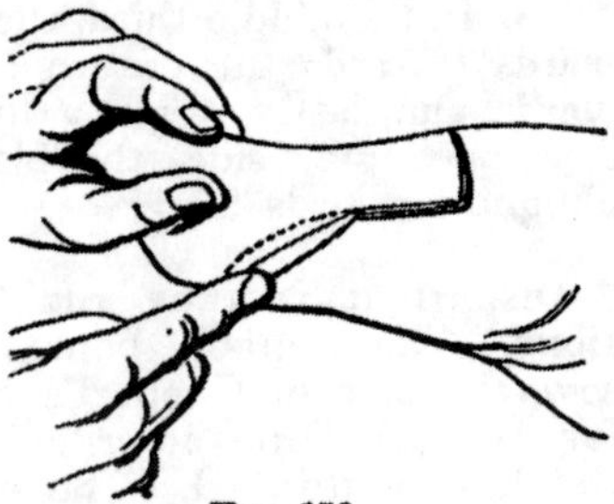

FIG. 156.

Complications.—In passing the finger along the internal surface of the foot there is a liability of passing the slight tubercle on the base of the first metatarsal bone, and mistaking for it the prominence of the cuneiform bone; thus the operator may be led to look for the articulation behind, instead of in front of the internal cuneiform bone. If the right obliquity is not given to the knife in entering the articulations of the metatarsal bones, there is a liability of penetrating the corresponding tarsal bones. Difficulty of luxation depends upon the incompleteness of the separation of the second metatarsal bone. The sesamoid bones should not be included in the flap.

Disarticulation of Tarsal Joints.—(Fig. 144.) The mediotarsal articulation is formed by the astragalus, *c*, and os calcis, *d*, behind, and the cuboid, *f*, and scaphoid, *e*, in front; the dorsal and plantar ligaments are not important, but the interosseous ligament, extending from the os calcis and astragalus, to the scaphoid and cuboid bones, is very strong.

The precise location of the line of articulation is determined as follows:—1. On the internal side of the foot it lies one inch in front of the internal malleolus; or, the first tuberosity in front of the internal malleolus is the scaphoid, and the joint is just behind it; 2. On the external side it is half an inch behind the prominence of the fifth metatarsal bone; or, it is in front of the first tuberosity anterior to the malleolus, which is on the os calcis. 3. In the centre the articulation is immediately in front of the head of the astragalus, which is made prominent by extending and abducting the foot.

Malgaigne (*op. cit.*) gives the following guide as to the variations in the line of articulation:—

"1. It is important to know that it is changed according as the foot is flexed or extended. When the foot is flexed, the astragalus and calcaneum are almost in the same line; when it is extended, the calcaneum is at least a quarter of an inch in front.

"2. The scaphoid is so prolonged towards the internal malleolus, that, in order to penetrate between it and the astragalus, the handle of the knife must be carried towards the toes so as to form with the axis of the foot an angle of forty-five degrees, and it must follow the direction of a line passing from the internal posterior surface of the scaphoid to the junction of the posterior with the middle third of the fifth metatarsal bone.

"3. In its middle third, the articulation is slightly inclined backwards towards the external malleolus, then it turns a little forwards, and, lastly, again a little backwards; so that, to enter it from the outer side, the blade of the knife should be slightly oblique forwards."

Disarticulation of the Tarsus anterior to the Scaphoid Bone.—The scaphoid bone having accidentally been left in place several times in Chopart's operation, and the cases terminating favorably, Laborie described the method by which the operation should be performed. The internal commencement of the line of articulation is found just behind the prominence of the tubercle on the inner surface of the internal cuneiform. The steps of the operation are the same as in Chopart's method next described, except that greater length should be given to the flap.

Chopart's operation (*Malgaigne, op. cit.*)—"First recognise the three capital points of the articulation; then, holding the foot in the left hand, place the left thumb on the outside of the joint, and the index or medius on the tuberosity of the scaphoid. Make a semilunar incision between these two points, the middle of which is half an inch beyond the articulation; then, passing the heel of the knife under the nail of your left thumb, its handle having the above-mentioned inclination, open the joint in the direction pointed out. When the joint is half opened, carry the knife in front of the head of the astragalus, cut the dorsal ligaments without penetrating between the bones, and lastly, carrying the edge of the knife to the other side of the foot, the heel of its blade inclined towards the toes at an angle of ninety-five degrees, finish opening the external side of the joint marked out by the index finger.

"All the dorsal ligaments being thus divided, push the point of the instrument under the external and anterior side of the head of the astragalus, with its edge directed forwards, and cut the interosseous ligament in the direction of the articular surface of the calcaneum. The joint is then wide open. Then carry the knife under the plantar ligaments, and pass it under the bones, grazing them, to cut a sufficient flap, avoiding the protuberances of the scaphoid and cuboid, and further on of the first and fifth metatarsal bones. The foot, during this time, is kept in the horizontal position. You should raise the handle of the knife slightly, to follow more exactly the concavity of the tarsus and metatarsus."

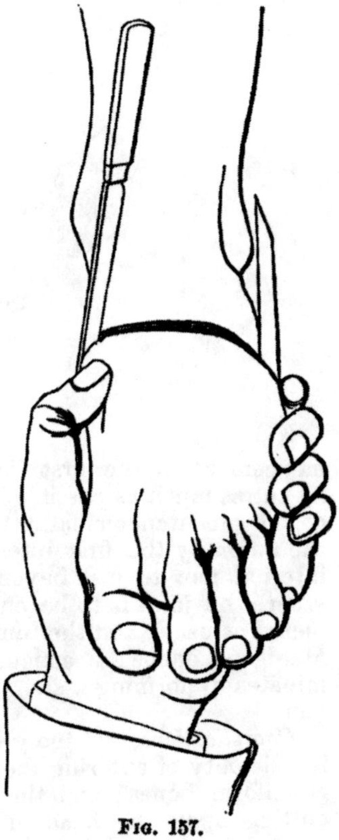

FIG. 157.

It is important to make the lateral incisions low down upon either side, and in order to this the knife should be held, according to Chassaignac, in a nearly perpendicular direction (Fig. 157), at the commencement and termination of the incision. It is important also to give an oval shape to the flap, and before its completion it may be necessary to apply the knife to the external part (Fig. 158) and shape it accordingly.

Modifications.—Sedillot operated as follows (*Bernard* and *Huette*):—"After determining the position of the articulation, and the foot being properly supported, a transverse incision is made, commencing a few lines in advance of the calcaneo-cuboid articulation, and terminating about the middle of the dorsum of the foot, on the outer side of the tendon of the tibialis anticus; from this same point a curved incision, with its convexity downwards, is then carried around the inner border of the foot, extending downwards to within two fingers' breadths of the metatarso-phalangeal articulation of the great toe, and thence across the sole to the com-

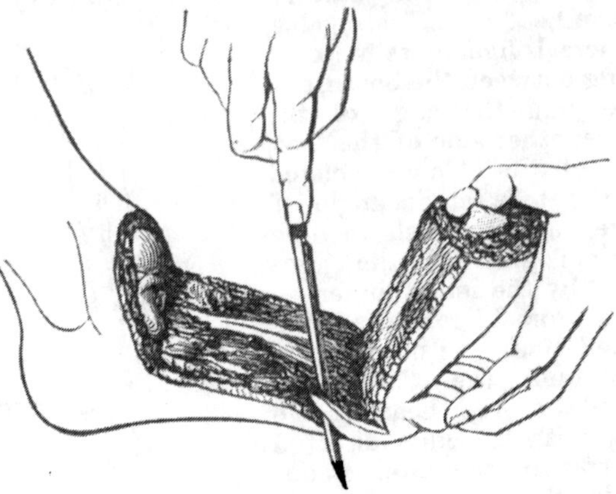

FIG. 158.

mencement of the first incision; the plantar integuments should be cut as much as possible in a slanting direction to rid their edges of the subcutaneous fat, the protrusion of which tends to prevent the union by the first intention; it remains now to dissect up the internal flap to just beyond the tuberosity of the scaphoid bone, where the joint is to be entered; the disarticulation is then completed as usual, and the remaining soft parts divided transversely." Manigault opens the articulation from the plantar surface, and terminates by forming a short dorsal flap. Baudens makes a dorsal flap.

Complications.—If too great convexity is given to the flap there is a liability of entering the articulation between the scaphoid and cuneiform bones; and the opposite error may be committed of cutting upon the head of the astragalus unless the foot is well extended; in dividing the interosseous ligament care must be taken to hold the knife sufficiently vertically, in order to make it enter the calcaneo-scaphoid space.

DISARTICULATION OF THE TARSUS UNDER THE ASTRAGALUS.—The astragalus articulates with the os calcis by two surfaces, separated by a groove; the posterior is the larger, and is oblong, and deeply concave from side to side; the anterior is oval, elongated, convex from side to side, and sometimes divided into two by a ridge; the two articular surfaces are separated by a very strong interosseous ligament.

Malgaigne's Process.—The operator holding the foot in the left hand, makes a horizontal incision over the tendo-achillis, dividing at one stroke the skin, tendon, and cellular tissue, down to the calcaneum, cutting a little more freely on the outer than on the inner side; this incision is continued around the external part of the foot, one-third of an inch below the external malleolus; then passing abruptly upon the dorsum of the foot, about an inch and a half in front of the tibio-tarsal articulation, continue on that level over the dorsum, and descend, without changing the direction, to the middle of the sole of the foot; a second incision commences at the internal extremity of the first incision, behind the malleolus, and is carried obliquely to the sole of the foot, at an angle of about forty-five degrees, and joins the other incision, forming thus an internal flap of from four to five inches in width at its base, and from two to three inches at its summit, which terminates in a curve; this flap is raised, including all the soft parts, over the sole, side, and dorsum of the foot, as far as the articulation to be entered; the flap being raised, the operator with the thumb and finger of the left hand ascertaining the lateral limits of Chopart's disarticulation, makes a large opening in the scaphoido-astragaloid articulation, passing around the head of the astragalus so as to divide at the same time the external calcaneo-astragaloid ligament, and also the synovial membrane of the small articulating surface of the calcaneus; now divide the internal ligament and posterior membrane, guided by the points given above; cut the tendons attached to the internal surface of the calcaneum, then divide the interosseous ligament by carrying the knife flatwise, the edge backwards in the small anterior articulation of the calcaneum, and following the direction of the articulation cut all that obstructs its passage; on the division of the first fibres the bones separate readily, and the operation is readily completed.

Modifications.—Roux commenced an incision on the posterior and external face of the calcaneum, and carried it forward below the external malleolus to a point half an inch anterior to the articulation of the astragalus in front; it was then carried to the internal border of the foot, and from thence it passed obliquely backwards across the plantar surface to the point of departure; the flap is thus made from the entire integument of the heel. Verneuil commenced the incision at about the same point, and carried it forward to within one inch of the posterior and internal extremity of the fifth meta-

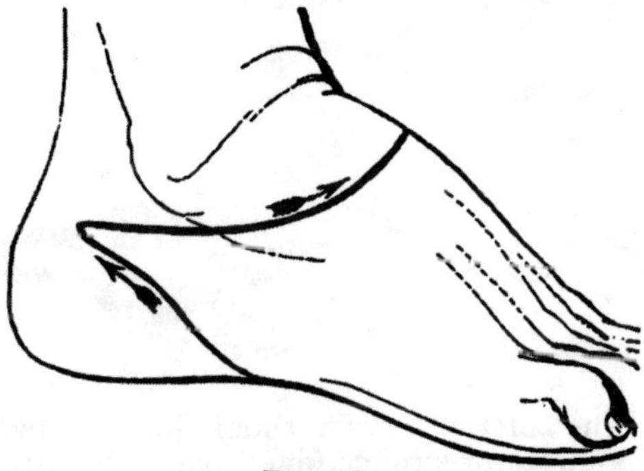

FIG. 159.

tarsal bone, thence with a downward curve across the dorsum of the foot to the middle of the internal cuneiform bone, thence across the sole of the foot from within outwards, and from before backwards to the commencement. Nélaton makes the same incision until he reaches the internal border of the foot; he then carries it transversely across the plantar surface to the posterior extremity of the fifth metatarsal, then backwards and obliquely upwards along the external surface of the foot to the point of departure. The course of this incision is seen in Fig. 159; it may be reversed, passing in the opposite direction, under the foot, from the external to the internal side. In the dissection care should be taken to avoid injuring blood-vessels high in the flap by turning the edge of the knife to the bone. Simon proceeded as in amputation at the ankle-joint.

Disarticulation of the Ankle-Joint.—The articulation at the ankle is a perfect hinge joint, there being only an antero-posterior motion.

The broad articular surface of the lower extremity of the tibia with its internal projection, the internal malleolus, and the large projecting extremity of the fibula, the external malleolus, form a mortise to which the lateral and upper surfaces of the astragalus are so accurately adapted that there can be no lateral motion, and disarticulation can only be accomplished when the foot is firmly extended, and the knife penetrates the anterior part of the articulation.

Syme's Method (*Contributions to Surgery*).—The foot being placed at a right angle to the leg, a line drawn from the centre of one malleolus to that of the other, directly across the sole of the foot, will show the proper extent of the posterior flap. The knife should be entered close up to the fibular malleolus (Fig. 160), and carried to a point on the same level of the opposite side, which will be a little below the tibial malleolus (Fig. 161).

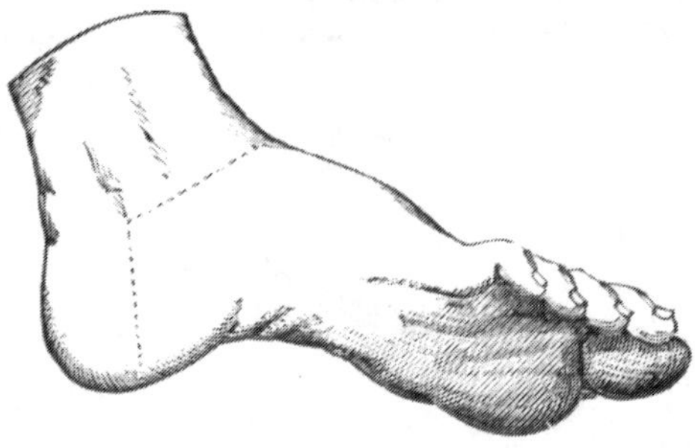

FIG. 160.

The anterior incision should join the two points just mentioned in a direct or straight line, over the instep, as represented in Figs. 160 and 161. In dissecting the posterior flap, the operator should place the fingers of his left hand upon the heel, while the thumb rests upon the edge of the integuments, and then cut between the nail of the thumb and tuberosity of the os calcis, so as to avoid lacerating the soft parts, which he, at the same time, gently but steadily presses back until he exposes and divides the tendo-achillis. The foot should be disarticulated before the malleolar projections are removed, which it is always proper to do, and which may be most easily effected by passing a knife around the exposed extremities of the bones, and then sawing off a thin slice of the tibia connecting the two processes. The method of dissecting the flap on the anterior and lateral part of the ankle is represented in Fig. 162.

Modifications.—Quain advises "after the incision from malleolus to malleolus, under the os calcis, to make a straight incision at right angles with the first, to the back part of the heel, on the outer side of the foot, a little above and parallel with its outer margin."

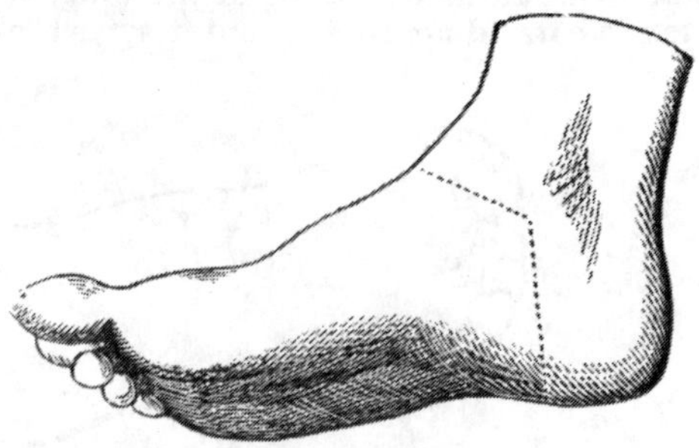

FIG. 161.

Handyside recommends antero-lateral flaps. A strong bistoury is entered in front of the joint, midway between the malleoli; from this point an incision is carried forwards, over the side of the instep, in a semicircular direction, and then downwards to the middle line of the foot, terminating immediately in front of the ball of the heel; the extremities of this incision are met by another and a similar one on the outer aspect of the joint, the second one terminating where the first had been commenced; the flaps are dissected backwards, the tendo-achillis divided at its attachment to the os calcis, and the separation of the foot accomplished. The malleoli were removed by the saw, and along with them about one-eighth of an inch of the lower end of the tibia.

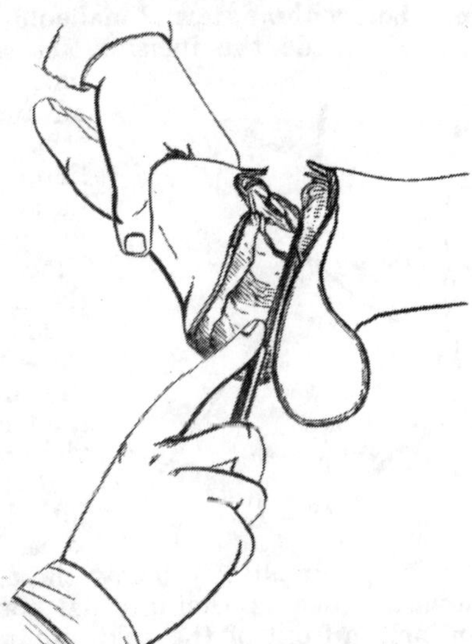

FIG. 162.

Mackenzie operated as follows (Fig. 163):—"The body reclining on the right side, and the foot and ankle projecting from the table with their internal aspect upwards, the point of the knife is entered in the mesial line of the posterior aspect of the ankle, on a level with the articulation, carried downwards obliquely across the tendo-achillis towards the external border of the plantar aspect of the heel, along which it is continued in a semilunar direction. The incision is then curved across the sole of the foot, and terminates on the inner side of the tendon of the *tibialis anticus*, about an inch in front of the inner *malleolus.* The second incision is carried across the outer aspect of the ankle in a semilunar

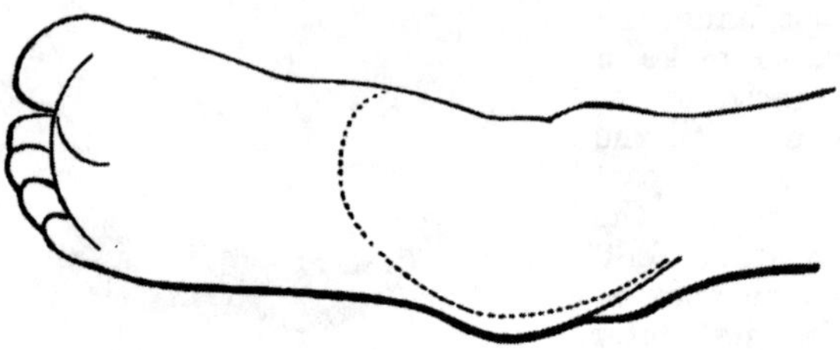

FIG. 163.

direction, between the extremities of the first incisions, the convexity of the incision downwards (Fig. 163), and passing half an inch below the external malleolus."

Teale made the incision across the sole of the foot, the extremities of which were three-quarters of an inch in front of the malleoli; a second incision was made in the median line, commencing over the tendo-achillis, and meeting the first at right angles in the sole of the foot. This method allows the removal of one or more of the tarsal bones if required.

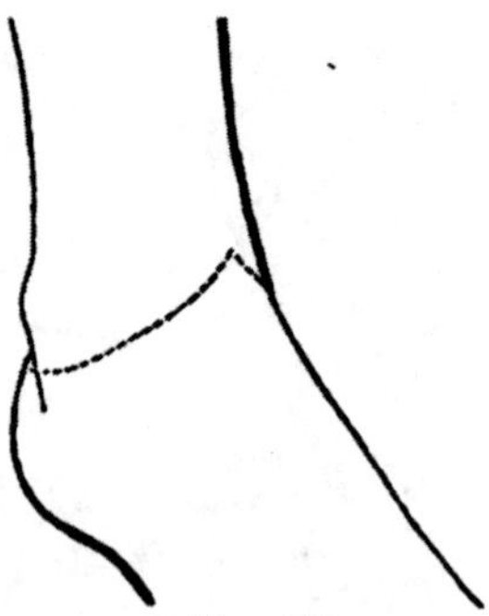

FIG. 164.

These and the following modifications show how variously the soft parts about the ankle may be usefully adapted in the form of flaps in amputations in this vicinity.

Roux made an incision from the junction of the tendo-achillis with the os calcis around the external surface of the foot, immediately below the external malleolus, then carried it inwards towards the internal border, curved forwards, and about an inch in front of the ankle-joint; it then passed along the internal border of the foot to the point of departure; the inner side of the removed foot is represented in Fig. 165, and the stump in 166.

Baudens made two horizontal incisions, commencing at the insertion of the tendo-achillis and meeting a little behind the commissure of the toes; Sédillot made an incision comprising the semi-circumference of the anterior part of the foot, about three fingers' breadth in front of the malleoli, then from the external extremity of the wound he carried horizontally around under the external malleolus to the internal border of the tendo-achillis, which was divided; disarticulation was effected, and a quadrilateral flap made from the internal and plantar part of the heel.

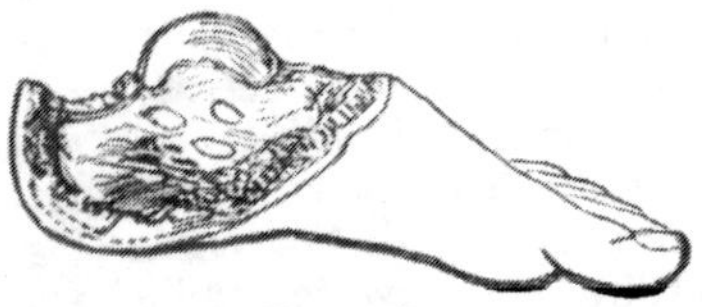

FIG. 165.

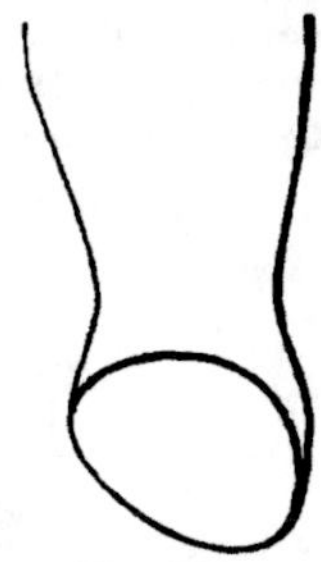

FIG. 166.

Pirogoff's Method.—Spencer Wells, of London, gives the following description of this method (*Med. Times and Gazette*), translated from the author:—"I commence my incision close in front of the outer malleolus, carry it vertically downwards to the sole of the foot (Fig. 160), then transversely across the sole, and lastly obliquely upwards to the inner malleolus, where I terminate it a couple of lines anterior to the malleolus (Fig. 161). Thus all the soft parts are divided at once quite down to the os calcis. I now connect the outer and inner extremity of this first incision by a second semilunar incision, the convexity of which looks forward, carried a few lines anterior to the tibio-tarsal articulation. I cut through all the soft parts at once down to the bones, and then proceed to open the joint from the front, cutting through the lateral ligaments, and thus exarticulate the head of the astragalus. I now place a small narrow amputation saw obliquely upon the os calcis behind the astragalus, exactly upon the sustentaculum tali (Fig. 167), and saw through the os calcis, so that the saw passes into the first incision through the soft parts. Saw carefully, or the anterior surface of the tendo-achillis, which is only covered by a layer of fat and a thin fibrous sheath, might be injured. I separate the short anterior

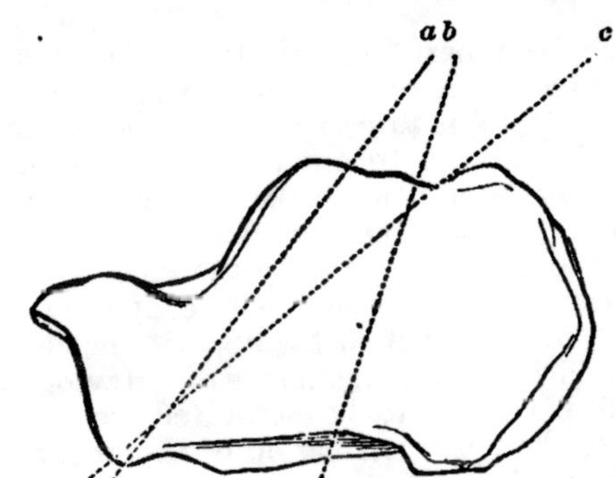

FIG. 167.

flap from the two malleoli, and saw through them at the same time close to their base. I turn this flap forwards, and bring the cut surface of the os calcis in apposition with the articular surface of the tibia. If the latter be diseased it is sometimes necessary also to saw off from it a thin slice with the malleoli." When the dissection has reached the posterior part of the os calcis (Fig. 168), the saw is applied and section of the bone is made. The lines drawn in Fig. 167 represent the different sections of the bone by operators; *b*, *f*, is nearly that made by Pirogoff. He directs that the tendons be not cut off too short; in other words, "not too near the spot where their synovial sheaths are cut through; their ends should rather project a little. If they are cut too short they conceal themselves in the fibrous canal, or what is worse, when the limb is moved they slip upwards out of their sheaths."

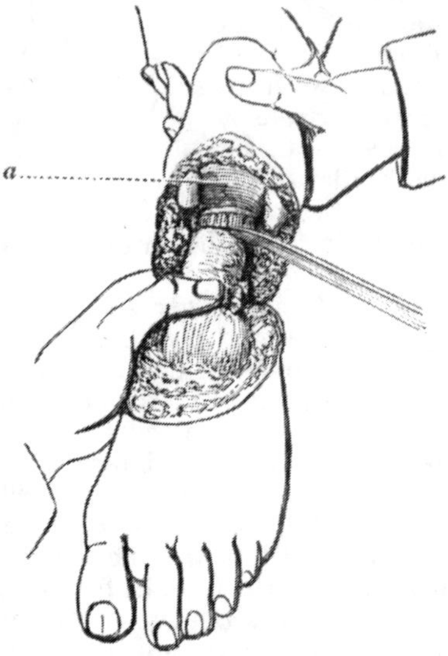

FIG. 168.

Modifications.—Croft (*London Lancet*), one of the surgeons of the Dreadnought Hospital, where the operation had, at that date, been performed six times, describes the operation as follows: —"The mode of operation, as performed by Mr. Busk, Mr. Tudor, and myself, is to grasp the projecting portion of the foot with the left hand, then to enter the point of the knife *immediately* behind the malleolus, and make a semicircular incision in front of the point, terminating at a corresponding point behind the opposite malleolus; next, to carry the incision downwards and slightly forwards to the edge of the sole of the foot, straight across the sole, and terminate it at the opposite malleolus, or the point at which the incision was commenced. Having disarticulated the foot, the soft parts are to be separated from around the os calcis in a line from the posterior margin of the upper articulating surface to the under edge of the articulating surface of the cuboid, and the mass in front of this line to be removed by the saw. The ends of the tibia and fibula are sawn off in the way usual in Syme's operation. During the process of separating the soft, or rather tough parts about the os calcis, care should be taken to keep the edge of the knife close to the bone, in order to avoid wounding the posterior tibial or plantar arteries. The portion of the os calcis left on the flap should be placed in contact with the end of the tibia, and if the saw has been entered well behind the calcaneo-astragaloid articulation, and brought out at the under margin of the calcaneo-cuboid articulation, the contact will be accurate.

Pierrie and Watson modified the operation by sawing the os calcis from below upwards, before disarticulation. Pierrie thus describes the procedure:—"The patient being laid on the table, the surgeon—whichever foot be the subject of the operation—being placed on the left side of his patient, with the heel, in the first step of the operation, directed towards himself, and having with his left hand taken hold of the soft parts, and drawn them a little backwards, so as to secure greater breadth of flap, inserts the knife on one side in front of the malleolus, carries it down across the sole of the foot, and upwards to the corresponding point just at the front and upper part of the other malleolus, taking care to direct the incision so as to pass opposite to the part where the posterior portion of the astragalus rests upon the calcaneum, and to use the knife energetically, so as to cut through all tissues down to the bones. By this single movement of the knife, a clearance is made for the saw, by a few movements of which the portion of calcaneum behind the astragalus is speedily cut off from the rest of the bone, the section being from below upwards, and a little backwards, so that the portion remaining in the flap will be a little longer from behind forwards, below than above. The assistant having slightly changed the position of the leg, so as to make its posterior part rest upon the table, the surgeon, by a second movement of the knife, unites the extremities of the first incision by a slightly semilunar incision, using the knife boldly, so as to cut through every tissue in front of the bones, and then, by a few touches below, admits of the flap being brought back, and makes a clearance for the saw. By a few movements of the saw the bones are cut through immediately above the ankle."

Bontecou, Brigade Surgeon U. S. Army, proposes the following modifications:—"Make an incision from the posterior margin of one malleolus to the other, by cutting from within outwards, closely hugging the os calcis, and transfixing the plantar mass; then raise a flap from the dorsum of the foot of sufficient size, and reflect it as far as the articular extremity of the tibia, which proceed to saw off *at once*, with the fibular projection; then pass the knife closely behind the ankle-joint, and clear the os calcis of soft parts, far enough back to saw obliquely forwards and downwards, and the bony flap will fit without force."

Amputation at the Base of the Malleoli.—Guérin performs amputation at the base of the malleoli by making the flaps of Roux in amputation at the ankle-joint (page 144), except that the incisions are prolonged upwards to the base of the malleoli, and the two extremities of the base of the flap are united by a transverse incision, slightly convex downwards; the soft parts are separated from the bones, and the tibia and fibula sawn through at the base of the malleoli, about an inch above the articular surface.

Amputation above the Malleoli.—The soft parts of the leg at its lower part are meagre, and for the most part tendinous; the arteries requiring ligature are the anterior and posterior tibial and peroneal.

Circular Method.—The circular operation is not readily performed in this situation owing to the conical shape of the limb, which renders it difficult to retract the skin. Lenoir has modified it as follows:—The operator stands on the inside of the limb, makes a circular incision through the skin, one and a half inches below the point where the bone is to be sawn; a second incision is made vertically down to it from the point where the bone is to be sawn, along the internal surface of the tibia, near its crest; the two flaps are reflected from the anterior third of the leg, as thick as possible, but the sides and back of the flap are untouched; he then makes another incision by placing the knife at the margin of reflection of the integument (Fig. 169), on the outside, and carries it around the limb along the edge of the flap; this makes an oval incision; the skin is retracted; the deep muscles are divided transversely to the bone; the interosseous space penetrated with the point of the knife, the retractor applied, and the bones sawn together; the vertical incision is held together with sutures, and the wound closed as in the circular incision.

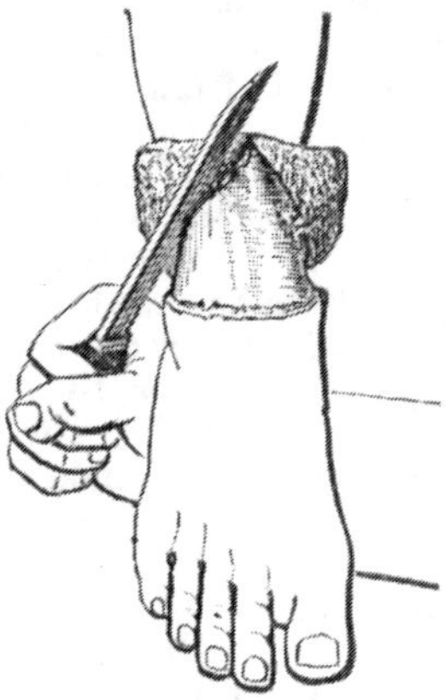

FIG. 169.

Flap Method.—Guérin describes the following method (*op. cit.*):—The operator standing upon the inner side, passes the knife immediately behind the tibia and fibula, and cuts a posterior flap (Fig. 170), four fingers' breadth in length; the knife is then applied in front and a second incision is made uniting the extremities of the first, and curved downwards, these flaps are dissected upwards, the point of the knife introduced into the interosseous space, and the bones sawn as before.

Lateral flaps may be made in this situation, or an anterior and posterior flap (Fig. 171).

Rectangular Flap.—(Fig. 172.) In this case the long flap is made from the anterior part of the leg as follows:—Make two parallel longitudinal incisions on either side of the leg, in length equal to two-thirds of the circumference of the limb; a second incision unites transversely their inferior extremities; this flap is dissected up from the bone, care being taken not to wound the anterior tibial artery at the upper part of the flap, by using the edge of the knife but little in this part of the dissection; the posterior flap, which should be about one-fourth the length of the anterior, is made by a circular incision down to the bone; this is

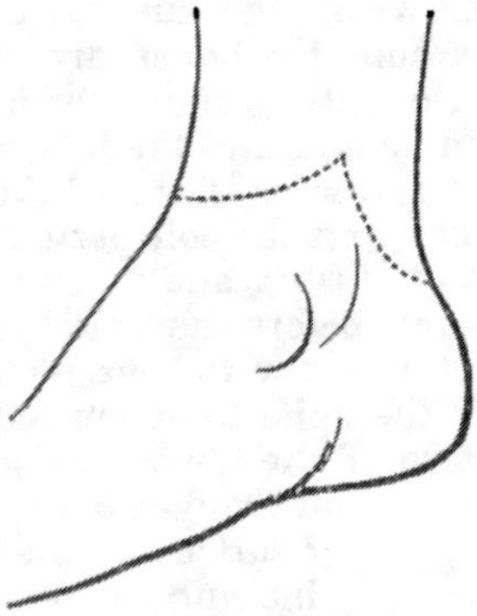

FIG. 170.

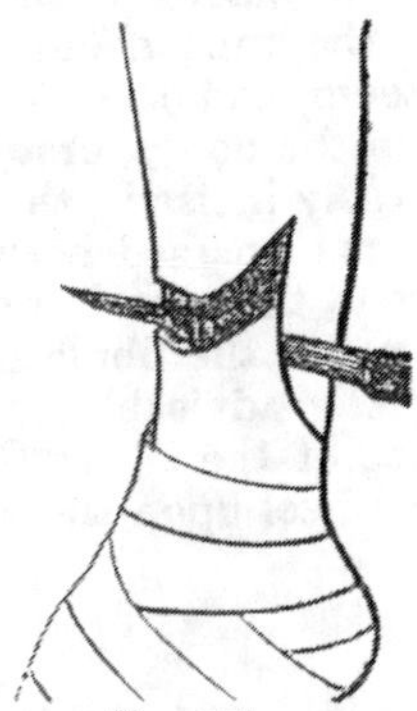

FIG. 171.

also dissected from the bone to the requisite height, and the bones are divided; the flaps (Figs. 173) are then brought together.

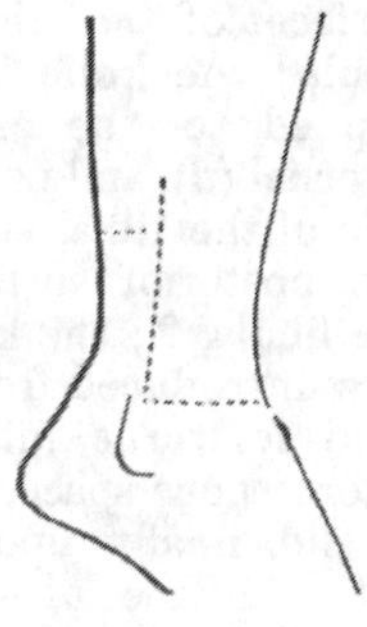

FIG. 172.

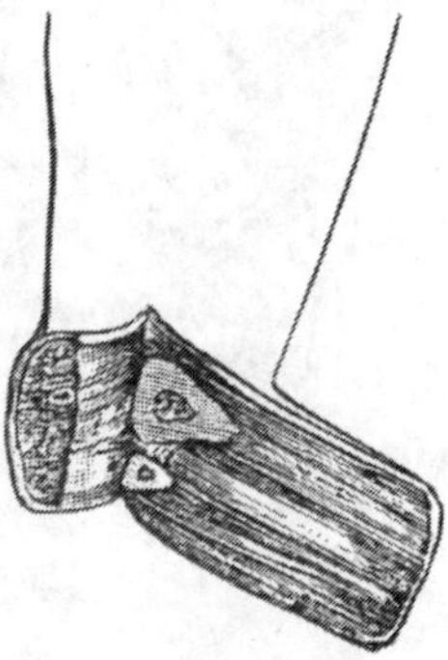

FIG. 173.

Amputation of the Leg at the "Place of Election."—The "place of election" in amputation of the leg is generally fixed at four inches below the patella; the principal change in the anatomical characters of the part is in the large increase of muscles upon the posterior part, the thick muscular structures that form the calf; the arteries are the anterior tibial, anterior to the interosseous ligament; and the posterior tibial, and peroneal, between and a little behind the bones; the following operations have been advised:—

Circular Method.—The patient is placed on the table and the leg brought to the edge; the operator standing on the inside of the limb, or, if he much prefer, upon the right, makes a circular incision (see page 92) through the skin, about three and a half inches below the point of dividing the bones, in a leg of ordinary size; the integuments are dissected and turned back like a cuff; a second incision is made on the level of the reflected skin, down to the bones; the knife should be carried around the bones dividing the periosteum, and then the point of the catling should be inserted between the bones, first in front, then behind, and the interosseous space freely incised; the three-tailed retractor is then taken, the middle part passed between the bones, and the soft parts forcibly retracted; the saw is now applied to the tibia, and when fixed in its substance the fibula should be divided, before the tibia begins to yield; it is advisable to remove with the saw the sharp angle of the spine of the tibia; Guérin directs the knife to be applied, first, with the heel upon the external surface of the fibula, *c* (Fig. 174), and brought over the upper surface of the bones, 1, incising the soft parts; then the point should be introduced into the interosseous space in the position of *a* and *b*, cutting upon the two opposed surfaces of the tibia and fibula; the knife is then applied to the anterior internal (*d*), and posterior face of the tibia, and also the posterior surface of the fibula, 2; the knife is now introduced from behind forwards into the interosseous space, *e*, and *g*, and finally upon the external face of the fibula, *f*.

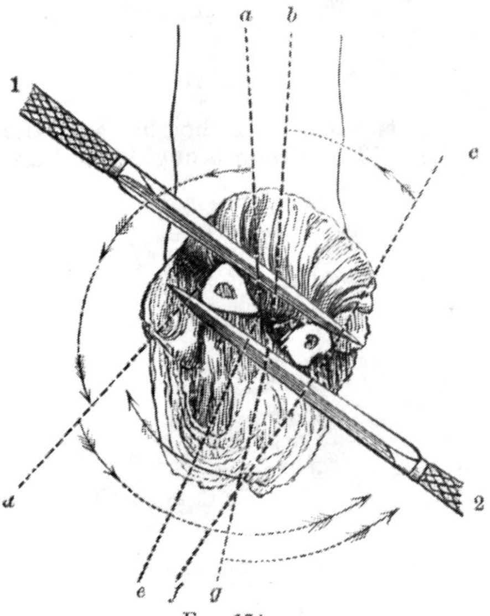

FIG. 174.

Malgaigne (*op. cit.*) remarks of the division of the bones:—"Whatever be the proceeding preferred for the section of the soft parts, some modification must be added in sawing the bone; for, if you saw off the bone on a level with the muscles, their retraction will leave it projecting. Velpeau advises, before applying the saw, to dissect the interosseous membrane from each bone. We much prefer the proceeding of Bell. Many surgeons considered that this projection of the bones was caused by their shape. On this account, Roux saws the fibula higher up than the tibia; a modification of doubtful utility, but almost all in France agree in cutting off the angle of the tibia. Béclard, after the incision of the soft parts, carried the saw obliquely on the ridge of the tibia, then withdrew the saw and applied it perpendicularly; but in this way you substitute for the anterior angle an internal one, almost, if not quite as bad. Sanson happily corrected this inconvenience, by placing the saw obliquely, not on the ridge, but on the internal surface of the bone."

Single Flap.—The operator grasps the limb with his left hand, the thumb and forefinger resting one on the edge of the tibia, and the other on the edge of the fibula; placing the heel of the knife on the opposite side, at the point of the forefinger, he draws it in a downward curve over the front of the leg, and terminates the first incision by bringing the point of the knife to the end of the thumb, over the margin of the bone, on the side next to him; he there transfixes the limb, remembering that the lower margin of the fibula is on a lower level than the tibia, the knife passing close behind the two bones, and cuts from the calf a flap, four or five inches long; the skin in front is now dissected upwards, the posterior flap retracted, the soft parts divided to the bone, and the operation completed as in the circular method.

Single External Flaps.—Sédillot operated as follows:—The leg being flexed, and the foot extended to relax the muscles of the calf, the operator, standing on the inner side of the limb, elevates with his left hand the muscles over the fibula; with a long, narrow knife, he then transfixes the limb, the point entering midway between the crest of the tibia and the fibula, and grazing the external surface of the latter emerges in the calf two fingers' breadth higher than it entered, and including as much of the calf as possible; the flap is then cut from the external surface of the leg; the knife is carried around the internal surface of the leg, making a short flap; the operation is then completed as in the circular method.

Double Flap.—The double flap method of Mr. Luke is recommended by English surgeons; it is as follows:—The patient being properly arranged on a table, the operator stands upon the right side of the limb, and grasping it above the point of the operation transfixes the limb, *c* (Fig. 175), the knife passing behind, but

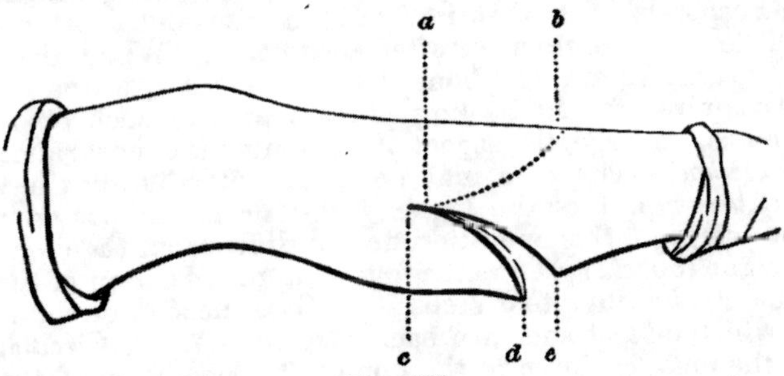

FIG. 175.

grazing the bones; he then cuts a flap from the calf (*d* and *e*, margins of flap,) of four or five inches in length; he now cuts an anterior flap, *b*, *a*, from without inwards, of the same length as the posterior; the operation is completed as in the circular incision.

Skey performs the following operation (Fig. 176):—"The operator stands on the right side of the patient. The leg being raised, the calf is supported on the palm of the left hand of the operator, by which it is flattened out considerably in breadth. The knife is then introduced through the skin at a depth of not more than half or three-quarters of an inch above the palm of the hand, and passed straight across to the opposite side, and the posterior flap, which in addition to the integuments will thus include a small thin portion of the gastrocnemius, is formed of sufficient length to pass forwards around the end of the tibia. The anterior flap is now cut, but of small dimensions. A circular sweep of the knife around

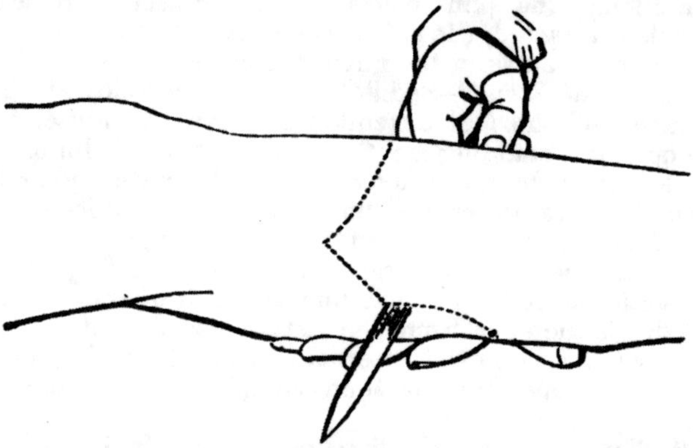

FIG. 176.

the limb is then made, which divides the rest of the calf, and the catling is introduced through the deep muscles and interosseous membrane. By this means a posterior flap is formed, which being thin corresponds with that in front, in size and substance, and leaves little or no muscle for after absorption. When the entire calf is brought round the bone, I have known upwards of three months required for the healing process, and in such operations, when the calf is large, the aspect of the stump is almost ridiculous."

Oval Method.—The oval may be made with the apex upwards, on the anterior part of the leg (Fig. 96), or on the posterior part, the other steps of this operation do not differ from the circular.

Malgaigne (*op. cit.*) prefers the following modification of the oval, which he divides into five steps:—1. Oval incision of the integuments, which dissect and turn back two inches. 2. Circular division of the muscles down to the bone. 3. Separation of the muscles half an inch up, according to the proceeding of Bell, grazing the tibia, fibula, and interosseous ligament with the knife. 4. Section of the flesh and interosseous ligament, by the figure-of-8, and application of the retractor. 5. Section of the bones. after the method of Sanson.

Amputation above the Place of Election.—Malgaigne (*op. cit.*) gives the following description of Larrey's method:—"The section of the bones should not be made above the tuberosity of the tibia, for fear of depriving the ligamentum patellæ of its attachments, of opening the synovial bursa placed behind, and even of entering the articulation. Assure yourself beforehand of the exact situation of this tuberosity: it presents a triangular surface, whose inferior angle is confounded with the crest of the tibia. The ligamentum patellæ is inserted into all this surface; but it may be without fear divided almost to its base, as only a small portion of its attachments need be left. Divide the skin as usual, preserving as much of it as possible. If the bone is to be divided very high up, having drawn back the skin, make a longitudinal incision on the fibula; dissect from both sides the muscles that are attached to it. By moving it, you recognise its articulation, which is formed of plane surfaces, easily separated; disarticulate it. The operation then resembles amputation of the thigh or arm, the tibia resting alone; divide the soft parts, and saw the bone. The saw, here, should act perpendicularly to the axis of the limb. If the dissection of the skin has not exposed the articulation of the fibula, cut it off: the operation is here easier than at the place of election, the interosseous space, so to say, no longer existing. Another advantage is that there is only one artery to be tied, the popliteal not dividing till further down. If the bone is diseased higher up, you may saw it obliquely upwards and backwards, preserving the attachment of the ligamentum patellæ in front."

Modifications.—Liston and Syme oppose removing the head of the fibula, owing to the danger of opening the knee-joint, and destroying the attachments of the external lateral ligament, and the biceps muscle.

Disarticulation of the Knee-Joint.—In this joint the condyles are not on the same level, the internal descending nearly half an inch lower than the external; the articular surface of the tibia presents two cup-shaped depressions into which the condyles are received. The joint is strongly bound by ligaments which are external and internal; the external are, anteriorly, ligamentum patellæ, *posteriorly*, ligamentum posticum Winslowii, *internal* lateral, and two external lateral; the *internal* are the external and internal crucial, transverse, and coronary. The popliteal artery, vein, and nerve, pass down behind the articulation, the artery being in contact with the joint.

The line of the articulation lies internally three-fourths of an inch above the prominence of the tibia; the lower border of the patella is on a line with the articulation; and externally it is three-fourths of an inch below the prominence of the condyle of the femur.

Oval Method.—(Fig. 177.) The leg being placed in a straight position, and the integuments firmly retracted by an assistant, the operator standing upon the right side of the limb, with a strong narrow-bladed knife, makes an incision, curved downwards, which passes from a point on the inside, two fingers' breadth below the line of articulation, to the same level on the external side, descending at its lowest point in the centre three fingers' breadth below the patella, *c;* the skin is then reflected to the line of articulation, the ligamentum patellæ and lateral ligaments divided, the leg bent at right angles, the knife, *b*, enters the joint, and disarticulation is completed by incising the internal ligaments, and finally the structures on the posterior part of the joint. Malgaigne prefers this method to all others.

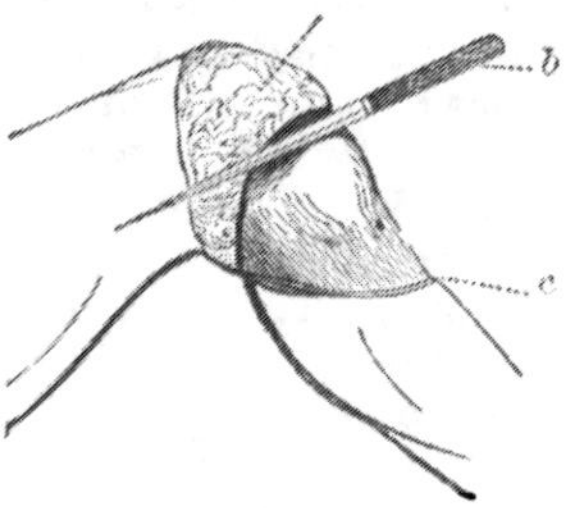

Fig. 177.

Circular Method.—Make a circular incision through the integument, three or four fingers' breadth below the patella, reflect it with the adipose tissue to the articulation; then bend the knee at right angles, and placing the left hand upon the upper part of the tibia with the knife held horizontally divide the ligamentum patellæ, the external ligaments, and with the point of the knife the internal (crucial) ligaments; the joint being well opened, the knife is passed behind the head of the tibia, and a flap cut from the posterior part.

Single Flap.—Fergusson (*Syst. Pract. Surg.*) approves the following operation of Syme, in which the condyles of the femur are also removed:—

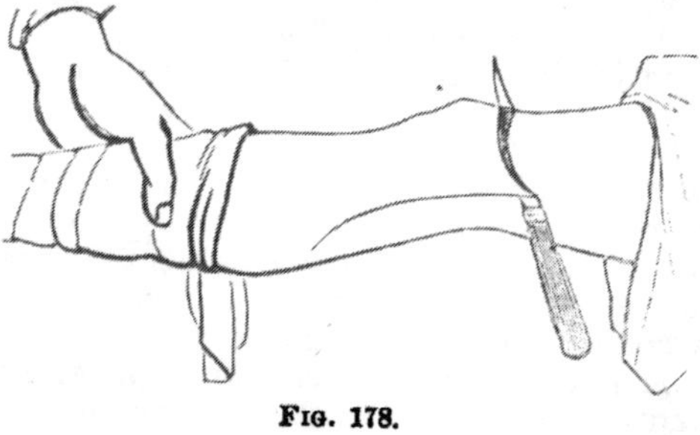

Fig. 178.

"The circulation being arrested as usual, the surgeon, standing on the outer or inner side of the limb as he may feel disposed, should lay the heel of an ordinary amputating knife, such as is used for the common operation in the thigh, over one condyle of the femur, draw the blade to the other condyle across the front of the joint in a lunated course, on a level with the middle of the patella, and divide the tissues down to the bones; the little flap should then be pulled upwards, and the knife should again be applied so as to cut the quadriceps extensor immediately above the patella; the point of the blade should then be pushed in at one end of the wound, thrust behind the femur, and made to appear at the other end, when it should be carried downwards in the line indicated on the drawing (Fig. 178), so as to make a flap from the calf of the leg, about six or eight inches in length, in proportion to the thickness of the limb; this flap should now be slightly retracted, when the knife should be carried round the bone a little above the condyles, to clear a way for the saw, which should then be applied to complete the separation. * * * The proceeding above described may be modified according to the taste or discretion of the surgeon: the posterior flap may be made first, as in the leg; but I imagine that it will be a little broader if the knife be first used in front, and the saw may be applied at the condyles, or higher, as may seem requisite. The point which probably most demands attention is, that the posterior flap be made sufficiently long: it appears almost absurd to recommend that the whole calf of the leg should be reserved for this object, yet I concur with the recommendation of Mr. Syme, that the flap in question should be 'to the full extent of the fleshy part of the gastrocnemii muscles, and therefore somewhat longer, even, than is indicated in the drawing.' The cicatrix should be in front; and it is, perhaps, one of the most striking features of this operation that the principal coverings to the stump in the thigh are reserved from the leg."

Double Flap.—Nathan Smith operated as follows:—"Mark two points, one on the out, and the other on the inside of the limb; the latter half an inch below the head of the tibia, and the other opposite to it. Then draw a semicircular line from one point to the other, over the anterior part of the leg, and in such a direction, that its lower part shall touch the lower part of the tubercle on the tibia into which the ligament of the patella is inserted, and then mark another circle on the posterior part of the leg exactly corresponding to the former. The above lines limit the two flaps, the former of which will be formed of the patella and its ligaments, and the latter of the head of the gastrocnemius, the tendons of the flexor muscles, and the popliteal blood-vessels and nerves. The operator should first raise the anterior flap with the patella, which will expose the anterior part of the joint, and render the division of the lateral ligaments easy. Two or three strokes of the knife will then complete the section of the lower flaps with the crucial ligaments."

Pancoast modified the double flap by dividing the posterior flap in the centre, as follows:—"The surgeon, placing his thumb and forefinger upon the condyles of the tibia, at the opposite sides of the leg, makes with a common scalpel on the front of the upper part of the leg, a semilunar incision, which extends as far as three inches below the tubercle of the tibia, one extremity resting on either side, an inch below the joint. The flap of skin is now to be rapidly dissected towards the joint. The leg is then to be extended and made horizontal. The point of the knife is next to be entered through the skin, at the middle of the back part of the leg, an inch and a half to two inches below the fossa of the popliteal space, and carried vertically downwards for the space of three inches. From the lower end of this, the knife is to be continued round, on one side, to strike the line of the first, or anterior incision, so as to mark out a second flap, convex downwards, and extending a little lower than that of the one in front. The lower end of the vertical cut is then united by a similar convex sweep of the knife to the other margin of the front incision, so as to form a third flap. The two posterior flaps are next to be dissected from the fascia up to their base. The leg is now to be again flexed, and from the general loosening of the flaps, already made, the insertion of the ligamentum patellæ upon the tibia will be exposed. This is to be divided across, and the joint opened upon the front and sides, so as to leave the semilunar cartilage on the head of the tibia; the crucial ligaments, as they become subsequently useful as a nidus for granulations, are to be divided at their connexion with the latter bone, and the posterior ligament lastly cut. The leg, which is now loose, is to be twisted on the thigh. An assistant grasps the popliteal artery with his thumb and finger, and the surgeon divides below at one stroke with the knife the remaining parts, consisting mainly of the two heads of the gastrocnemius, some of the hamstring tendons not previously cut, and the popliteal vessels and nerves. The patella is to be left in its position. The whole operation may be done with the scalpel; the femoral artery should be compressed with the tourniquet."

Markoe prefers the double flap, with a long anterior, and a short posterior flap:—"This has the advantage of throwing the wound on the most depending aspect of the stump,—thus allowing easy exit to the discharges; and it, moreover, brings the cicatrix so far back between the prominence of the condyles, that it is not exposed to pressure. By cutting short the gastrocnemius muscles, it diminishes the number, and concentrates the situation of the ligatures, so that they can be brought through the posterior flap directly, without traversing the face of the stump." He adds:—"It will, however, often happen, that the mode of operation will be determined by the condition of the integuments; and it is, therefore, fortunate that the success or failure of the case does not essentially depend upon the particular method adopted. In all cases, it must be borne in mind that a great deal more flap is required to cover the ends of the condyles, than to cover a bone sawed through its shaft; and the most common mistake, in performing this operation, has been the not making due allowance for this circumstance, and, consequently, cutting the flaps too short."

The patella is generally removed in this operation, but if it be allowed to remain it becomes anchylosed to the extremity of the femur, whether the condyles are removed or not.

Amputation of the Thigh.—The principal bulk of the thigh is muscular structure, which surrounds the femur in two distinct layers, the superficial and deep. Malgaigne (*op. cit.*) makes the following practical suggestions:—"As the superficial muscles all spring from the pelvis to go to the leg, the lower you cut them the more they retract, and *vice versâ*. Whence it results that, no matter where you amputate, you must leave nearly the same extent of soft parts to cover the stump; above, on account of the size of the wound—below, to make up for the increased muscular retraction. Moreover, the posterior part of the femur being almost uncovered by deep muscles, retraction is stronger there than on the other sides; the more so as the slightly flexed position of the thigh, by stretching the posterior muscles, favors still more their retraction, and leaves them, when cut, less real length than the others. The same thing takes place, but in a less degree, on the inside compared with the outside, the latter only offering muscles adherent to the bone, and the muscles on the inside being also extended by abduction. This explains why, after circular amputation, the cicatrix is almost constantly behind and inside, and puts us in the way of a more rational proceeding." The arteries to be secured in the thigh are, 1. The superficial femoral, which is on the inside, under the sartorius muscle, having the vein to its posterior and external aspect below, but above, to the inside, and the saphenous vein to its external side; 2. Muscular branches which vary according to the part amputated.

Circular Method.—The patient being properly arranged, the skin retracted by an assistant, the operator standing upon the right side of the limb, or on the outside, makes a first incision as already directed, page 93, through the skin; this is raised by dissection two inches and turned back; the superficial layer of muscles is then divided on a level with the reverted integument, and still further retracted; a third circular incision is made on the margin of the retracted muscle down to the bone, the muscle is dissected from the bone still higher, the periosteum divided, and the bone sawn through at the apex of the cone thus formed; the section of the bone should be about three and a half inches above the incision of the integument.

Single Flap.—The method by a single flap, already described, or a short anterior and long posterior flap, is especially adapted to the thigh. The patient being placed in the proper position, the operator standing upon the right side of the limb, grasps the thigh with the left hand, placing the fingers and thumb upon opposite points; he then applies the heel of a long amputating knife on the further side of the limb at the ends of fingers, and drawing it in a semicircular direction over the limb to the end of the thumb, with this single sweep divides all the soft parts down to the bone; without entirely removing the knife it is withdrawn sufficiently to enter the point at the angle of the wound, and is made to transfix the limb, passing under the bone, and emerging at the angle of the wound on the opposite side; a flap is then cut of the requisite length from the posterior part of the thigh; the flaps are retracted, the knife carried around the bone, and the saw applied at the highest part of the wound.

Double Flaps.—The patient being properly arranged, the operator standing upon the side of the limb, grasps the soft parts and brings them forward; he then transfixes the limb, the knife grazing the upper surface of the bone, and makes an anterior flap (Fig. 179); the knife is reintroduced, and passing under the bone a posterior flap is made longer than the anterior (Fig. 179), to com-

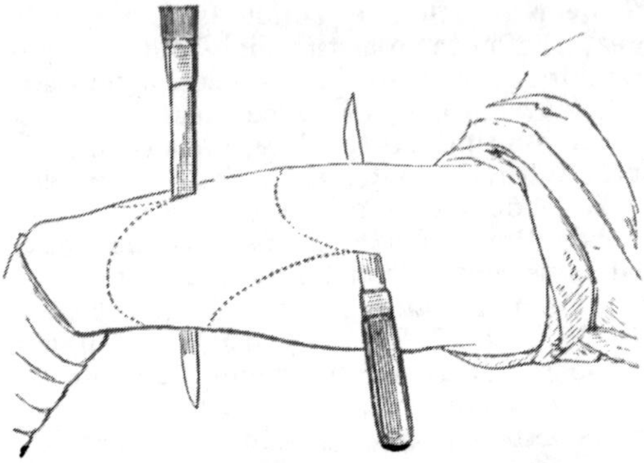

FIG. 179.

pensate for the greater retraction; the operation is completed as in the former method.

Flaps may also be made from the sides of the limb; the knife is introduced in the centre of the limb, directly down to the bone, on one side of which it is passed to the opposite side of the limb, and a flap is then formed (Fig. 179); the knife is then introduced and a flap made from the opposite side; the flaps are strongly retracted, and the bone sawed.

Guthrie advocates Luke's method, and gives the following description of the operation:—"The patient being placed so that the thigh projects beyond the table, the surgeon stands with his left hand towards the body, or on the outside when amputating the right, and on the inside when amputating the left thigh. The knife to be used ought to be narrow, pointed, and longer by two or three inches than the diameter of the thigh at the place of amputation. The point of the knife should be entered *mid*-distance between the anterior and posterior surfaces of the thigh, A (Fig. 180), which may be effected with accuracy, if the eye is brought to a level with the thigh, when the middle point is easily determined. The posterior flap, A, E, D, is to be formed first, by carrying the knife transversely through the thigh, so that its point shall come out on the opposite side, exactly midway between the anterior and posterior surfaces. In traversing the thigh, the knife should pass behind the bone, and will be more or less remote from it in different individuals, according to the greater or less development of the posterior muscles, when, by cutting obliquely downwards, to the extent of from four to six inches, according to the thickness of the thigh, a posterior flap is formed. The anterior flap, G, F, is effected, not by making a flap, but by commencing an incision through the integuments and muscles on the side of the thigh opposite to the surgeon, at a little distance anterior to the extremity of the posterior flap. This incision is made from without inwards, through the integuments, so as to form an even curve, and without angular irregularity, over the thigh, to near the base of the posterior flap on the side on which the surgeon stands. The length of this flap is determined by that of the posterior. It will therefore vary from four to six inches, as before stated; and for its completion will require a second, or perhaps a third, application of the knife. In the two flaps thus made, the division of almost all the soft structures is included, a few only immediately surrounding the bone remaining uncut. These are to be divided by a circular sweep of the knife, at the part where it is intended to saw the bone; in this way it is sufficiently denuded for the

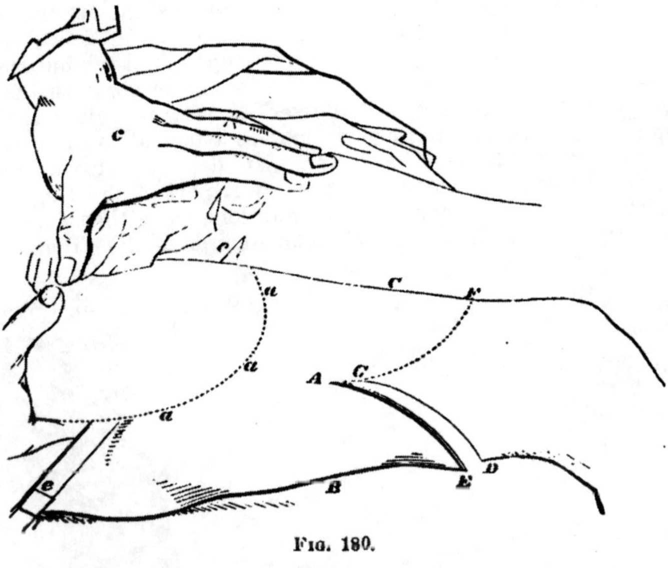

FIG. 180.

application of the saw. The flaps being held back by an assistant, the bone is to be sawn through in the usual way."

Double Flap of Integuments.—Skey remarks (Fig. 181):—"I prefer the double flap of the integuments, and the circular division of the muscles. The breadth of the limb should be calculated, allowance being made for the elastic recoil of the integuments when divided.

The flaps should be sufficient, and not more than sufficient, to meet without effort. They should correspond in size, and not be made too arched. In dividing the muscles, the knife, unless the thigh be of unusual dimensions, should be carried down to the bone at once, and this can only be effected by the application of considerable force, great care being taken that the muscular mass behind the bone be not pushed before the knife, but divided without displacement from its natural relations to the parts around. When the thigh is very large, it would be well if the looser muscles, such as the rectus, sartorius in front, the biceps, semi-tendinosus, and semi-membranosus behind, were divided separately, and allowed to retract, before the division of the remaining muscles which are attached to the bone."

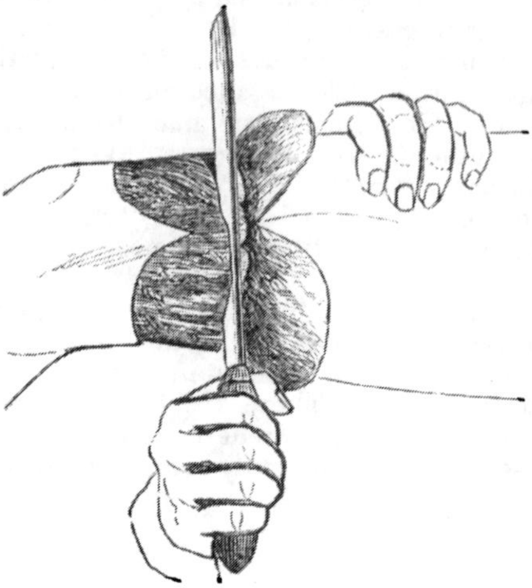

FIG. 181.

Rectangular Flaps.—The rectangular flaps are highly recommended by some surgeons for the lower part of the thigh. The operator makes two longitudinal incisions on either side of the limb (Fig. 182), in length equal to two-thirds of the circumference

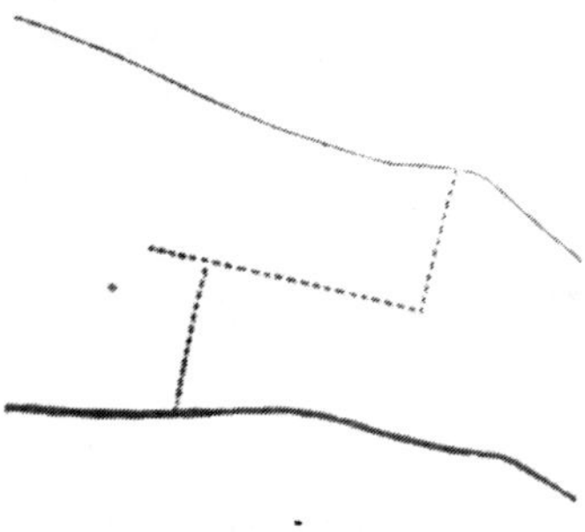

FIG. 182.

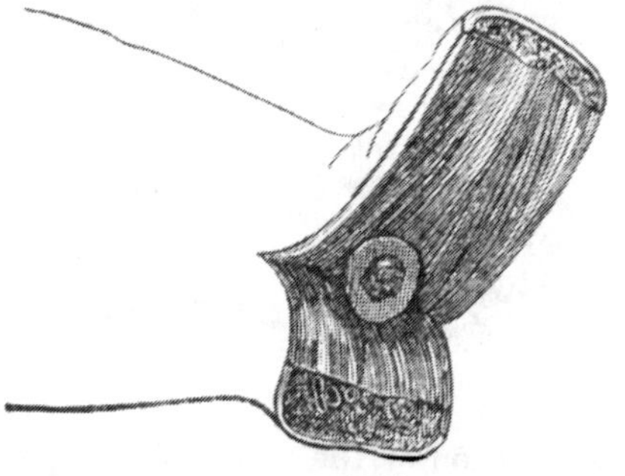

FIG. 183.

of the limb at this part; a second incision, extending to the bone, unites the lower extremities of these two incisions; this quadrilateral flap is raised from the bone; a third incision made transversely down to the bone, forms the posterior flap; both flaps are raised and firmly retracted (Fig. 183), the bone sawn at its point in the flaps, and the flaps united as seen in Fig. 95.

Disarticulation of the Hip-Joint.—The hip-joint is formed by the head of the femur and the acetabulum, into which it is received; its ligaments are the round ligament, which attaches the head of the bone to the bottom of the cavity, and the capsular ligament surrounding the joint; it is deeply situated under thick and powerful muscles, and can be felt only on the anterior part. The great trochanter projects upwards and backwards, three-quarters of an inch above the neck of the femur; the small trochanter projects six lines on the internal surface of the bone; the head of the femur being more than a hemisphere and not entirely received into the cavity, the capsule so envelops and binds it that the latter should be divided close to the margin of the cavity; in carrying the knife around the head of the bone it must be recollected that the plane of the margin of the acetabulum inclines downwards and forwards, projecting more posteriorly than anteriorly. The arteries to be tied are the femoral, the obturator, the ischiatic, and external and internal circumflex. The following anatomical guides to the joint are from *Bernard* and *Huette*:—

"1st. The anterior inferior spinous process of the ilium is three-quarters of an inch above the superior margin of the acetabulum; the anterior superior spinous process is about an inch and three-quarters above the same point, and three-quarters of an inch to its outer side;

"2d. The subject being erect, a line drawn from the anterior superior spinous process of the ilium to the tuberosity of the ischium, crosses the acetabulum at the junction of its posterior with its two anterior thirds;

"3d. The anterior border of the acetabulum is from an inch to an inch and a quarter to the outside of the spine of the pubes;

"4th. The axis of the horizontal ramus of the pubes, extended by an imaginary line, crosses the acetabulum at the junction of its superior with its middle third;

"5th. The superior border of the trochanter major is on a level with the upper third of the cavity of the joint."

Lisfranc gives the following indications:—

"1. Let fall from the superior spine of the ilium a perpendicular line one inch and five lines long; half an inch inside its extremity you will find the external anterior surface of the joint.

"2. From the anterior inferior spine of the ilium, let fall a perpendicular line, half an inch long; its extremity corresponds to the upper part of the joint.

"3. If you draw a line from the spine of the pubes, transversely outwards for two inches, a perpendicular a quarter of an inch long, descending from its extremity, will fall upon the joint.

"4. Lastly, draw upwards a perpendicular line half an inch long, from the anterior superior, and external part of the great trochanter, another line one inch long at right angles to its extremity, directed inwards, will reach the external side of the head of the femur; but this relation varies according to the length and inclination of the neck of the bone."—*Malgaigne.*

Amputation may be performed at the hip-joint by the following methods:—the single flap, anterior and internal; the double flap, lateral, and antero-posterior; the oval, and the circular. These different methods have been almost indefinitely modified.

Single Flap (Anterior).—(Fig. 184.) The single flap method is regarded by Malgaigne and Guérin as superior to all others: the following are the several steps:—The patient lying upon the edge of the table, the hip projecting, the artery is compressed upon the horizontal branch of the pubes; the operator then takes a position on the outside of the limb (the left), which is separated from the other and slightly flexed on the pelvis, and raising the soft parts, which cover the anterior face of the limb, enters a very long doudle-bladed knife midway between the great trochanter and the anterior superior spine of the ilium, directing it at first slightly from below upwards, and from without inwards, A, C, so as to reach the head of the femur, and open the capsule of the joint; he now elevates the handle, and carries the knife in the direction A, B, the point emerging about an inch below and in front of the tuberosity of the ischium; the knife is then carried downwards along the anterior surface of the bone, and a large semilunar flap is made, extending nearly half the length of the thigh, *c* (Fig. 185), or six inches; care should be taken that the flap is as long on the inside as on the outside; an assistant raises the flap, *a*, *e*, at the same time compressing the artery which it contains; the knife is now applied to the capsule, which is divided close to the acetabulum, as if about to cut across the middle of the head of the femur, D, and at least half of its circumference; the limb is then abducted to luxate the head of the bone, the knife passed behind it, and the soft parts on the posterior portion of the limb divided as in the circular operation.

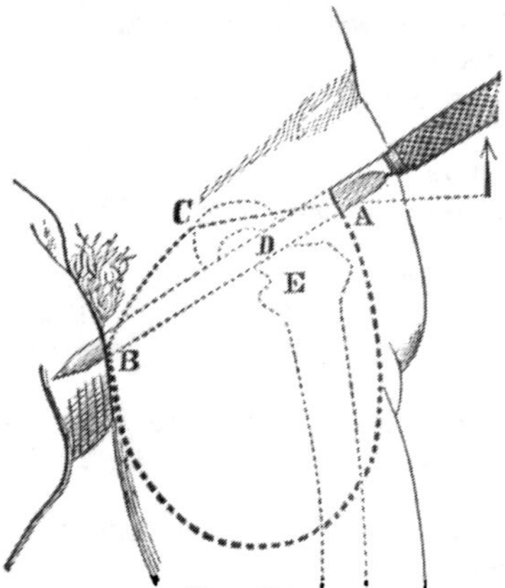

FIG. 184.

Modifications.—Guérin advises, after the articulation is opened, to cut the posterior part from within outwards, as in the circular operation, the knife being held in the position *b* (Fig. 185).

The method of Van Buren, of New York, is similar to that of Guérin:—"The patient, already under the influence of chloroform, being placed on his back upon a table, with the buttocks projecting beyond its edge, the limb to be removed is committed to an assistant previously instructed as to its management, the other limb to a second assistant, who carries it with the scrotum and penis as far as possible to the opposite side, and who also steadies the pelvis; the external iliac artery is then, at the word, forcibly compressed against the horizontal ramus of the pubes, by the principal assistant; and the surgeon, standing on the outer side of the limb, transfixes it with a straight narrow knife, ten inches long, entering its point about an inch above the great trochanter, grazing the head or neck of the femur, if possible, as it passes in front of it, and pushing it through the integuments near the anus, at a point diametrically opposite to its entrance, cuts out an anterior flap in the usual method, at least six inches in length. Meanwhile the principal assistant, passing one hand into the wound behind the knife, grasps the flap, and with it the artery before it has been divided, and as soon as the division is completed, with both hands carries the flap upwards as forcibly as possible. The surgeon then, slightly kneeling, carries the knife beneath the thigh to its inner side, as in a circular amputation, and placing its heel on the integuments, at the internal angle of the wound, sweeps it firmly across the tissues on the back part of the thigh, cutting with a slightly sawing motion down to the bone, and joining the two extremities of the first incision. The long knife is then immediately relinquished, and with a large straight scalpel, the femur being forcibly abducted, the capsule of the joint is laid open as near as possible to the acetabulum, the round ligament divided with the rotator muscles inserted into the trochanter, and the fossa at its base, the assistant managing the limb so as to keep these parts successively on the stretch, and the operation is completed."

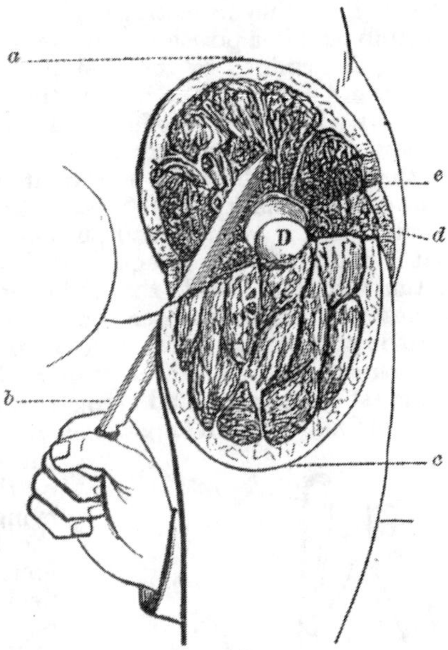

FIG. 185.

Modifications.—Larrey and Delpech tied the artery before the operation; Plantade cut the flaps from without inwards; Lenoir made a circular incision posteriorly; Lalouette made the flap from the antero-interior part of the thigh; Delpech recommended a single internal flap.

Double Flaps (Lateral).—Lisfranc's method (Fig. 186) is as follows:—"The patient must be laid upon his back with the tuberosities of the ischia projecting slightly beyond the edge of the bed, and the limb held in a position between abduction and adduction. Then having determined by the anatomical rules laid down, the anterior and external side of the articulation, the operator holding perpendicularly a long double-edged knife, introduces it at this point, with its lower edge looking downwards towards the great trochanter. As the point of the knife enters, it should be carried around the head of the femur, on its outer side, whilst its handle is inclined upwards and outwards, and pushed steadily on in this direction so that it perforates the integuments a few lines below the tuberosity of the ischium. While this is being done, an assistant grasps the tissues over the trochanter and carries them outwards, in order to assist in the formation of the external flap, and the knife is carried downwards and outwards with a slightly sawing motion, around the great trochanter, and along the femur, cutting out a flap from three to four inches in length, *a*, *b*, *c*. The first flap being thus made, the operator grasping the tissues on the inside of the thigh and carrying them inwards, introduces the knife below the head of the femur, and on the inner side of its neck, holding it in a perpendicular position. As it enters, the point of the knife should pass around the neck of the femur and come out at the lower angle of the wound already made, without coming in contact with the bones of the pelvis; it is then carried downwards along the femur, and avoiding the lesser trochanter, so as to make an internal flap of the same length as the external, *e*, *f*. The flaps being drawn aside by the assistants, and the arteries tied, the surgeon grasps the femur with his left hand, and holding the knife perpendicularly on the inner side of the head of the bone, cuts the capsular ligament without attempting to penetrate the articulation. The joint being opened, the disarticulation is concluded by cutting the fibrous and muscular tissues which remain.—*Bernard* and *Huette.*

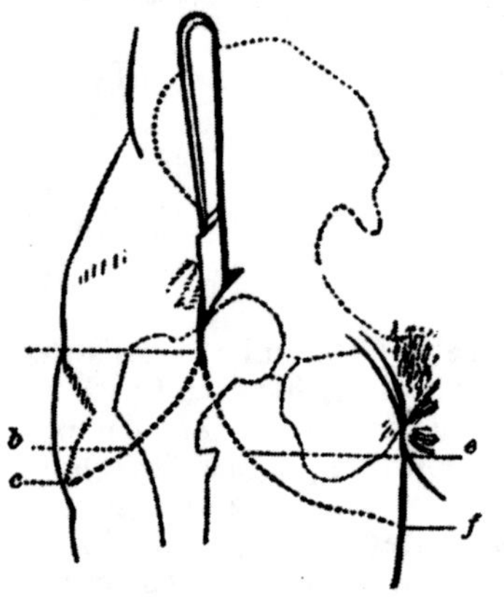

FIG. 186.

Modifications.—Larrey first tied the femoral artery and vein, then transfixed the limb, formed the internal flap, and, disarticulating, made the external flap; Mott tied the artery first, then made the external flap from without inwards; Blandin transfixed the limb through the incision for tying the artery, and made an internal and external flap before disarticulating; Dupuytren made an incision from near the anterior superior spine of the ilium to the tuberosity of the ischium, with its convexity downwards, through the skin only, which was then retracted, after which he divided the muscles forming the internal flap, opened the joint, and made the external flap; Langenbeck made the external flap first, outside of the femoral artery, dislocated the hip outwards, and completed with the internal flap.

Double Flaps (Antero-Posterior).—This method is thus described by Fergusson (*Syst. Pract. Surg.*):—(Fig. 187.) "The surgeon, standing on the outside of the limb, should insert the point of a long catling about midway between the anterior superior spinous process of the ilium and trochanter major, keeping it rather nearer the former than the latter; he should then run it across the fore part of the neck of the bone, and push it through the skin on the opposite side, about two or three inches from the anus; next, he should carry it downwards and forwards, so as to cut a flap from the anterior aspect of the thigh, about four or six inches in length When the blade is entered, the limb should be held up, and even slightly bent at the joint; the instrument will then pass along more readily than if all the textures were thrown on the stretch; moreover, there is greater certainty of passing it behind the main vessels, and even dividing some of the fibres, if not the whole, of the iliacus internus and psoas muscles. As the knife is carried downwards, the assistant who stands behind the operator, should slip his fingers into the wound and carry them sufficiently far across to enable him to grasp the femoral artery between them and the thumb: this he may do from the inside or outside at will, and with the right or left hand, as may be most convenient, the same grasp enabling him to raise the flap as soon as it is completed. The flap being raised, the point of the knife should then be struck against the head of the bone, so as to divide the anterior part of the capsular ligament and any textures in this situation which may not have been included in the flap. To facilitate this part of the operation, the knee should be forcibly depressed by the assistant who holds it; the head of the bone will thus be caused to start from its socket, and if the round

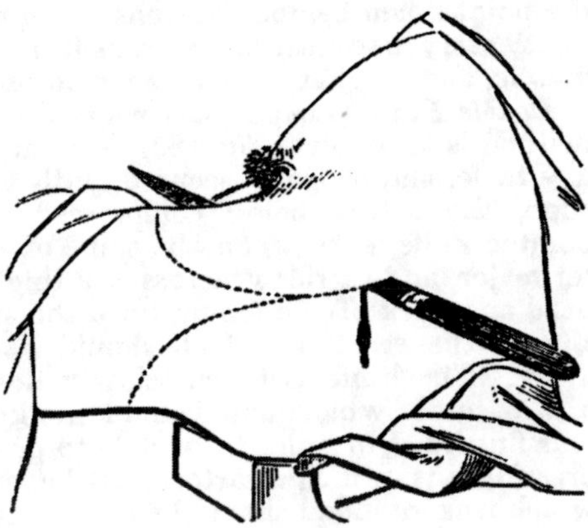

FIG. 187.

ligament is not ruptured by the force, a slight touch with the edge of the knife will cause it to give way. At this period, depression being no longer required, the assistant should bring the head of the femur a little forwards, to allow the knife to be slipped over and behind it, and when it is in the position represented in the design, it should then be carried downwards and backwards, so as to form a flap somewhat longer than that in front, the last cut completing the separation of the limb.

"I have not inculcated the necessity of introducing the point of the blade a certain number of lines distant from the spine of the ilium, nor have I been very precise as to the exact distance from the anus at which it should protrude, for I believe that the operator, instead of limiting himself to lines here, may actually take the freedom of inches: his object should be to make as broad a flap in front as the method by transfixion will admit of; but whether he pushes in the knife, or brings it out, an inch above or the same length below certain given distances, seems to me of very little consequence: if he begins low down, he has to cut out so much deeper, as it were, ere he reaches the capsule, and if this is a disadvantage, it is, perhaps, compensated by the wound on and near the surface being a little further from the trunk: if he introduces the point much behind the tensor vaginæ femoris, he cannot with safety carry it so near the anus as if it were pushed in front of that muscle, and so what he strives for on one side is lost on the other."

Double Flaps (Long Anterior and Short Posterior).—Brownrigg's method is as follows (Fig. 180):—"The patient is to be placed on a low table, and properly secured, with the nates projecting over its edge, the artery being compressed. The surgeon enters the pointed knife, *e*, between the spine of the ilium and the trochanter major, and carries it across the thigh, as near as may be to the head and neck of the femur, until the point appears on the inside, *e*, near the scrotum, which should have been previously drawn away. The knife is to cut slowly downwards, to make a flap, *a*, *a*, *a*, under which, and behind the knife, an assistant inserts his four fingers, *d*, in order to be able to grasp the flap and aid in compressing the principal artery, as the operator completes the flap, which it is intended should be a large one (Fig. 185). The assistant holding up the flap, the surgeon cuts the attachment of the gluteus medius muscle, from the upper edge of the trochanter, if it has not been already done, opens the capsular ligament of the joint, and divides the ligamentum teres. The head of the bone can then be readily withdrawn from the acetabulum. The knife being placed behind the head of the bone and the trochanter, should be carried obliquely downwards and backwards, so as to form a shorter flap behind than was made before."—*Guthrie.*

Mr. Skey advises the method of making double flaps of the skin, and circular divisions of muscles:—"The dimensions of the limb should be measured. The circumference of a well-sized thigh is about twenty inches, and its diameter therefore about seven. The flaps from the centre of their arch to their base should therefore be full three inches and a half to four inches in length; but it should be recollected that they have no projecting central bone to invest, but rather that of a flat surface, and also that the circumference of the limb is not circular, but irregular in form, being flat in front and projecting further from the centre in some parts than in others. The flaps, therefore, should not be made too arched, and no integument should be wasted at their angles or points of junction. Their proposed line should be marked in ink before the operation is begun. The instrument employed should be a common strong amputating knife of the largest size, turned up at the end, and sharp to the point. The first flap may be commenced about one inch below the anterior superior spine of the ilium, and carried straight down for about an inch and a half, and then inclined inwards, nearly following the line of Poupart's ligament, and about four inches below it. Reaching the adductor longus muscle, descending from the os pubis, it should be carried round in a gentle curve to a point about two inches below the tuber ischii. The second or outer flap should cross the shaft of the femur immediately below the trochanter major, and run almost circularly backwards to the same point as the former. The flaps being reflected high, the muscles may be divided by a circular sweep, applied with great force of pressure, commencing with the adductors on the inner side, keeping the knife close to the bone both at *their* origin, and also on the division of the flexors of the leg arising from the tuber ischii. The circle should be completed in front, when the femoral artery will be divided, and should be immediately tied, if the pressure by the assistant fail to arrest the hæmorrhage. In dividing the muscles, the limb should be made to follow the application of the knife to each surface, abducted in division of the muscles of the inner side, elevated for the flexor behind, and adducted for the glutei. The capsule being bared should be divided in front, the head disarticulated, and the ligamentum teres cut asunder, during powerful abduction by the assistant, and the arteries tied *to the smallest size.*"

Oval Method.—Cornuau's method is as follows:—"1st. The patient being placed on the healthy side, the surgeon enters the point of the knife an inch above the great trochanter, and from this point makes an oblique incision backwards, outwards, and downwards, to a point below the tuberosity of the ischium. 2d. The knife placed in the superior angle of the wound, makes a similar incision forwards and inwards. 3d. The muscles are divided on the outside as deeply as possible, and the limb being luxated outwards, the knife enters the articulation externally and is carried through the joint to the inner side of the femur. One assistant compresses the artery in the anterior flap, another lifts up the flesh on the external side, while the surgeon terminates the operation by dividing the soft parts between the two incisions in the form of a V."—(*Bernard* and *Huette.*)

Guthrie performed the oval operation as follows (Fig. 188):—"The patient is to be laid on a low table, or other convenient thing, in a horizontal position; an assistant, standing behind and leaning over, compresses the external iliac artery, becoming femoral as it passes over the head of the pubes. The surgeon, standing on the inside, commences his first incision some three or four inches directly below the anterior spinous process of the ilium, *a*, carries it across the thigh through the integuments, inwards and backwards, in an oblique direction, at an equal distance from the tuberosity of the ischium to nearly opposite the spot where the incision commenced, *c;* the end of this incision is then to be carried upwards with a gentle curve behind the trochanter, until it meets with the commencement of the first, *b;* the second incision being rather less than one-third the length of the first. The integuments, including the fascia, being retracted, the three gluteal muscles are to be cut through to the bone. The knife being then placed close to the retracted integuments, should be made to cut through everything on the anterior part and inside of the thigh. The femoral or other large artery should then be drawn out by a tenaculum or spring forceps, and tied. The capsular ligament being well opened, and the ligamentum teres divided, the knife should be passed behind the head of the bone thus dislocated, and made to cut its way out, care being taken not to have too large a quantity of muscle on the under part, or the integuments will not cover the wound, under which circumstance a sufficient portion of muscular fibre must be cut away. The obturatrix, gluteal, and ischiatic arteries are not to be feared, being each readily compressed by a finger until they can be duly secured. The capsular ligament, and as much of the ligamentous edge of the acetabulum as can be readily cut off, should be removed. The nerves, if long, are to be cut short. The wound is then to be carefully cleansed, and brought together by three or more soft leaden sutures in a line from the spine of the ilium towards the tuberosity of the ischium. This mode of proceeding is more certain of making good flaps where integuments are scarce. Where the integuments will admit of the anterior flap being made by the sharp-pointed puncturing knife dividing the parts after it has been passed across from without inwards, there is no objection to this proceeding, and some prefer it."

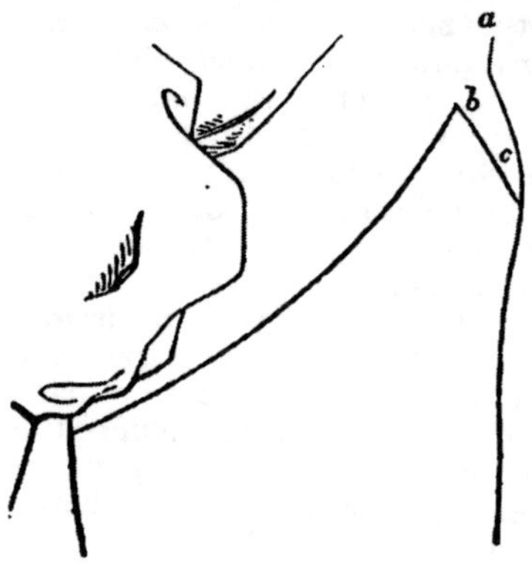

FIG. 188.

Modifications.—Larrey tied the artery first, then made a circular incision; the incision for ligating the artery formed the apex of the oval in the dissection; Sanson began the incision four fingers' breadth below the perineum, and extended it over the front of the joint to the great trochanter, a second began at the inner angle of the first and passed around the outer part of the limb to unite with the former at the trochanter; Scoutetten cut from the trochanter downwards, and carried the incision around the thigh to the point of beginning.

Circular Method.—This operation was first performed by Aber nethy. The incision is made perpendicular to the axis of the femur, four or five fingers' breadth below the great trochanter; the remaining steps of the operation are the same as in circular operations elsewhere.

Modifications.—Veitch proposed the following:—The integuments being retracted by an assistant, make a circular incision through the skin and fascia, freely into the muscles; these parts are retracted, and the operator divides the muscles to the bone; the bone is then sawed an inch or two below the circular incision, by raising the soft parts from it, aided by two lateral incisions; the blood-vessels are now secured, and the patient being turned upon the sound side, an incision is made from two inches above the trochanter, in a direct line over its projection, to the extremity of the stump, the soft parts are now detached, and the bone removed.

Kerr bent the thigh at a right angle with the trunk, made an incision from the top of the trochanter, obliquely downwards and backwards to the inside of the thigh, and then obliquely upwards, to within two inches of the femoral artery; a second, beginning at the same place as the former, but carried in an opposite direction, over the upper extremity of the trochanter, and from thence obliquely downwards and forwards, to within the same distance as the former incision; the muscles were then divided, the bone dislocated, and lastly the parts containing the vessel were severed.

Graefe made the circular incision through the skin, three or four fingers' breadth below the trochanter; this is retracted and another incision is made down to the first, carried over the front to the inner side, along the neck, close to the thigh; the muscles are now divided, the bone dislocated, and the operation completed.

CHAPTER V.

ON RESECTIONS.

RESECTIONS IN GENERAL.

RESECTION, or excision of bones, belongs strictly to the department of Conservative Surgery, the design being to preserve limbs in more or less integrity, and avoid the total destruction which follows its alternative—amputation. The operation has for its object the removal of diseased or injured bones from their connexions, either entire, or such portions as are destructive of the functions of the limb. This branch of operative surgery has assumed the highest importance within the past few years, owing to the recognition of the fact that when the osseous substance is removed, and the periosteum is left in position, new bone is formed, and often in sufficient perfection to restore the symmetry as well as the function of the part.

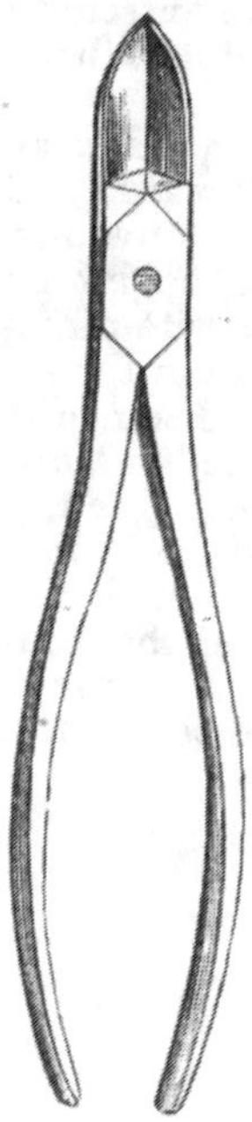

FIG. 189.

Instruments.—Resection, like many other operations, may ordinarily be successfully performed with but few instruments; if, however, the surgeon desire to provide himself with a well-appointed case, which would comprise not only the usual instruments, but those designed for special purposes, he should obtain the following list, which forms a complete exsecting case:—One straight, and one curved bone-gouging or gnawing forceps; one drill bow, to which is attached a number of drills, with guards, to fit the depth to any distance and avoid the danger of slipping into the soft parts after perforation; one set drills, with burr and antrum hook; two retractors or spatulas; one lead hammer, with German silver plate around; one large bone forceps; one necrosis forceps, parrot beaks; one lion-jawed bone-holding forceps; two chisels; one cartilage knife, heavy, with steel blunt handle, for scraping bone; one elevator and lenticular knife; one chain saw, with rotating handles; one narrow bone saw; one instrument for carrying chain saw under the bone; one bayonet shaped forceps for sequestrum; one rasp, and concave bone scraping knife; one right and left curved narrow bone saw; one Symanowsky saw; one set cautery irons; ligature silk; iron, lead, silver, and zinc wire.

Forceps.—(Fig. 189.) The straight bone forceps of Liston is the most useful instrument of the kind yet devised; in the section of the small bones, and in the division of osseous tissue, wherever it can be brought to bear, it cannot be superseded. But frequently it is quite difficult to reach the part which may be more readily divided with the forceps than the saw, unless the blades are curved at a considerable angle; in such cases a forceps curved as in Fig. 190, or Fig. 191, will be found serviceable.

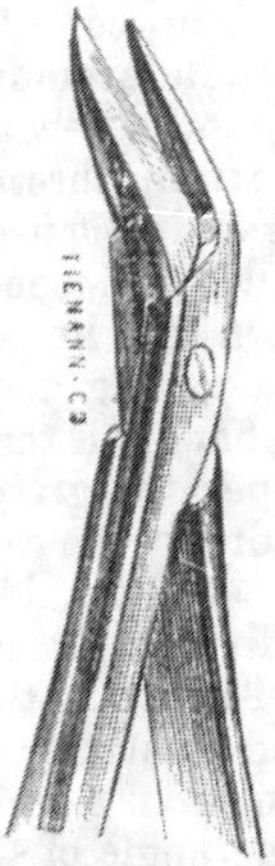

FIG. 190.

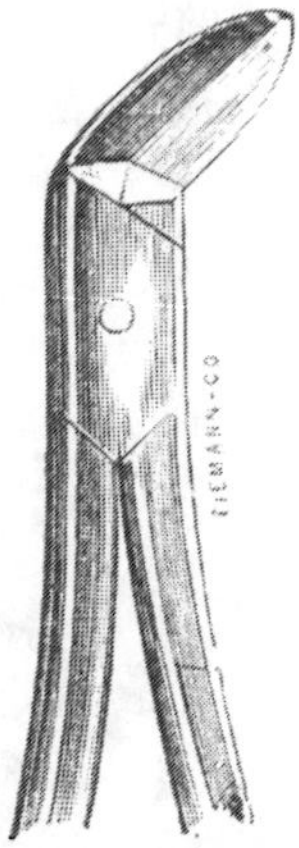

FIG. 191

A great variety of forceps for seizing the bone in removing it have been devised. The small dressing forceps are always useful, but for large bones the forceps of Chassaignac (Fig. 192), which resembles the lion-jawed forceps of Fergusson, is most useful. Halstead, of New York, has enlarged

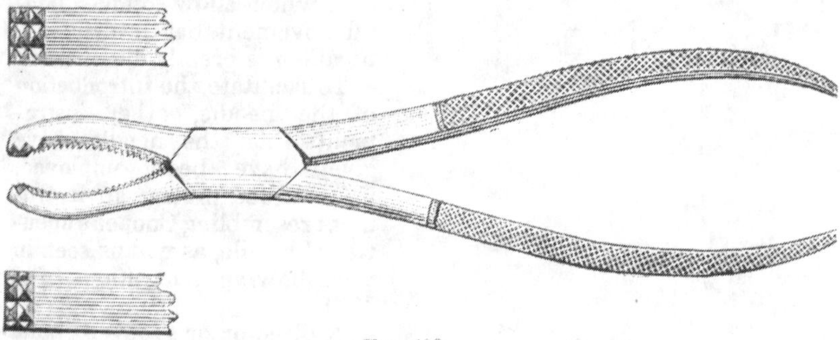

FIG. 192.

the curve of the beaks, and made the inner surface rough for the purpose of grasping large pieces of bone—a most useful improvement.

Drills.—(Fig. 193.) The bone drills of Brainard, *a*, *b*, *c*, are the best form in use; they are used with the handle, *a*, or with a drill bow, for the removal of portions of large flat bones. In cases of carious bone, the burr, *e*, proposed by Isaacs, is very useful. The drill, *d*, was designed by Parker, of New York, to enlarge the antrum.

Pope, of St. Louis, has added a bone drill (Fig. 194), resembling a small trephine, which may be used in penetrating bony cavities.

Saws.—The chain saw (Fig. 195) is an indispensable instrument in resecting; it is formed of a large number of pieces, with movable articulations, and is terminated at each extremity by handles, with which it is worked. To use this saw one handle is removed by a hook, B, and a needle, C, armed with a strong thread, is attached to this end; the needle is passed under the bone, and the saw drawn into its position, with the cutting edge upwards, and the handle is then reattached; the operator, grasping the handles, draws the saw alternately from side to side, until the bone is divided. There is great danger of breaking this saw if it is worked carelessly; it should be drawn from side to side steadily, at an angle of 45° to the long axis of the bone. This saw has lately been improved by Mr. Tiemann, of this city, who has given it rotating handles, which allow so much lateral movement that the danger of breaking is greatly diminished.

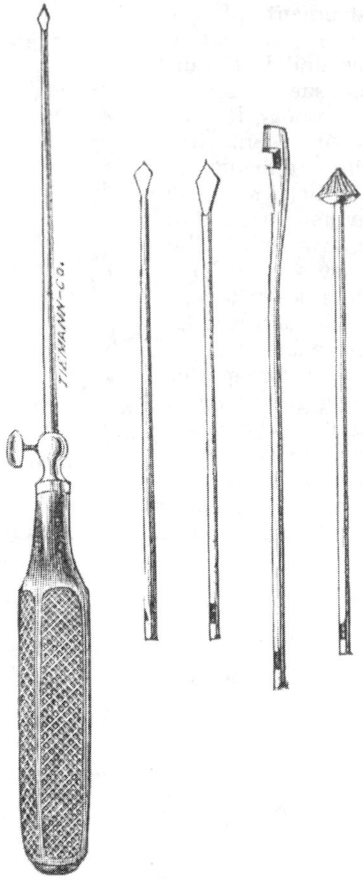

a b c d e
FIG. 193.

To facilitate the introduction of the needle, other instruments than the needle above given have been employed. Chassaignac prefers an instrument resembling Cooper's aneurismal needle, as will be seen in the following illustrations (Fig. 197).

A director or grooved sound (Fig. 197), articulated at A, has been invented; the end being passed under the bone, the needle

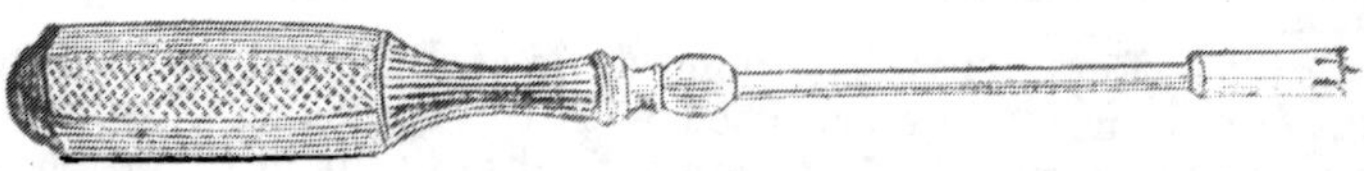

FIG. 194.

is carried along the groove. Prince, of Illinois, Brigade Surgeon U. S. Army, has improved this instrument by terminating the end with a slender spring, having a rounded extremity.

Post, of New York, has recently devised an instrument for passing the saw under the bone. It consists of a staff (Fig. 198), to the end of which, at right angles, is attached a semicircular needle.

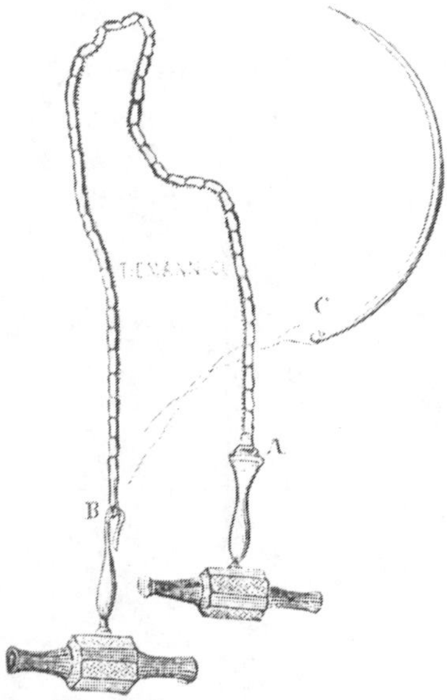

FIG. 195.

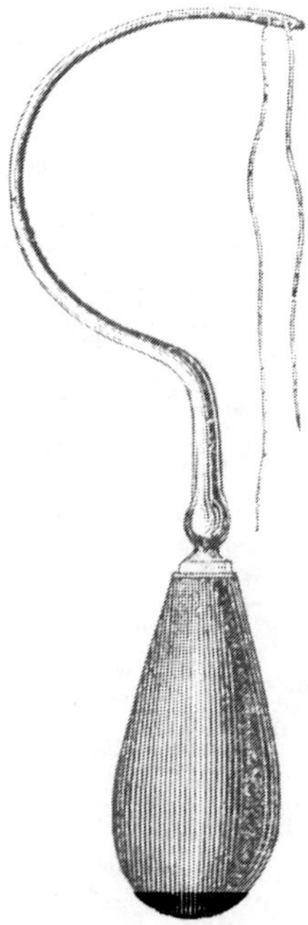

FIG. 196.

b, *c*. The extremity of the staff is split longitudinally, and has a horizontal perforation through each division, for the reception of the attached end of the needle. The needle is by this means made to revolve describing a circle; and can be fixed at short intervals in its course by means of the following contrivance:—The needle is prevented from slipping from the perforations by means of a small cross-piece (after the plan of a lynch-pin in the axle-tree) in the situation between the two separated portions of the end of the staff. This little cross-piece, as the needle is caused to revolve around its axis, is made to correspond to little grooves on the internal aspect of the split ends, and when it is necessary to fix the needle in any one position, the two ends pinched together by means of a ring slide, *a*, on the staff, the two extremities of the cross-piece fitting in one or other of the grooves. The free extremity of the needle is blunt, provided with a hook, and is also perforated; the staff is provided with a suitable handle.

The delicate saw of Butcher, represented in general outline in Fig. 199, answers admirably in many resections; it is, however,

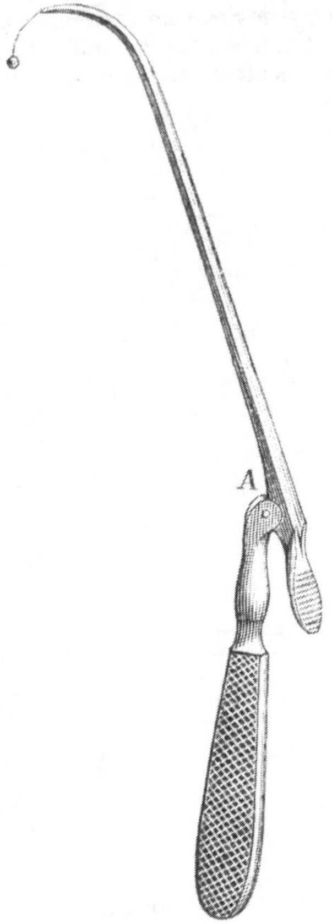

Fig. 197.

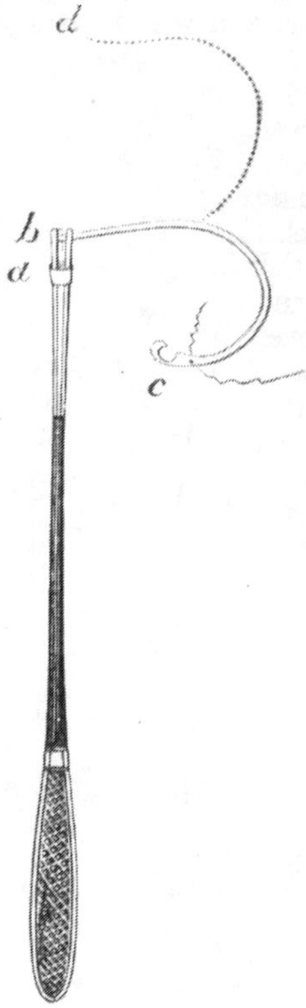

Fig. 198.

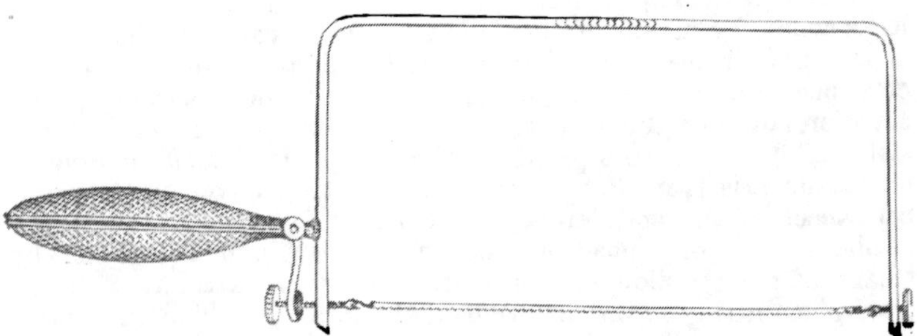

Fig. 199.

surpassed by the saw of Symanowsky (Fig. 199), which combines the advantages of a chain and fixed saw; the saw may be taken from its position, where it is firmly held by a spring (Fig. 200), connected with the handle, and passed under the bone, if required, and the ends, being reattached in the frame, the bone is as readily divided from beneath as from above. The saw may be turned laterally also, or be made to cut in a curve. The spring which regulates the tension of the saw is seen (Fig. 200) inclosed in the handle.

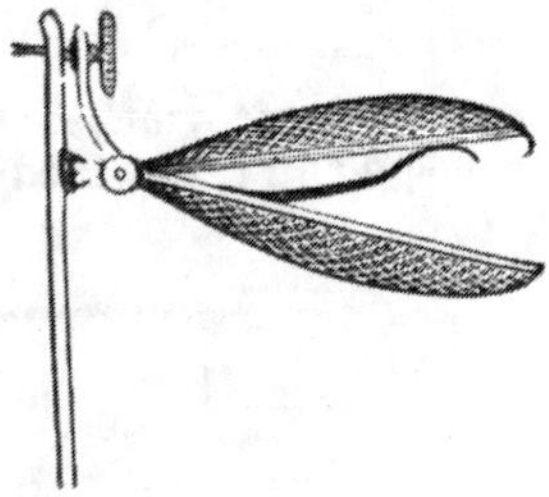

FIG. 200.

Other saws, of peculiar shape, are found useful in the removal of certain bones, though not absolutely essential. The articulated saw (Fig. 201), having a movable back, may be used to advantage in most resections of bones of the extremities. In the removal of the superior maxilla, the right and left bone saws (Figs. 202, 203) enable the operator to separate its superior attachments with great facility. A small

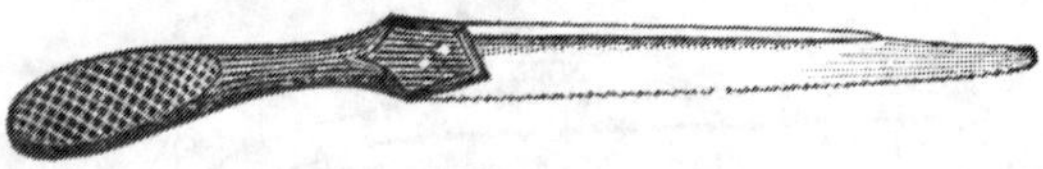

FIG. 201.

straight saw (Fig. 204) is often required, and when it is necessary to use a part of the edge, Detmold, of New York, has suggested

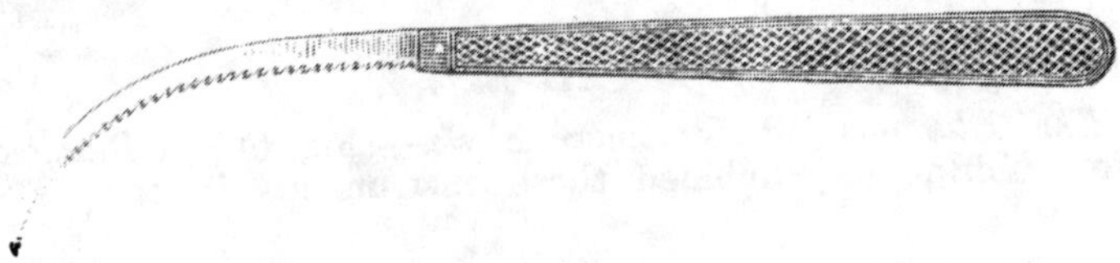

FIG. 202.

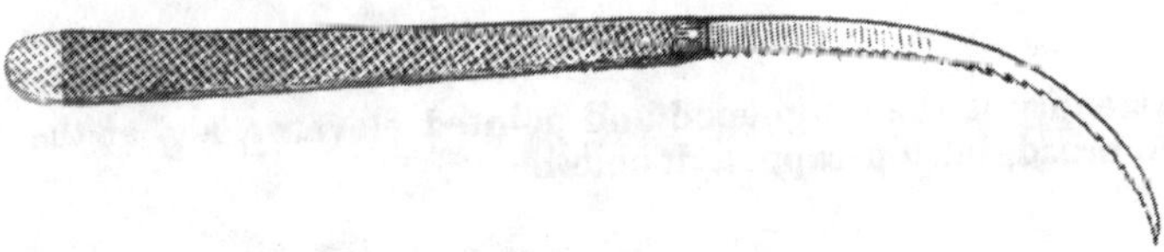

FIG. 203.

drawing an india-rubber tube over the part unused to prevent its injuring the soft parts. Hey's saw, or some of the various modifications (Fig. 205), is frequently used for delicate bones. For the same purpose the reverse saw is used (Fig. 206); it consists of two

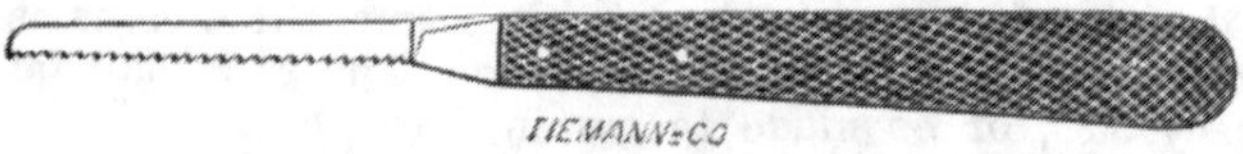

FIG. 204.

circular saws worked by the lever, *a*, which acts upon the two arms, *b* and *c*, attached to the saws; in using it the saw is placed

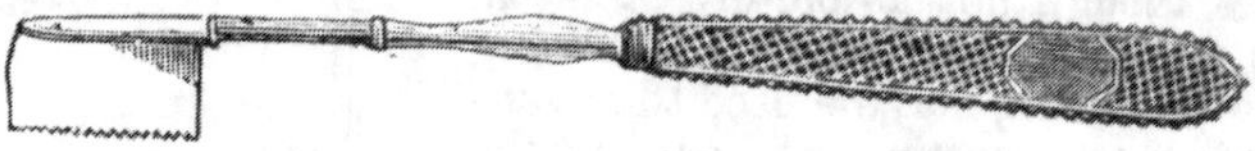

FIG. 205.

upon the bone, the left hand grasping the handle, and the lever, *a*, is worked with the thumb and finger of the right hand.

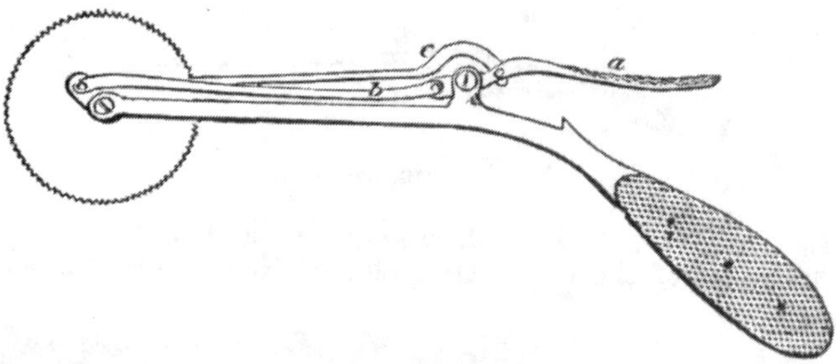

FIG. 206.

The Elevator and Lenticular Knife.—(Fig. 207.) Detmold, of New York, has combined these instruments in one; at one

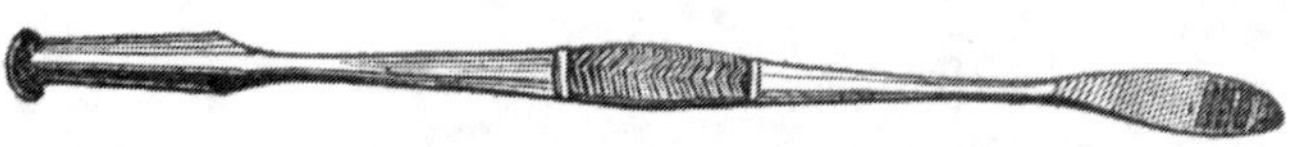

FIG. 207.

extremity is the roughened and pointed elevator, and at the other the broad, button-capped double blade.

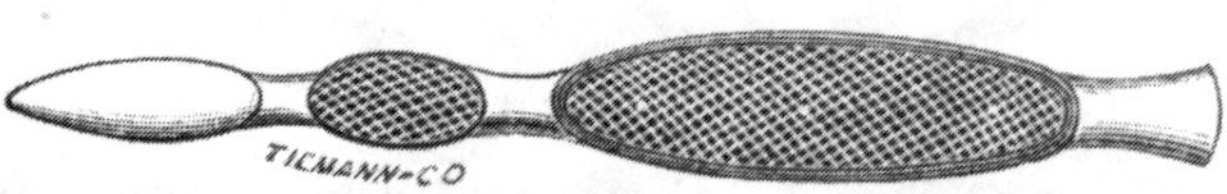

FIG. 208.

Bone Scraping Knife.—(Fig. 208.) Sands, of New York, has recently devised a knife, having a double, obtusely-pointed blade, and a stout, rough handle, terminating in a broad blunt extremity for denuding bone.

Arrangements.—The arrangements for the operation of resection are not unlike those preceding an amputation, and do not require repetition.

Operative Procedure.—Chassaignac lays down the following very rational propositions as the basis of his *Nouveau Systéme de Resection*:—1. Make but a single integumentary incision in all resections, whatever they may be; 1. In all cases make a section of bone before disarticulation; 3. Isolate and separately remove each articular extremity, always commencing with that which is the most easily extracted, and making it thus an aid to the extraction of the other.

In the following descriptions of the different operations for resections of bones, the above rules will be recognised as correct in their general application; but various other methods, adopted by eminent operators, will also be given, as has been done in the preceding chapters on the ligature of arteries and amputations, to enable the surgeon to exercise his judgment intelligently in individual operations.

Incision.—Various incisions have been recommended by different operators, of which the following are the principal:—The straight, ———; the crucial + or ×; the H; the T; the L; the V; the elliptical, ⬭; the quadrilateral, ▭; the elongated, |———|; the |———, &c. &c. Of these incisions the straight is adapted to the greatest number of cases, and by many surgeons of great experience in resections is exclusively made. The straight incision certainly has the advantage over all others of not dividing the tendons, and but slightly exposing the blood-vessels and nerves to injury. There are instances, however, in which a combination of the forms given will be found useful in order to completely expose the parts to be removed.

The incision should in general be made as nearly as possible over the bone to be removed, and distant from important blood-vessels and nerves; the soft parts should not be destroyed, except so far as they have undergone degeneration, or interfere with the proper closure of the wound. Injuries to blood-vessels and nerves lying in the track of the incision should be scrupulously avoided by drawing them aside. Muscles and tendons should not be divided, and their attachments to bones should not be incised, but separated to the least practicable extent with a blunt instrument, as the handle of a scalpel.

Isolation of the Bone.—The bone being exposed to the desired extent, the next care of the operator should be to preserve in the wound, and as far as possible in its original position, the periosteum of the bone to be removed, in order to the reproduction of sufficient new bone to preserve the function of the part; in this manner the lower jaw may be completely excised, and subsequently sufficiently reproduced to preserve nearly the original contour of the jaw, and in part its function. The periosteum is best preserved by first incising it to the extent of the bone to be removed, and then separating it with the handle of the scalpel carefully inserted between it and the bone.

Removal of the Bone.—The periosteum being separated, the bone, if short or flat, may be removed with the forceps; but if a long bone, it must be divided in its shaft by cutting forceps or the saw, and each portion separately removed; before the saw is used the soft parts should be carefully protected by compresses or a spatula introduced underneath it.

In removing diseased bone Sédillot recommends scooping out the affected parts, and leaving the cortical portion in preference to the removal of its entire structure; the reproduction of bone is much more rapid and complete when this portion is left than when only the periosteum remains.

Dressings.—If any considerable vessel is divided, and continues to bleed, it should be ligated, as subsequent hæmorrhage will greatly interfere with the process of repair. When short or flat bones and the shafts of long bones are removed, in whole or part, the wound is generally at first filled with lint to promote granulation from the bottom; and when the articular extremities are excised, and it is desirable to obtain subsequent motion or anchylosis, other dressings are to be employed. These special dressings for individual cases must be left entirely to the discretion of the surgeon.

Classification.—Resections may be divided into resection in the continuity and resection in the contiguity, or, which is more practical, partial and complete resections; the former term implies the removal of but part of a bone, and the latter the extirpation of the entire bone.

Partial Resection.—In long bones partial resection may be made, as of a portion of the shaft, or of the extremity; in flat bones portions are removed with the trephine or the gouge; and in short bones processes may be excised, as in the vertebræ.

Complete Resection.—Total resection, or the extirpation of entire bones, has been practised on some of the larger and more important bones in the skeleton; thus the radius, ulna, tibia, fibula, clavicle, and scapula, have been successfully removed, the patients not only recovering from the operations, but in many cases the reproduction of bone has been so complete as to restore to a considerable extent the function of the part.

RESECTIONS OF THE UPPER EXTREMITIES.

General Principles.—Resection is preferable to amputation in the greater number of lesions of the upper extremities, as the principal function is that of mobility.—*Sedillot.*

Resections of the Phalanges.—Resection of the phalanges, in whole or part, is occasionally required as the result of deep-seated inflammation. As the usefulness of the fingers depends upon their mobility, the stiffness, shortening, and deformity, which have hitherto followed resection of the phalangeal bones, have been strong objections to this operation. Recently, however, efforts have been made to preserve the periosteum with a view to the production of new bone in the shafts of the bones that have been removed, and when the articulations have been excised the cut surfaces of bone have been kept apart, and passive motion has been easily instituted in order to the formation of an artificial joint. This treatment has been followed by the happiest results; bones have been reproduced, and artificial joints formed, which have restored in a greater or less degree the usefulness of the limb. The true principles of treatment of these operations are forcibly stated by Butcher, of Dublin, who excised the entire first phalanx of the thumb, and "the power of flexing the unguinal phalanx was nearly complete" at the termination of the cure. Of the treatment, he says:—There are two points which I would strenuously urge as conspiring to the favorable issue in this case: *First,* The restraining of the unguinal phalanx from the end of the metacarpal bone, until the exuded fibrin thrown down in the bed from which the phalanx had been taken, acquired sufficient consistence to resist any great amount of shortening; and, *Secondly,* when this object was accomplished, removing restraint, and favoring gentle passive motion."

Resection of the Shaft.—A longitudinal incision is made on the dorsal or lateral aspect of the phalanx, the tendons are detached; the operator, with Liston's bone forceps, held at right angles to its long axis, divides the shaft in two places equally distant from its extremities, and then with forceps removes the fragment, the articular surfaces being preserved.

Resection of the Interphalangeal Articulations.—An incision is made over the articulation, or on its side, the tendons carefully pressed aside; with the bone forceps, or what is better, with a fine watch-spring saw, the operator divides the bone, and seizing it with forceps removes the articulating portion.

Resection of the Entire Phalanx.—An incision is made over the shaft of the bone on the side, and the tendons being raised, the bone forceps are introduced, the bone divided, and the two halves separately removed at their articulation. In removing the third or unguinal phalanx, Guérin makes on the palmar surface a T incision, double, one end corresponding to the articulation, the other to the extremity of the finger; the phalanx should be denuded from the end towards its base, the nail remaining intact.

Butcher excised the entire unguinal phalanx of the thumb as follows:—An elliptical incision was made corresponding to the phalangeal articulation, the two arms of the ellipse embracing the anterior extremity of the first phalanx, its most convex portion being a little behind the matrix; the flap was dissected back, the joint opened, and a very narrow sharp-pointed knife passed along the first phalanx, without perforating in front, and keeping its edge to the surface of the bone; it was then liberated from the soft parts, and removed with dressing forceps.

Resection of the Metacarpo-Phalangeal Articulation.—This resection may be limited to the articular extremity of the metacarpal bones, or may include also that of the first phalanx, when it is called a total resection of the joint.

In resection of the phalangeal extremity of a metacarpal bone, an incision is made on its dorsal surface, the extensor tendons carefully drawn aside, the bone cleared of the soft parts and then divided with a chain saw at the required point; the diseased portion is seized with the forceps (Fig. 209) and brought forward, exposing the articular extremity to the point of the knife, by which it is readily disarticulated.

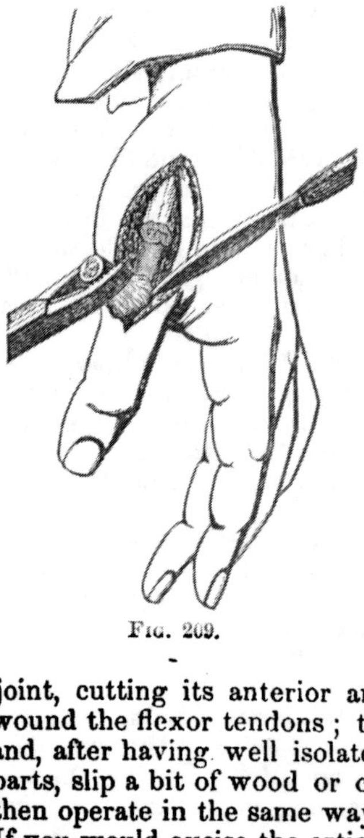

Fig. 209.

Modification.—Malgaigne (*op. cit.*) operates as follows:—"Make an oblique incision, commencing half an inch beyond the point at which you wish to apply the saw, from the middle of the dorsal surface of the metacarpal bone to the commissure of the finger, then another from the same point to the next commissure on the other side; thus circumscribing a V-shaped flap, with its base next the finger. Dissect back this flap, turn aside the extensor tendon, detach the interossii from the sides of the bone, and open the joint, cutting its anterior and lateral ligaments carefully, not to wound the flexor tendons; then dislocate the phalanx backwards; and, after having well isolated the diseased portion from the soft parts, slip a bit of wood or card-board beneath it, and saw it off; then operate in the same way on the head of the metacarpal bone. If you would excise the articulation of the index, thumb, or little finger, it would be easier to cut the flap on the free side of the joint; and we might, according to the condition of the parts, make the base inferior or superior. In this way we need not put the extensor tendon so far aside to make room for the saw."

In total resection the incision should be dorsal, except, according to Chassaignac, for the first, second, and fifth metacarpo-phalangeal articulations; in opening these the incision should be lateral, as the operator will thus avoid exposing the extensor tendons; the two articular surfaces being exposed, the ligaments are incised, and the bone either sawn with the chain saw, or divided with the bone forceps (Fig. 210).

Malgaigne operates as in the former case, viz.:—Make two incisions, beginning at the middle of the dorsal face of the metacarpal bone, diverging on either side to the commissure of the finger, and forming a V-shaped flap, with its base towards the finger; this flap is dissected up, the extensor tendon drawn aside, the sides of the bones laid bare, the ligaments divided, and the joints opened without wounding the flexor tendons, the phalanx is then dislocated backwards, and being isolated from the soft parts, is divided with the saw or forceps; the extremity of the metacarpal bone is then similarly removed; if the operation is on the thumb, index, or little finger, this flap should be on the lateral free surface of the joint.

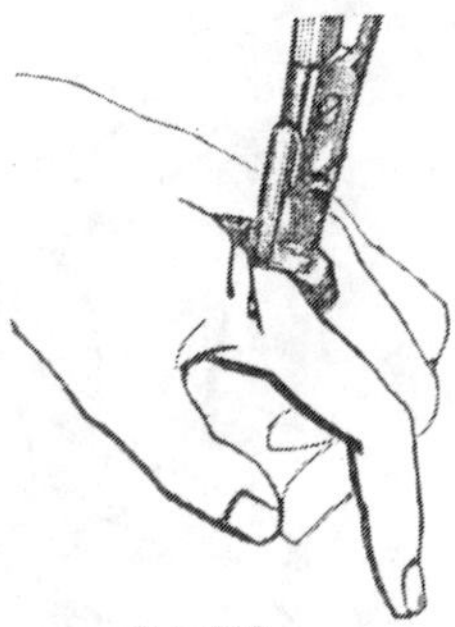

FIG. 210.

Resections of Metacarpal Bones.—The superficial condition of the dorsal aspect of the metacarpal bones, and the important anatomical relations of their palmar surface, require that all operations for their excision be commenced on the posterior part.

RESECTION OF THE SHAFT.—A longitudinal incision is made on the radial border of the first and second, on the ulnar border of the fifth, and the dorsal surface of the third and fourth; the extensor tendons are carefully avoided, the bones denuded, and with a chain saw divided at two points, and the isolated portion is readily removed.

After Treatment.—It is quite as desirable at this articulation to preserve mobility as at the phalangeal articulations, and numerous cases prove that this result may be obtained by proper after treatment. The cut surfaces of bone should not be placed in direct and permanent apposition, but be supported, as in excision of the phalangeal articulations, so that the fragments are slightly separated; as soon as the inflammation subsides sufficiently, passive motion should be cautiously commenced.

RESECTION OF THE CARPO-METACARPAL ARTICULATION.—This resection may be partial or complete. In partial resection a longitudinal incision is made over the upper extremity of the metacarpal bone, the extensor tendon avoided, the soft parts separated from the sides of the bone; the bone is then divided at the requisite point with bone forceps, or with the saw, after being isolated from the soft parts, and as far as possible from the periosteum; the fragment is then seized with the forceps, raised from its bed (Fig. 211), and the joint is disarticulated with the point of the knife.

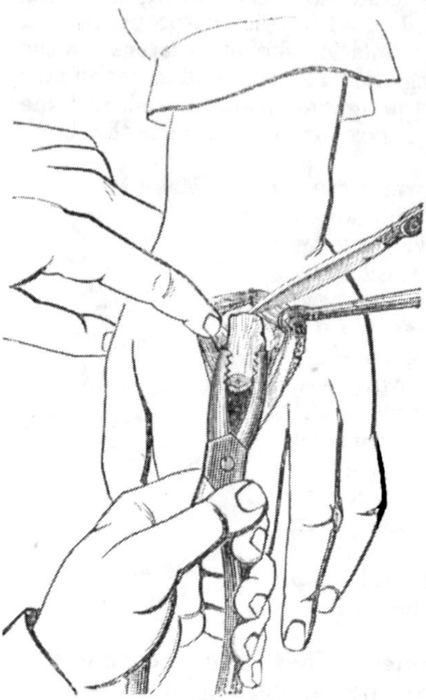

FIG. 211.

In complete resection the extremity of the metacarpal bone is removed and its corresponding carpal bone; a simple longitudinal incision is made in the direction of the superior extremity of the metacarpal bone, which is denuded of soft parts, and sawn at the proper point; this part is removed at its articulation, and then the carpal bone is extirpated.

RESECTION OF AN ENTIRE METACARPAL BONE.—An incision is made along the dorsal surface of the third and fourth metacarpal bones, and on the radial side of the second and ulnar side of the fifth, the extensor tendon drawn on one side, and the sides of the bone relieved of the soft parts; the bone is then isolated from its periosteum as much as possible, and divided in the centre with the bone forceps (Fig. 212), or with the chain saw, the soft parts being protected by a compress or spatula; the fragments are then separately elevated, and disarticulated with the point of the knife.—*Chassaignac.*

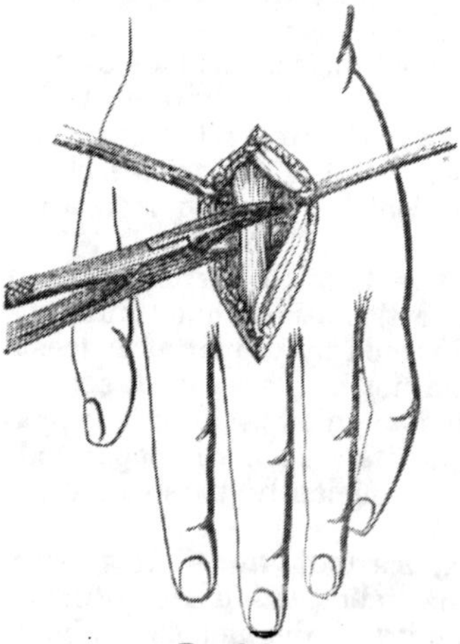

FIG. 212.

Modifications.—This operation is variously modified, according to the condition of the part. The following are the most important general methods:—

Sédillot suggests making a short lateral incision at each extremity of the longitudinal incision, when there is much tumefaction; Guérin notices the position of the tendons of the long and short extensors on the posterior part of the thumb, and the thenar eminence on the palm, and directs that the incision be made between the two along the radial border.

In resection of the fifth metacarpal bone, Sédillot advises a T or L incision.

Resections of the Carpus.—The resections in this region are numerous; the carpal bones have been removed singly, and with individual metacarpal bones; they have all been removed at a single operation, as also with several of the metacarpal bones below, and with the extremities of the radius and ulna above. The result has generally been so far successful, as regards the usefulness of the limb, as to make these resections legitimate operations.

The articulation of the carpal bones with each other is arthrodial; the synovial sacs are so arranged that their communications are limited (Fig. 213); this anatomical peculiarity should be remembered in the effort to remove portions of the carpus, as it is

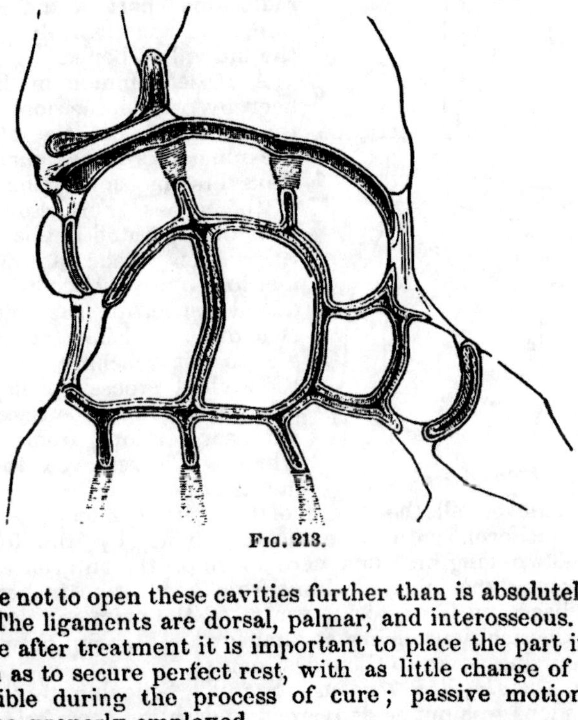

FIG. 213.

desirable not to open these cavities further than is absolutely necessary. The ligaments are dorsal, palmar, and interosseous.

In the after treatment it is important to place the part in such a position as to secure perfect rest, with as little change of position as possible during the process of cure; passive motion should finally be properly employed.

RESECTION OF SINGLE CARPAL BONES.—The carpus is composed

of two rows of bones, of irregular articulations, and firmly held in position by ligaments; they are accessible only upon the posterior or lateral part; resection of individual bones of the carpus may be successfully accomplished as follows:—

Operation.—The following is the method by a single incision:—Make a longitudinal incision on the dorsal surface of the carpus, over the bone which it is desired to remove; draw aside the tendons which are met with in the dissection, divide the lateral ligaments, and seize the bone; if it is necessary divide the bone, and draw it outwards, at the same time separating its attachments on the palmar surface; for this purpose a short and strong scalpel should be employed.

Resection of the Entire Carpus.—(Fig. 214.) The operations proposed for the removal of all the bones of the carpus are numerous, and may be divided into those in which the tendons are preserved, and those in which they are divided.

Methods, Preserving the Tendons.—Chassaignac operates with a single curved incision, the convexity being downwards; he commences disarticulation on the radio-ulnar part of the articulation, and successively removes the individual bones.

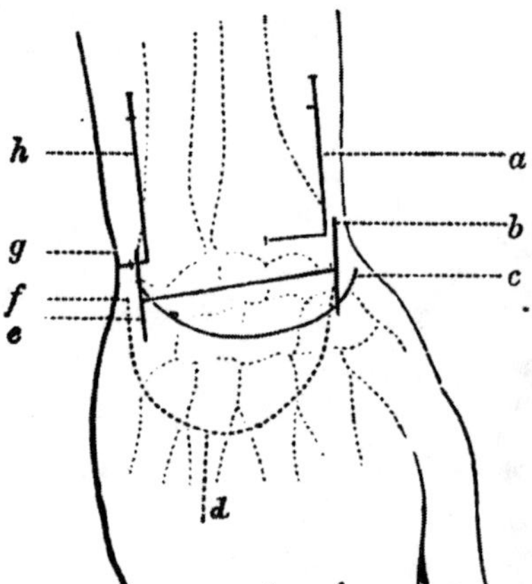

Fig. 214.

A more common method has been by parallel incisions, one on the radial, *b*, and the other on the ulnar border, *e*, joined by a transverse incision on the dorsum of the carpus; Fergusson has repeatedly operated in this manner.

Erichsen made a transverse incision over the centre of the dorsal aspect of the joint, and two other incisions at right angles to this, reaching from above the styloid process; a flap being then raised on the surface of the extensor tendons, from between which were removed the fragments of bone.

Simon removed all the bones of the carpus, except the trapezium and pisiform, with a metacarpal bone, by the following method:—Two long incisions were made on the anterior and posterior aspects of the joint, reaching from about two inches above the wrist, back and front, to the centre of the palm and dorsum of the hand, the incisions being so managed as to run between the tendons coursing down to their destination.

Methods, Dividing the Tendons.—Stanley, believing that division of the tendons was not as dangerous as drawing them aside, made a free semicircular incision above the wrist, turning back a considerable flap, together with tendons and integuments.

Butcher divided the tendons, but left those of the thumb intact. He says:—"The forearm, placed in a state of pronation, was grasped and supported above the wrist by an assistant, while the hand was steadied by a second. Standing on the right side of the patient, I thrust the knife down to the carpal bones, two lines to the ulnar side of the extensor secundi internodii pollicis, from a quarter to half an inch below the radio-carpal articulation, *c;* from this point it was swept in a curvilinear direction, downwards, close to the carpal extremities of the metacarpal bones, and carried up to a point just below the end of the ulna, *g,* and fully half an inch higher than that where the knife was first laid on. The flap thus marked out, *c, g,* was rapidly dissected up, and consisted of the integuments, areolar tissue, and extensor tendons of the four fingers. * * * By the elevation of these soft parts, *en masse*, the diseased bones were at once brought into view; the flap being turned up to its base, which was oblique, the scalpel was passed further, higher up under it, liberating the soft parts from the back of the radius and ulna, together with the second extensor of the thumb, from the osseous groove in which it lay: thus the tendon remained undisturbed in its superior and part of its lateral connexions. The liberation of the tendon being accomplished after this manner, it was an easy proceeding to divide the ligamentous shreds which bound the diseased bones together; and by forcing down the hand the carious ends of the radius and ulna were made to project; a few cautious touches of the knife, carried close to the base of the styloid process of the radius, left uninjured and undisturbed the radial artery in its near proximity: while a similar guarded proceeding on the ulnar side and in front preserved the ulnar vessels. The next proceeding was to remove the protruded bones, which was accomplished with facility, by passing the fine blade of my own saw (as set for resection) in front of the bones and cutting backwards."

In a second case Butcher removed all the carpal with the fourth and fifth metacarpal bones by the following method:—"I raised a flap from the dorsum of the hand, beginning a little below and outside the second extensor of the thumb, over the junction of the first and second carpal range, and carried the knife in a semicircular manner, downwards and outwards, over the posterior thirds of the third, fourth, and fifth metacarpal bones, and from this upwards to a point nearly opposite to where the incision commenced, *f;* the flap thus formed, including the external tendons, was dissected up, and the diseased carpus fully brought into view. In order to expose the metacarpal bones sufficiently, a straight incision had to be carried along the fourth, *d,* and a flap dissected outwards."

Resections of the Radius.—The radius may be excised in part or whole. The lower extremity has frequently been removed with almost complete recovery of the natural motions of the part. The upper extremity and shaft have also been excised, giving good results. Carnochan exsected the entire bone, and even in this case the functions of the wrist and fingers were for the most part recovered.

Resection of the Lower Extremity.—The lower extremity of the radius is broad, of a quadrilateral form, having two articular surfaces, one concave, on the lower part, for articulation with the scaphoid and semilunar bones; the other on the inner side, narrow and concave, to articulate with the lower end of the ulna; the anterior and posterior ligaments are attached to the margin of the joint, and the lateral ligament to the styloid process; the posterior surface has three grooves for the passage of the tendons of extensor muscles; the outer surface of the styloid process has two grooves for tendons, and its base gives attachment to the supinator longus muscle; the pronator quadratus muscle occupies the lower fourth of the anterior surface.

Operation.—A straight incision is made along the radial border, over the part parallel with its long axis, the bone is then denuded and divided with the chain saw (Fig. 215); the bone being divided is raised by the left hand, and disarticulated with the point of the knife at the articulation, *b* (Fig. 216), avoiding the artery, *a*, and preserving the tendons.

Modifications.—Roux and others

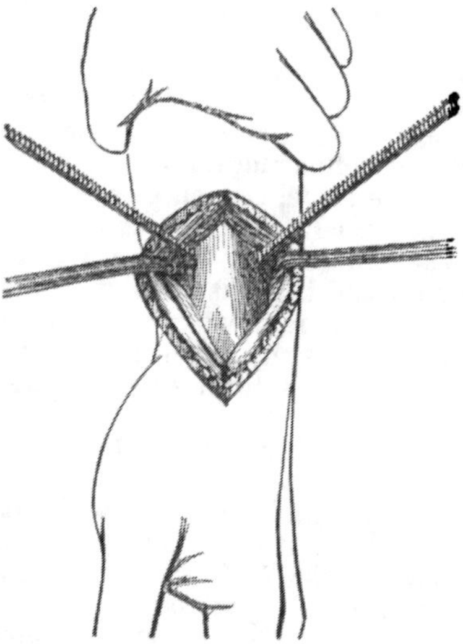

Fig. 215.

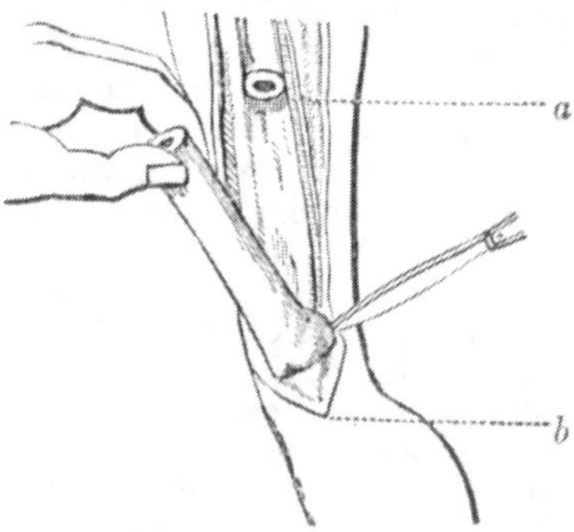

Fig. 216.

add a transverse incision, as seen at *a* (Fig. 214), and raise a flap. Carnochan removed the lower four-fifths of the radius as follows:—"The arm, supported by assistants, was placed so that the ulnar border of the forearm rested firmly upon the edge of the table, in a state of semi-pronation. A longitudinal incision was made in the direction of the radius, on its external anterior border; commencing about two inches below the head of the bone, and extending downwards to a point opposite, and a little behind, the styloid process. Two terminal incisions were then made at the extremities of the first one, extending transversely backwards, about three-quarters of an inch. The bone was laid bare a short distance below its middle, and the dissection carried upwards to within three-quarters of an inch below the bicipital tuberosity, so as to expose the bone on its different aspects; at this part the radius was perfectly sound, and its section was easily effected by means of the chain saw. The remaining steps of the operation consisted in separating the diseased portion from the soft parts, and in isolating the lower part of the radius from its attachments at the radio-carpal articulation, without injury to the arteries, nerves, or tendons. The humeral artery was compressed, during the dissection, by an assistant; the interosseous artery and a small branch only requiring the ligature."

Resection of the Upper Extremity.—The head of the radius is quite superficial on its posterior part; it is surrounded by the orbicular ligament, which retains it in the lesser sigmoid cavity of the ulna; below the head, on the inner aspect of the bone, is the tuberosity which gives attachment to the tendon of the biceps muscle.

Operation.—A straight incision is made on the posterior and external part of the arm over the bone to be removed; the soft parts are separated, the bone divided and raised from its articulation by dividing with the point of a knife its ligaments.

Resection of the Shaft.—The shaft of the radius is enveloped with muscles; on its anterior surface are the flexor longus pollicis and the pronator quadratus; on its posterior surface the extensor ossis metacarpi pollicis, and extensor primi internodii pollicis; and on its external surface the pronator radii teres.

Operation.—Make a long straight incision on the external aspect of the bone, parallel with its shaft; separate the muscles, and, drawing the lips of the wound apart, denude the bone; the chain saw is passed, the bone divided at the two points selected, and the fragment raised from its bed.

Resection of the Entire Radius.—The entire radius was resected by Carnochan, the operation leaving a useful hand and wrist, and a somewhat useful arm.

Operation.—"An incision was made in the direction of the axis of the radius, commencing at a point immediately below the external condyles of the humerus, and extending downwards to a point opposite and a little behind the styloid process of the radius; next, two other incisions were made at the extremities of the first one, extending transversely backwards, about three quarters of an inch. These incisions extend through the integuments, and subcutaneous cellular tissue and fascia; the middle third of the radius was now easily reached, and made bare on its outer aspect by dividing the inter-muscular tissue, behind the extensor carpi radialis brevior. The tissues were separated from the posterior aspect of the bone at this place, the edge of the knife being kept close upon the bone. The knife was now carried along the anterior surface of the bone, laying it bare as far as the interosseous ligament; the upper part of the radius was next denuded, and then the lower part, care being taken to raise the tendons from their grooves without injury. The bone was divided at its centre, and each part raised, and in turn disarticulated; the upper fragment had formed bony attachments to the humerus, and required a chisel to separate it; the carpal articulation was separated with the point of the bistoury."

Resections of the Ulna.—The upper and lower portion of the extremities of the ulna, and different portions of its shaft, have frequently been removed with the happiest results. Jones and Carnochan have excised the entire bone with success.

RESECTION OF THE LOWER EXTREMITY.—The lower extremity of the ulna articulates on its external surface with the radius, being excluded from the articulation of the wrist joint; it has an anterior and posterior ligament uniting it to the radius, and a lateral ligament connecting the styloid process to the carpus.

Operation.—The hand being carried outwards, make a longitudinal incision over the lower extremity of the ulna; dissect the soft parts from the bone to the required height, and carry the chain saw under the bone (Fig. 217); having divided the bone, proceed to dissect it from its articular connexions.

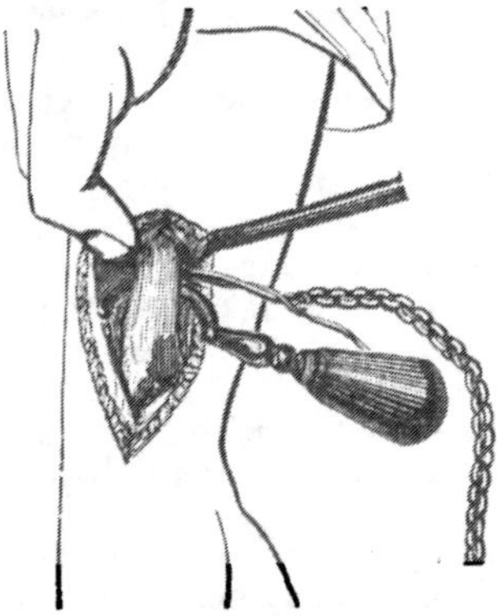

FIG 217.

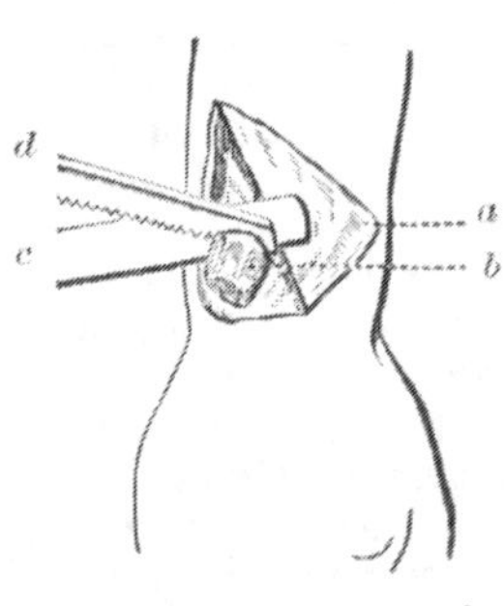

FIG. 218.

Modifications.—(Fig. 218.) The hand being carried outwards, a longitudinal incision is made along the internal border of the ulna, and terminated by a transverse incision outwards, *a*, or inwards, *b* (Fig. 214). A triangular flap is then carefully dissected up, and the tendons being drawn aside, and the vessels carefully avoided, the bone, *b*, is denuded of its soft parts and disarticulated with the bistoury. A small slip of wood, *c*, is passed beneath the extremity of the bone, which is then sawn through, as at *d*.—(*Bernard* and *Huette*.)

RESECTION OF THE SHAFT.—Make a longitudinal incision on its posterior part, parallel with the shaft, and external to its border; separate the soft parts and periosteum from the bone; make a section of the bone at the two points selected, and remove the included portion. Chassaignac advises, when a large portion of the bone is to be removed, to make two or three separate incisions instead of one, and remove the bone in pieces.

Modifications.—Velpeau directs as follows:—" The most convenient process here, consists in making two very long and slightly curved incisions, with their concavities facing each other, as in circumscribing an ellipse. The lips of these incisions are then dissected in front and behind, as far as the radial border of the bone. The section of the bone may then be effected by means of the chain saw."

RESECTION OF THE UPPER EXTREMITY.—A straight incision is made over the part, the soft parts and periosteum separated, and the bone divided with the chain saw at the proper point; the bone is removed from its articular connexions with the point of the knife; the ulnar nerve lying along the inner side is carefully protected by keeping the edge of the knife turned to the bone, and if exposed by drawing it inwards.

RESECTION OF THE OLECRANON.—Make a straight incision along the posterior part of the bone; separate the soft parts, and make the section with the chain saw, or divide it as far as possible, externally, with a small saw, and complete the section with the bone forceps; care should be taken to divide the tendon of the biceps to as small an extent as practicable, and the operator should, as far as possible, enucleate the process from its fibrous investments, with the handle of the scalpel, with a view to the future efficiency of the extensor muscle.

Modifications.—Velpeau made a crucial incision, bent the arm, and was enabled with two cuts of the saw to excise a cuneiform fragment corresponding with the length of the olecranon. Gross advises a T incision. Buck operated as follows:—" A longitudinal incision, five inches in length, was made over the middle of the olecranon, extending three inches above and two below it, penetrating to the bone; the triceps tendon was then divided at its insertion towards either edge, care being taken to avoid cutting across the aponeurosis, which is continuous from the edges of the tendon over the muscles lying on the posterior part of the forearm, and inserted into the edges of the olecranon; these insertions of the fascia, as well as the origins of the muscles beneath it, were dissected up from the bone to the extent of nearly two inches, which allowed the olecranon to be exposed, when the edges of the incision were drawn asunder over the condyles. Broad, curved spatulæ were used for this purpose, and with the amputating saw one-half the thickness of the bone was cut through with great facility; further progress was made in the section with Hey's saw, after which the separation was easily completed with a chisel and mallet."

Resection of the Entire Ulna.—Carnochan operated as follows:—" One assistant held and supported the upper arm of the diseased limb, compressing at the same time the humeral artery; and then seizing the hand and wrist, rotated inwards the limb from the shoulder-joint, and carried the pronation of the forearm so far as to cause the palm of the hand to look directly outwards. The elbow-joint was now slightly flexed, and the hand elevated. This twisted position of the vena upon the radius placed the ulna upon the posterior and outer aspect of the forearm, and rendered it more easily accessible. The limb thus placed, the assistants maintaining the arm and forearm steadily, standing upon the right side of the patient, and placing the fingers of the left hand upon the integuments of the forearm, towards the elbow, with a strong, straight, sharp-pointed bistoury, I made an incision along the posterior and inner aspect of the ulna; commencing at the lower part of its superior third and extending downwards to a point over the extremity of the styloid process. This divided the tegumentary layer and fascia, which were found dense, matted, and infiltrated. The tendon of the extensor carpi ulnaris was pulled back, and the bone exposed. * * * At the carpo-ulnar articulation, a transverse incision, about an inch long, parting from the lower extremity of the first incision, was made across the back of the wrist. The superficial tissues were here reflected, and the tendon of the extensor carpi ulnaris carefully detached from its groove on the lower part of the ulna. The dissection was now carried along the anterior surface of the lower portion of the ulna, and the soft parts were detached from the bone as far as the interosseous ligament, the ulnar artery and nerve being carefully avoided. The soft parts were now detached from the posterior surface of the ulna, avoiding injury to the extensor tendons. The bone was divided at the lower part of the middle third. The lower fragment was then separated from its articular connexions. The incision was then prolonged upwards, along the posterior surface of the ulna, terminating at the upper part of the olecranon, opposite its outer edge; to this a terminal incision was joined, which extended transversely across the back of the elbow-joint, as far as the inner margin of the ulna. The soft tissues were now dissected from the bone, upon its posterior and anterior aspects, as far as the interosseous ligament, and as high up as the insertion of the brachialis internus muscle. The bone was next seized and pulled from the radius, and a knife, curved flatwise, was passed close upon its interosseal margin, grazing the bone, and dividing the interosseal membrane upwards; the soft parts being held apart, and the interosseous and ulnar arteries protected. The elbow-joint was now flexed, and opened behind, by entering the bistoury close to the inner edge of the olecranon. The attachment of the triceps extensor was next divided, by cutting directly outwards. The ulnar nerve was found and hooked aside, the lateral ligament divided, the ulnar carried backwards, and the attachments of the brachialis anticus muscle divided; the coronary ligament was cut, and the bone removed from its articulation.

RESECTION OF THE INFERIOR EXTREMITIES OF THE RADIUS AND ULNA.—Make incisions on the radial and ulnar border of the lower part of the forearm, as in the method of operating for the removal of either bone singly (Fig. 214); divide the bones with the chain saw, and separate their carpal articulations with the point of the knife; the tendons anteriorly and posteriorly must be carefully displaced, and the radial and ulnar arteries avoided.

Modifications.—(Fig. 219.) 1st. The hand being pronated and held firmly upon some solid surface, two longitudinal incisions are made along the borders of the radius and ulna, *a b*, *c d*. A transverse incision across the back of the joint unites the lower extremities of these, *b d*, and (2d) the quadrilateral flap, *a b*, *c d*, thus circumscribed, is dissected up and turned backwards. 3d. The disarticulation is then effected, the tendons surrounding the two bones being detached with as little injury as possible (*Bernard* and *Huette*); Roux made two transverse incisions, extending from the lower extremity of the longitudinal incisions, across the dorsum of the wrist, to the edges of the extensor tendons, leaving the central portion of integument undivided; Velpeau dissected the flap from above downwards.

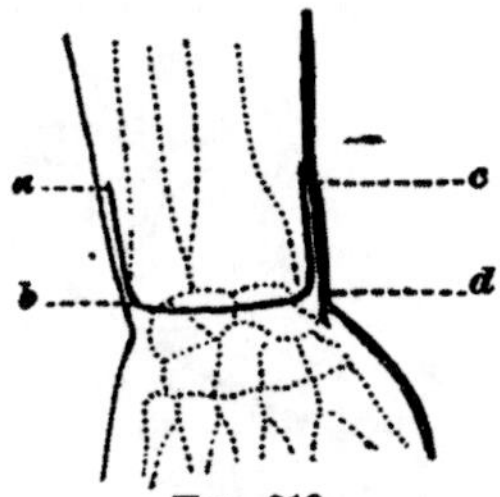

FIG. 219.

RESECTION OF THE SUPERIOR EXTREMITIES OF THE RADIUS AND ULNA.—The operation may be performed as in resection of the lower extremities by lateral incisions; the radius is first removed; the bone being denuded with the chain saw, the head is disarticulated by dividing the attachment of the biceps, and the orbicular ligament; the ulna is divided in a similar manner, and its disarticulation effected, carefully guarding against injuring the ulnar nerve on its inner aspect, the artery in front, and preserving if possible the attachments of the brachialis anticus muscle.

Modifications.—Moreau's method was to join the extremities of the lateral incisions (Fig. 219) and dissect up the flap; a crucial incision, lateral incisions with a transverse in the middle, or H, and other methods have been proposed.

RESECTION OF THE RADIUS AND ULNA.—Compton, of New Orleans, excised the entire ulna and all but a portion of the entire radius, for a severe compound fracture. A straight incision was made the whole length of the inner side of the radius, and a counter opening opposite the olecranon process; both bones were carefully dissected out, with the exception of a portion of the lower end of the radius; the periosteum was mostly detached.

Resection of the Elbow-Joint.—A great variety of methods of performing this operation have been devised, of which we mention the following:—

SINGLE STRAIGHT INCISION.—Chassaignac describes this method thus (Fig. 220):—A single straight incision, *a*, *c*, is made on the external and slightly posterior part of the elbow, commencing four fingers' breadths above the joint, and extending to a proper dis-

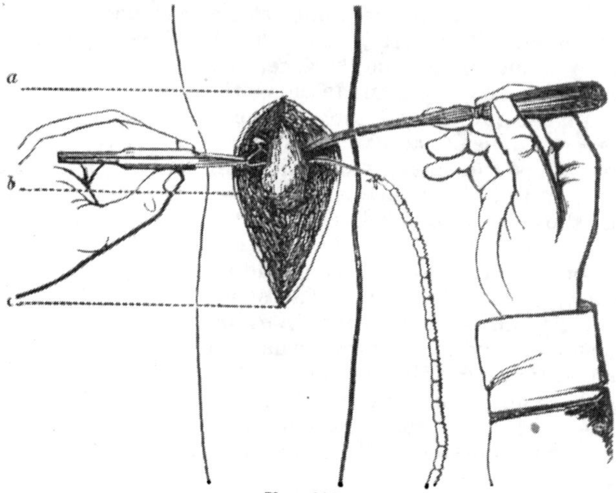

FIG. 220.

tance below; the head of the radius is first exposed, the shaft divided with the chain saw, and the upper extremity removed; the humerus, *b*, is now laid bare at the proper point above the articulation, and divided with the chain saw; the lower fragment is then readily made to protrude from the wound, and disarticulation is effected, care being taken to protect the ulnar nerve; the upper extremity of the ulna is now denuded, and readily sawn.

Modifications.—Park made a single straight incision in the axis of the limb, upon the median line of the dorsal surface of the joint, extending two inches above and below the olecranon, the biceps was cut, the lateral ligaments divided, and the bones exposed.

TWO QUADRILATERAL FLAPS—H INCISION.—Moreau operated as follows (*Malgaigne, op. cit.*):—"Place the patient on his belly opposite a well-lighted window, on a table three feet ten inches high, covered with a mattress, so that his arm rests on one of the edges of the table, and presents to the operator the posterior and internal part of the articulation. You may also operate on the patient sitting; but the position is not so favorable. The tourniquet should be first applied on the upper third of the arm. The arm being semi-flexed, plunge a scalpel or bistoury down to the ridge of the internal condyle, about two inches above its tuberosity, and prolong the incision longitudinally to the articulation; do the same on the other side; then unite these two wounds by a transverse section, dividing the skin and triceps brachialis, immediately above the olecranon. The result is a quadrilateral flap, which dissect up, and cause an assistant to hold back; then, with the point of the bistoury directed on the left index-finger, detach the soft parts from the anterior surface of the bone, opposite where you would carry the saw. When the way is clear, pass the handle of a scalpel under the bone, and saw upon it; turn back the fragment cut off, and you may easily detach it from the joint, which may be opened from before backwards; then go to the bones of the forearm. Prolong the external lateral incision along the radius as far as necessary, separate the head of this bone from the neighboring soft parts and ulna, pass a compress under it, and cut it off, trying to preserve all or part of the attachment of the biceps; then lay bare the ulna, prolonging downwards the internal incision, and turning down the second quadrilateral flap that results. Isolate the portion to be cut off; put it aside from the soft parts with a compress or protecting guard and saw it, preserving, if possible, the attachment of the brachialis anticus."

Modifications.—Dupuytren, after raising the flaps, removed the olecranon, and dissected the ulnar nerve from its groove, and drew it aside.

Two Semilunar Incisions and Excision of the Flap.—Manne made two semilunar incisions, on the posterior part of the joint; these were joined by longitudinal incisions, external and internal, and the inclosed integument was raised with the bone.

The T Incision.—Roux made a T incision, the longitudinal branch being placed on the external part of the limb, and the transverse branch commencing at the olecranon and crossing the first at right angles; two triangular flaps are thus formed, which being raised permit the removal of the three articulating surfaces.

Resections of the Humerus.—The humerus is excised only in part, as follows:—

Resection of a Single Condyle of the Humerus.—The condyles of the humerus give origin to the flexor and extensor muscles of the carpus, hand, and fingers; to the internal are attached the pronator radii teres and flexor muscles, and to the external condyle the anconeus, supinator brevis, and extensor muscles.

Operation.—An incision, either straight, curved, or crucial, is made on the posterior part of the condyle to be removed, the soft parts dissected from the bone, and with the saw having an articulated back, or Symanowsky's saw, the condyle is divided and removed; a section of bone may be removed by first making a hole for the chain saw with the bone drill, and then cutting out such a section as is desired.

RESECTION OF THE LOWER EXTREMITY OF THE HUMERUS.—The lower part of the humerus presents on its anterior and posterior surfaces, depressions for corresponding prominences on the ulna; the articular surface is very irregular, being divided by a groove into two parts; it is on a lower plane than the condyles, and the inner part descends lower than the outer; the flexor and extensor muscles of the hand arise from its condyles: it has anterior, posterior, and lateral ligaments; the brachial artery lies in front, and the ulnar nerve passes over the inner condyle on its posterior and external part.

Operation.—(Fig. 221.) Resection of the lower extremity of the humerus may be effected through a straight incision made on the posterior and external part of the arm; the incision should be

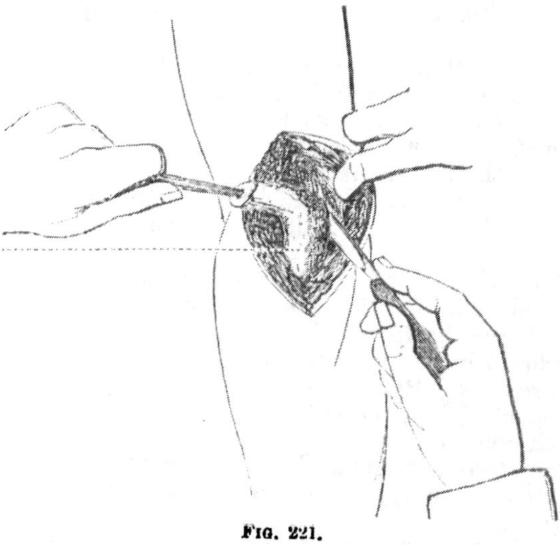

FIG. 221.

sufficiently extensive to make a free exposure of the bone, *a*, when the wound is separated; the bone is denuded and divided with the chain saw; raising the cut end with the left hand, or with forceps, the operator proceeds to disarticulate with the point of the knife, carefully avoiding the brachial artery in front, and the ulnar nerve behind and at the inside.

Modifications.—Moreau operated as follows (*Bernard* and *Huette*):—(Fig. 222.) 1st. The arm being semiflexed, and the posterior face of the articulation turned towards the surgeon, two longitudinal incisions, each about two inches and a half in length, should be carried upwards along the humerus, one from the outer side of the external condyle, the other from the inner side of the internal condyle; 2d. These two incisions should then be united by a transverse section through the skin and triceps muscle, immediately above the olecranon; a quadrilateral flap is thus formed, which being dissected from below upwards, must be supported by an assistant; 3d. The surrounding parts, and the ulnar nerve divested of its fibrous sheath, should then be carefully isolated from the bone, and drawn inwards by an assistant; 4th. The bone being carefully denuded, a slip of wood or metal is slid under it to protect the soft parts from the saw; the separated portion of the bone is then cut loose from its various adhesions, and the joint opened from behind."

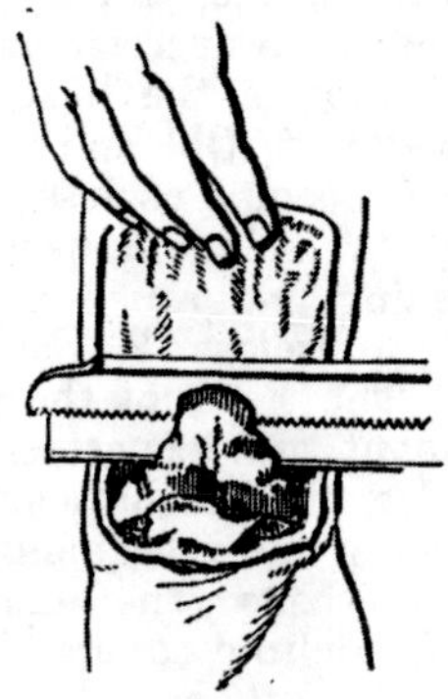

FIG. 222.

Various incisions have been made in this operation, as the H, the crucial, a straight incision with one lateral incision, etc.

RESECTION OF THE SHAFT.—The lower half of the shaft of the humerus is closely invested with muscles, as the brachialis anticus and triceps; the upper half gives attachment principally to the muscles from the shoulder, chest, and back, as the deltoid, pectoralis major, latissimus dorsi, and rotators; the brachial artery, with the median and ulnar nerves, passes along the posterior margin of the biceps muscle, and the superior profunda artery and musculonerve wind around the posterior and external part of the upper and middle portion of the shaft.

Operation.—If the upper portion of the shaft is to be removed, a straight incision is made on the external part of the deltoid muscle, care being taken not to extend the incision upwards so as to involve the circumflex artery and nerve; when the lower part of the shaft is excised, the incision should be along the outer border of the brachialis anticus muscle, avoiding the external cutaneous nerve. The bone is readily exposed and removed to the required extent.

Velpeau recommends at the upper part of the arm a semilunar incision, with its free border outwards and backwards.

RESECTION OF THE UPPER EXTREMITY.—Chassaignac gives the following indications for the operation:—1. Compound fracture of the superior extremity, with protrusion of the shaft through the wound of the soft parts, rupture of the capsule, and destruction of the periosteum; or, 2. Fractures of the head of the bone from gunshot wound, necessitating the removal of splinters of bone; 3. The lodgment of foreign bodies, balls, or projectiles, in the head of the humerus, resulting in a comminution of the bone, rupture of the capsule, and the final development of an inflammation terminating in necrosis and caries; 4. Compound dislocation with projection of the head of the bone through the wound of the soft parts; 5. Old and irreducible luxations, especially when the limb has become useless; or, when the head of the bone presses upon the vessels and nerves, causing violent pains, paralysis, or threatening gangrene; 6. True anchylosis, in a manner to render the limb useless; 7. Caries and necrosis of the head of the bone.

The head of the humerus is surrounded by the capsular ligament, and has attached to its upper extremity the following muscles, viz. the subscapularis inserted into the lesser tuberosity, the supra and infra spinatus and teres minor, inserted into its greater tuberosity; the long head of the biceps runs through the capsule; the deltoid covers the external surface of the joint.

Operations.—A straight incision is made, commencing between the acromion and coracoid processes, and half an inch below the clavicle, and is carried downwards to the requisite extent along the deltoid muscle on the anterior part of the joint; the bone is here quite superficial, and is most readily exposed; the bicipital groove being found, the long head of the biceps muscle is dislodged and drawn aside, *b* (Fig. 223), and the tendons of the rotator muscles of the head of the bone are divided, being first

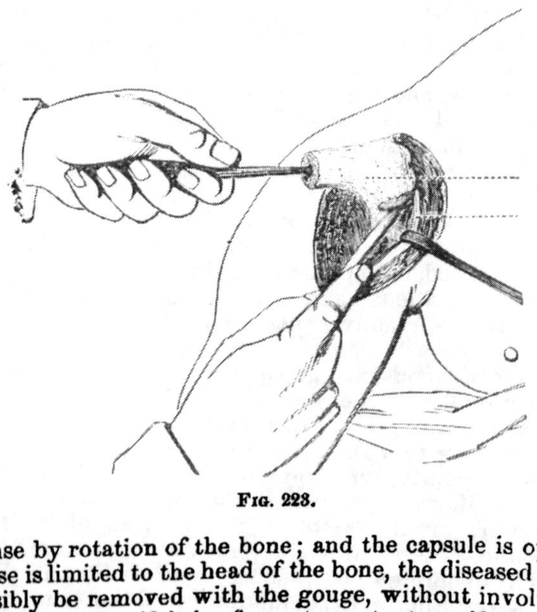

FIG. 223.

made tense by rotation of the bone; and the capsule is opened. If the disease is limited to the head of the bone, the diseased structures may possibly be removed with the gouge, without involving parts beyond the capsule; if it is of greater extent, or if the operation is undertaken for fracture involving the upper part of the shaft, the bone should be exposed at the proper place and divided with the chain saw; being now elevated, *a*, with the forceps or the elevator (tirefond, Chassaignac), the upper extremity is disarticulated with the point of the knife.

Modifications.—The methods of performing this operation are numerous; White made the single straight incision; Baudens made, in addition, a lateral subcutaneous division of the deltoid; Moreau made a quadrilateral flap, including the deltoid: Sabatier made a V incision (Fig. 224), having its base upwards; Monel made a semilunar flap, with its base above; Malgaigne recommends Lisfranc's lateral and posterior flap in amputation; Syme made a triangular flap on the external part of the deltoid; Nelaton commences the incision half an inch within and below the acromio-clavicular articulation, follows the anterior curve of the acromio-clavicular border, and terminates behind, at the angle formed by the acromion with the spine of the scapula; Stromeyer made a semicircu-

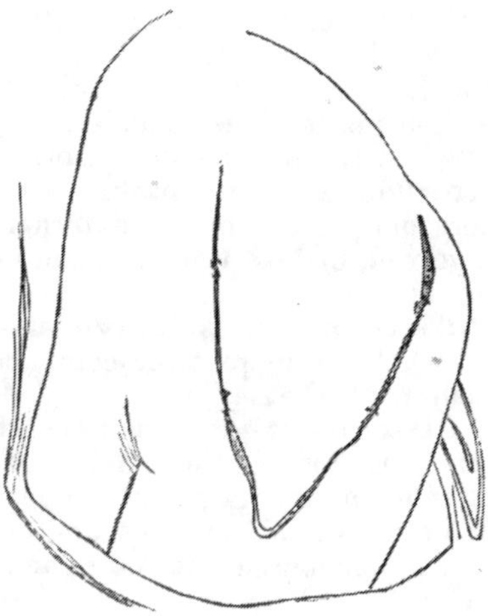

Fig. 224.

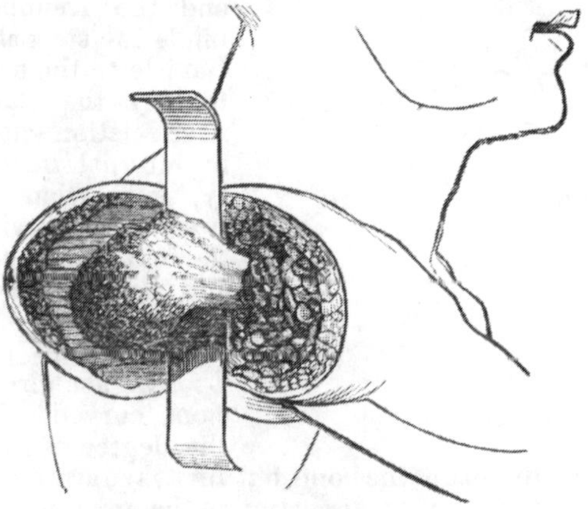

Fig. 225.

lar incision, commencing at the posterior margin of the acromion, and passing downwards and forwards, five inches, and opened the articulation above and behind to avoid the tendon of the biceps; Blackman made the triangular flap; Erichsen recommends a U-shaped incision (Fig. 225), which includes the deltoid muscle, the isolation being effected with a spatula.

Resection of the Shoulder-Joint.—The removal of the upper extremity of the humerus with the glenoid cavity may be accomplished by the methods already given for excision of the head of the former. Chassaignac directs a longitudinal incision on the anterior part of the shoulder, opening into the joint; if the disease involves the scapula, join a horizontal incision backwards under the acromion, and turn backwards and downwards the flaps; if the coracoid process, or the external extremity of the clavicle is also involved, make a third incision inwards.

Resections of the Clavicle.—The clavicle may require excision in whole or in part for complicated fractures, luxations, necrosis, malignant diseases, &c.

RESECTION OF THE STERNAL EXTREMITY OF THE CLAVICLE.—The inner portion of the clavicle is of a triangular form, and gives attachment on its postero-superior surface to the sterno-mastoid and sterno-hyoid muscles, and on its anterior surface to the pectoralis major muscle; it is directed inwards, and slightly downwards and forwards, and articulates with the sternum; its ligaments are the anterior and posterior sterno-clavicular, the interclavicular, and the rhomboid, which binds the sternal end of the clavicle to the first rib; posteriorly the clavicle is in near relation with the pleura, internal mammary artery, subclavian vein, and transverse cervical artery; the innominata on the right, and the thoracic duct on the left side.

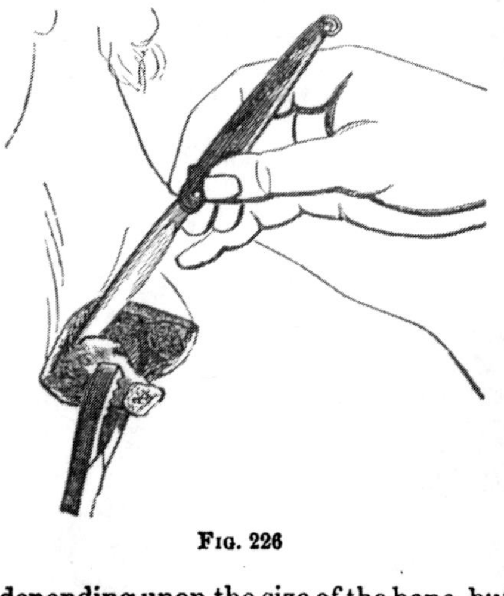

FIG. 226

Operation.—(Fig. 226.) Chassaignac directs an incision curved downwards, the degree of the curvature depending upon the size of the bone, but always so arranged as to enable the operator to raise it by dissection to the upper part; after raising the flap, instead of separating the muscles, a chain saw should be passed at the point where the bone is to be divided; the fragment is then removed by carefully disarticulating it with the point of the knife, and avoiding wounding the important parts posteriorly.

RESECTION OF THE SCAPULAR EXTREMITY OF THE CLAVICLE.—The outer portion of the clavicle is broad and flat, and gives attachment on its posterior part to the trapezius, and on its anterior to the deltoid; it is bound to the acromion by a superior and inferior ligament, and to the coracoid process by the coraco-clavicular, or coracoid and trapezoid ligaments.

Operation.—Velpeau removed the outer third of the clavicle for necrosis by a crucial incision, each about four inches in length; the flaps were raised, the attachments of the deltoid and trapezius divided, and the acromio-clavicular ligaments cut; a wooden lever was introduced into the articulation, the bone raised and detached.

Travers removed all the scapula but the sternal extremity for a tumor by the following method:—A crucial incision was made through the integuments and the platysma myoides, one limb of which was nearly in the line of the clavicle, and the other at right angles, and the flaps and facial coverings successively dissected, down to the external basis of the tumor. The pectoralis and deltoid muscles were then carefully detached from their clavicular origin, avoiding the cephalic vein, and the fibres of the trapezius and cleido-mastoid muscles divided on a director. One considerable vessel, in the situation of the transversalis humeri, required ligation. Disarticulation of the scapular extremity of the bone was next effected without difficulty, and the mobility thus communicated to the mass, facilitated the completion of the operation. A director was now worked beneath the bone, as near to the sternal articulation as practicable, and with a pair of strong bone nippers thus introduced, it was completely divided. The subclavius muscle and rhomboid ligament were detached, and the operation completed.

Chassaignac advises a curved incision, with its convexity forwards and a little outwards, which, reflected backwards, completely exposes the bone; this is divided with the chain saw, and being seized with the forceps, is raised, and the ligaments divided.

Syme removed the external extremity for a tumor by making an elliptical incision from the middle of the clavicle backwards, over the most prominent part of the tumor.

Mott exsected all but the scapular portion of the clavicle, for a tumor, as follows:—A semilunar incision, exposing the pectoralis major muscle, was made from the sterno-clavicular articulation, to near the junction of the clavicle with the acromion; owing to the extent of the tumor it was impossible to get under the clavicle from below, and an incision was made from the outer edge of the external jugular vein, over the tumor, to the top of the shoulder, the platysma myoides and a portion of the trapezius divided, the bone exposed external to the coracoid process, and divided with the chain saw. Another incision was made over the tumor from the sternal extremity of the clavicle to the termination of the first incision at the external jugular vein; in the subsequent dissection, owing to the large size of the tumor, and the incorporation of the structures with it, the external jugular vein and a large number of vessels required ligature, and the outer portion of the sterno-mastoid muscle was divided.

Bartlett, of Missouri, made an incision from the sternal articulation to the base of the tumor, and thence on either side towards the acromion, the bone was divided near the sternum with the chain saw, and the external portion dissected out.

Resection of the entire Clavicle.—Warren, of Boston, operated as follows for osteo-sarcoma:—An incision was made from the acromial extremity of the clavicle to the external extremity of the clavicle of the opposite side; this was crossed by an incision at right angles with it, beginning just below the middle of the sterno-mastoid muscle, and extending to the face of the pectoralis muscle below the middle of the clavicle; the four flaps were then dissected from the surface of the tumor; the outer extremity of the clavicle was laid bare by dissecting the deltoid muscle from its anterior edge, and the trapezius from its posterior edge, and the division of the corneo-clavicular ligament; the chain saw was passed and the bone divided by means of the needle for resection (Fig. 195); the fragment is seized with the forceps and the detachment of the soft parts effected with the point of the knife, the edge being kept constantly turned towards the bone, in order not to make the slightest wound of the soft parts.

Davie made an incision of from two to three inches in extent on the sternal extremity of the clavicle, in a line with the axis of that bone; the ligamentous connections were divided; a piece of sole leather was introduced under the bone, and the bone sawed through one inch from its sternal extremity; the fragment was then detached by tearing through the inter-clavicular ligament.

Sédillot, operating on the left clavicle, made a crucial incision through the integuments, detached the soft parts, sawed through the bone, upon the handle of a scalpel; passed behind it; the muscular and ligamentous attachments were divided; difficulty was experienced in disarticulating, owing to the proximity of the subclavian artery.

Wedderburn, of New Orleans, removed the entire clavicle for necrosis, as follows:—An incision was made down to the clavicle, over its entire length, and sufficiently far beyond its articulating points to enable the disarticulation to be effected. The soft parts attached to the upper surface and the anterior border of the bone, were separated—next the separation of the acromion effected—the dissection was then continued close to the bone beneath, whilst the parts were kept on the stretch by elevating the bone from the point just indicated.

Blackman, of Cincinnati, removed the entire clavicle for necrosis and exostosis by an incision commencing at the middle of the sternum.

Velpeau (*op. cit.*) gives the following method of resecting the clavicle:—"An incision parallel to its cutaneous border, and which extends a little beyond its extremities, will ordinarily answer for this purpose, or we may make two vertical incisions, of one to two inches in length, one on the outside, the other on the inside of the first incision, the flap resulting from which divisions, on being raised up, completely lays bare the bone. We then disarticulate either the sternal or acromial extremity, and grasp it with the left hand in order to raise it up, while with the right we detach with the bistoury the adhesions upon its lower border. We might also saw the bone through its middle and remove the two halves separately."

Chassaignac directs an incision parallel to the clavicle, isolation of the bone at its middle portion, and division by the chain saw; the fragments are then separately removed.

Guérin advises a longitudinal incision, upon the upper surface of the clavicle, extending beyond either extremity; if there is a large tumor, vertical incisions may be made on the first, giving the form of a double T.

RESECTION OF THE SHAFT OF THE CLAVICLE.—The central portion of the clavicle has attached to its under surface the subclavius muscle, while its anterior and upper portions are nearly subcutaneous.

Operation.—The methods of operating on this part of the clavicle are the same as are given for the extremities; the incision may be straight, curved, or crucial.

Resections of the Scapula.—The scapula may be removed in part or totally as follows:

RESECTION OF THE ACROMION PROCESS.—The acromion, the external termination of the spine of the scapula, articulates on its inner border with the outer extremity of the clavicle; it affords a partial origin to the deltoid and trapezius muscles, and its under surface overhangs the shoulder joint; it is united to the clavicle by a superior and inferior ligament, and to the coracoid process by the coraco-acromial ligament.

Operation.—Chassaignac directs a semilunar incision at the posterior part of the shoulder with the convexity downwards, the passage of the chain saw under the narrow part of the neck of the acromion, division of the bone at this part, and disarticulation. Others prefer the crucial or T incision. Fergusson followed the track of sinuses.

RESECTION OF THE SPINE OF THE SCAPULA.—The posterior border or crest of the spine of the scapula is superficial; it gives origin by its upper surface to the trapezius and supraspinatus muscles, by its inferior surface to the deltoid and infraspinatus muscles.

Operation.—The bone may be readily exposed, owing to its superficial position, by an incision made parallel to its border; if required, the incision may be curved downwards so as to raise a flap; the bone being denuded, the diseased portions may be removed with a strong cutting forceps. Chassaignac directs to perforate the bone with a drill, pass the chain saw, and separate the diseased part.

RESECTION OF AN ANGLE OR BORDER OF THE SCAPULA.—In resection of the *superior angle*, Velpeau directs a transverse incision which would involve a portion of the trapezius and levator anguli scapulæ, and in resection of the *inferior angle* a transverse incision below the spine through the latissimus dorsi; the bone should be removed with Liston's forceps or the chain saw. Chassaignac recommends a V incision in resection of the inferior angle, the branches of which are parallel to the borders of the scapula. Von Walther removed the lower angle and part of the body of the scapula by a crucial incision over the part, turning back the flaps, separating the attachments of the muscles to the outer and inner edge, and sawing through the bone transversely. In resection of a border the incision is made parallel with the part to be removed.

RESECTION OF THE BODY OF THE SCAPULA.—(Fig. 227.) The body of the scapula may be removed to a greater or less extent. No general method of operation can be given.

Velpeau operates by making three incisions, one over the whole length of the spine, A, *d*, and the other two extending from its extremities, one upwards to the root of the neck, A, *i*, the other downwards to the angle, *d*, F; the triangular flaps are dissected from the supra and infra spinatus fossæ, the root of the acromion sawed through, and the posterior and anterior surfaces of the bone denuded; the body of the scapula is then reversed from within outwards, and the part divided at the proper point with the chain saw or hand saw.

Reid proposed a longitudinal incision extending from the superior to the inferior angle along the vertebral border, F, *b*, a second parallel incision is made extending from the neck of the acromion to the middle of the external border, A, B, a transverse incision unites these along the spine; the flaps are then dissected, the muscles detached, posteriorly and anteriorly, and the bone divided with the chain saw, or forceps.

Chassaignac makes a single incision, but strongly curved downwards so as to permit raising a flap which will allow the division of the bone into fragments by the saw, perforator, or forceps, and the extraction by pieces of the portion to be removed.

Gross, operating for an osteo-sarcomatous affection, made an incision, sixteen inches in length, commencing at the superior angle of the scapula in a direction obliquely downwards and inwards; a second incision began five inches below the upper end of the first, and having a curvilinear direction terminated about the same distance from its lower end; the integuments were dissected towards the axilla and spine, the muscles detached, the acromion, and afterwards the neck of the scapula separated, and the bone removed.

Walter, of Pittsburgh, removed the body of the scapula for a tumor, by an incision extending from the acromion horizontally backwards to the posterior border of the scapula, and another from the centre of the first directly downwards below the margin of the tumor.

South made a curved incision from the acromion to the lower angle of the scapula.

Resection of the Entire Scapula.—The scapula gives attachment to a large number of muscles, by some of which it is principally maintained in its position. To the anterior surface is attached the sub-scapularis; to the anterior, the supra and infra spinatus; to the spine, the trapezius and deltoid; to the superior border, the omo-hyoid: to the vertebral border, the serratus magnus, levator anguli scapulæ, rhomboideus major and minor; to the axillary border, the triceps, teres major and minor; to the glenoid cavity, the long head of the biceps; to the coracoid process, the short head of the biceps, coraco-brachialis, and pectoralis minor. It articulates with the humerus and clavicle.

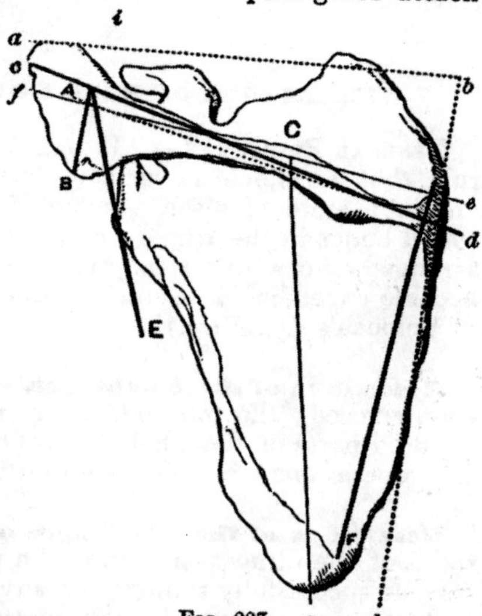

Fig. 227.

The subscapular artery, the largest branch of the axillary, descends along the outer border of the scapula.

Operation.—Syme operated as follows:—The patient being fully under the influence of chloroform, and placed on her right side, I made an incision from the acromion process to the posterior edge of the scapula (*f*, *e*,) and another from the centre of this one downwards, below the lower margin of the tumor (*c*, *g*). The flaps thus formed being reflected without much hæmorrhage I separated the scapular attachment of the deltoid, and divided the connexions of the acromial extremity of the clavicle. Then wishing to command the subscapular artery, divided it with the effect of giving issue to a fearful gush of blood, but fortunately caught the vessel and tied it without delay. I next cut into the joint, and round the glenoid cavity, hooked my finger under the coracoid process, so as to facilitate the division of its muscular and ligamentous attachments, and then pulling back the bone with all the force of my left hand, separated its remaining attachments with rapid sweeps of the knife.

The entire scapula may be removed by any of the methods given for the excision of a part of the body; other methods have been adopted, viz. a flap formed by the incisions *a*, *b*, and *b*, *h*; or A, *d*, joined at the extremities by *b*. *h*, and A, E; Chassaignac makes a single curved incision.

Resection of the Scapula and Part of the Clavicle.—No single method of performing this resection can be given: the steps of the operations which have been performed are, for the most part, the same as for the removal of the body of the bone, with a simple extension of incisions to include the external portion of the clavicle.

RESECTIONS OF THE LOWER EXTREMITIES.

General Principles.—"It ought to be laid down, as a general rule, that we should never amputate any parts except those that are in a state of disease, even if there should remain but two sound bones in the whole foot; for, by means of a shoe, properly arranged, and with a strong sole, a very small part of the foot may become exceedingly useful."—(*Encyclop. Meth.*, part Chir. quoted in Velpeau's *Op. Surg.*)

Resections of the Phalanges.—The four last toes have seldom been excised; the methods of operating in resections of corresponding parts of the phalanges of the fingers may be adopted, if such operations are undertaken on the phalanges of the toes.

Resections of the Phalanges of the Great Toe.—The great toe is of the utmost importance in progression, and diseased bone may be successfully removed at any point.

Resection of the Articulations of the Phalanges.—Chassaignac advises an incision curved downwards, on the internal aspect of the toe, over the phalangeal articulation; the flap is dissected, and the ends of the bone divided with the chain saw, or bone forceps.

Resections of the Shafts of the Phalangeal Bones.—A straight incision may be made on the dorsum, the extensor tendon being drawn aside; or, as in the last operation, the incision may be curved downwards; the bone may be divided with the forceps.

Resections of the Metatarsal Bones.—The individual metatarsal, like individual metacarpal bones, may be exsected in part or entire.

Resection of the Phalangeal Extremity of the Metatarsal Bones.—A straight incision is made on the dorsum of the toe, over the part to be removed, avoiding the extensor tendons, division of the bone with forceps or saw, and disarticulation; in operating upon the first and fifth, the incision may be upon the free lateral surface, and it may be straight, or curved, as recommended by Chassaignac.

Malgaigne (*op. cit.*) remarks of resection of the extremity of the first metatarsal bone—"The operation is similar to that for amputation of this-bone. Cut a flap on the inside with its base posterior, denude the bone to the point at which it is to be cut, and saw it *perpendicularly* to its axis; then detach it from the soft parts, proceeding from behind forwards, and finish by separating it from the phalanx."

Blandin recommends a quadrilateral flap, with its base posteriorly on the inner side of the foot.

RESECTION OF THE SHAFT OF METATARSAL BONES.—The same incisions are practised on this part of the metatarsal bones as at the extremities; in removing the body of the first and fifth, a curved incision more completely exposes the bone (Fig. 228); the chain saw should be used to divide the shaft of the first metatarsal bone.

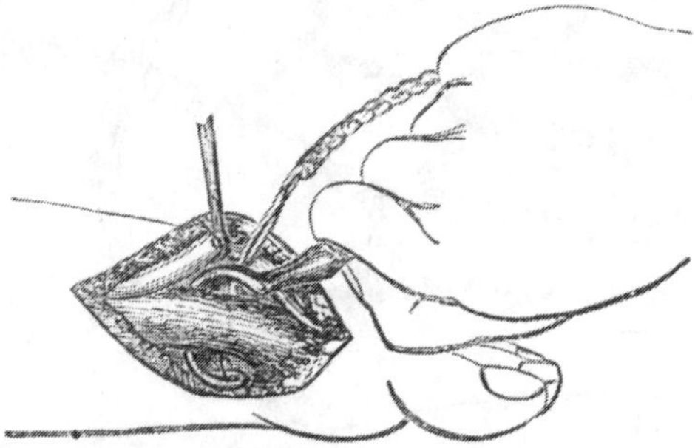

FIG. 228.

RESECTION OF THE TARSAL EXTREMITY OF THE METATARSAL BONES.—The same incisions may be made in resections of the tarsal as in the phalangeal extremities of the metatarsal bones. The chief difficulty in the disarticulation is the interosseous ligaments which unite the metatarsal bones together. The incision should freely expose the articulation, and the bone being divided, it should be raised with the forceps, and disarticulation effected with the point of the knife.

RESECTION OF ENTIRE METATARSAL BONES.—For the removal of the first and fifth metatarsal bones a curved incision should be made with its convexity downwards, *a*, *b*, *c*, (Fig. 229), and extending beyond the articulation; the bone being exposed, the middle of the shaft should be divided with the saw, and the fragments separately disarticulated. In the removal of the three middle metatarsal bones, a long straight incision should be made, the bone divided in its centre, and the operation completed as in the preceding case.

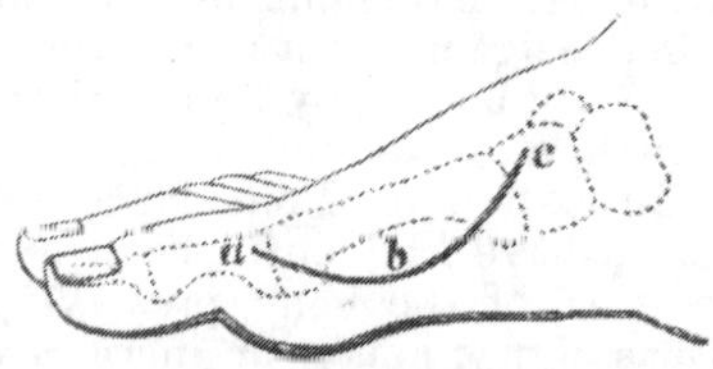

FIG. 229.

Resections of the Tarsal Bones.—The tarsal bones have all been exsected, either alone or in connexion with others. These operations have never been performed according to any prescribed rules, but each operator has adapted his incisions to the exigencies of the individual case in hand. In many cases the bones have not been removed entire, but the portion of bone diseased has been removed with a gouge. In the exsection of the bones of the

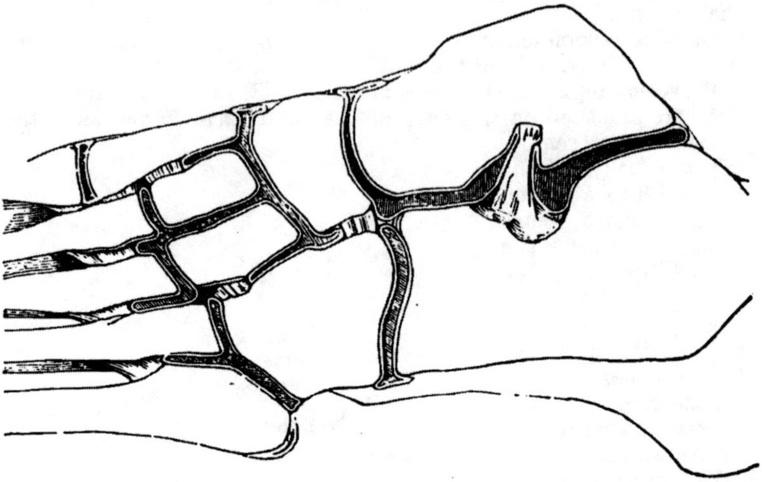

FIG. 230.

tarsus, care should be taken not to involve the synovial membrane of adjacent articulations, which, in the section of the tarsus, from Gray (Fig. 230), it will be seen, do not all communicate.

Several operations for the excision of single tarsal bones, and also of two or more bones at one operation, are given in illustration of the methods that have been pursued.

Resection of the Os Calcis.—The os calcis articulates above with the astragalus by two articular surfaces having an interosseous ligament; it articulates in front with the cuboid, to which it is firmly bound by four ligaments, two plantars, which are very strong, a dorsal, and interosseous.

RESECTION OF PORTIONS OF THE OS CALCIS.—Portions of the os calcis have frequently been excised; Moreau removed the inner portion of the bone, preserving the attachments of the muscles. Chassaignac makes an incision with a large inferior curve on the internal or external aspect of the bone, dissects off the soft parts, and perforates the bone with the drill at the proper points; through these holes the chain saw is passed and excision effected (Fig. 231).

RESECTION OF THE ENTIRE OS CALCIS.—The following are some of the methods which have been adopted:—

Anterior Flap.—Guthrie directed as follows:—Make a semilunar incision down to the bone from the posterior angle of the inner malleolus, the convexity of the flap being forwards. This flap being turned back, the tendo-achillis is brought into view, and is to be separated from its attachment or cut across above it. The point of junction between the os calcis and astragalus having been ascertained, the ligamentous fibres are to be cut through, and the joint between those opened, then the knife is to be carried from behind forwards in order to divide the inter-osseous ligament between them. Some ligamentous fibres passing between the os calcis and cuboid bones are then to be cut through, when the os calcis may be dissected out without difficulty. The posterior tibial artery and nerve will be divided."

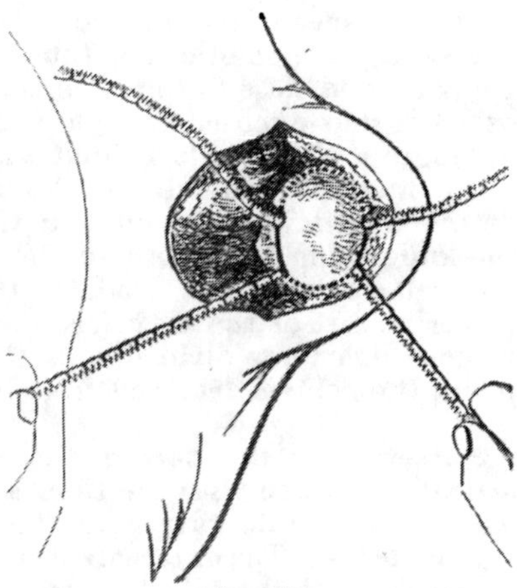

FIG. 231.

External Lateral Flap.—Guérin gives the following method, which he declares to be long and difficult:—The incision commences on a level with the internal border of the tendo-achillis at the point where it is inserted into the calcaneum, and passes horizontally below the external malleolus to a point half an inch in front of the calcaneo-cuboid articulation; from this point the incision passes at right angles over the external part of the foot and upwards of an inch across the sole; this flap is detached, the tendo-achillis divided, the calcaneo-cuboid articulation opened, the ligaments divided, and the bone, separated from the soft parts, removed.

Square External Lateral Flap.—Morrogh, of N. J., operated as follows:—A vertical incision over the posterior extremity of the os calcis, extending from the superior to the inferior surface, then continued along the inferior surface of the bone to its articulation with the cuboid, taking care to keep outside of the plantar artery; the incision was then carried upwards to a short distance above the inferior surface of the bone, without wounding the peroneal tendons; this incision described a square flap on the outside of the foot, which was dissected up, and the tendo-achillis separated close to its attachment. A strong narrow scalpel was then introduced underneath the peroneal tendons and made to separate the calcaneo-cuboid articulation without serving the tendons or the artery beneath; the knife was then introduced between the upper surface of the bone and the astragalus, and made to cut the inter-osseous ligament, and gradually separate the articular surfaces; the calcaneum was then rotated so as to bring its upper surface outwards till the internal made its appearance, when the soft structures were carefully separated, principally by the handle of the scalpel, thus completing the operation.

Plantar Flap.—Erichsen gives the following method:—The patient lying on his face, a horse-shoe incision is carried from a little in front of the calcaneo-cuboid articulation around the heel, along the sides of the foot, to a corresponding point on the opposite side. The elliptic flap thus formed is dissected up, the knife being carried close to the bone, and the whole under surface of the os calcis thus exposed. A perpendicular incision about two inches in length is then made behind the heel through the tendo-achillis in the mid line and into the horizontal one. The tendon is then detached from its insertion, and the two lateral flaps dissected up, the knife being kept close to the bones from which the soft parts are well cleared. The blade is then carried over the upper and posterior part of the os calcis, the articulation opened, the interosseous ligaments divided, and then by a few touches with the point, the bone is detached from its connexions with the cuboid.

Resection of the Astragalus.—The astragalus is very firmly articulated above with the tibia and two malleoli, below with the os calcis, and anteriorly with the scaphoid. It has the following ligaments:—1. The external calcaneo-astragaloid, uniting the external surfaces of the two bones; 2. The posterior calcaneo-astragaloid, uniting the under surface of this bone to the calcaneum; 3. The superior and inferior astragalo-scaphoid, which support the articulation of these two bones.

Operation.—Guthrie thus describes Statham's operation:—"An incision, four and a half inches long, is to be commenced within the anterior edge of the fibula, and carried down in a straight line beyond the anterior end of the metatarsal bone of the little toe; a second incision, about an inch in length, should then be made from the centre of the wound downwards towards the sole of the foot, for the purpose of giving room. The integuments are then to be raised from the bone, from the upper edge of the first incision, carrying with them the extensor tendons towards the inside of the foot, to give more room for ulterior proceedings, without injuring them. The under joint of a pair of short, strong scissors, such as are supplied in the capital cases of instruments, ought then to be pushed under the neck of the astragalus, at the hollow, where it is attached by a strong interosseous ligament to the os calcis. The upper blade being then closed upon the bone, it may be divided, but not without considerable force. The articulating end of the astragalus with the os naviculare can then be easily removed by a strong pair of forceps, its ligamentous attachments being first divided by the knife. In order to extract the remaining portion of the bone, the under blade of the strong scissors must be again pushed under it from before backwards, and made to cut it in two. The outer part being now separated from the internal end of the fibula, care being taken not to injure the perpendicular ligament going from that bone to the os calcis, this piece should be forcibly removed by strong forceps—an operation which could not be easily borne unless chloroform were used. The remaining piece or pieces must follow, when an examination should be made by the finger to ascertain that none remain."

Guthrie also gives the following method, which resembles the flap operation on the wrist in which the tendons are (Fig. 232) divided:—"The astragalus may be removed by a flap operation dividing the extensor tendons of the toes, commencing on the outside of the fibula, and being carried round in front, but not so far as to injure the tibialis anticus tendon, nor the anterior tibial artery and nerve; or, when the incision reaches the edge of the outer extensor, the whole of them are to be separated from the parts beneath, and drawn inwards, when the operation of removing the bone is to be completed, as in the former instance. But many surgeons believe that when tendons are forcibly drawn aside, after being separated from their attachments, they are apt to slough, and that their division would, in most cases, be less injurious. In neither operation need tendon, artery, vein, or nerve of any importance be divided."

Resection of the Calcaneum and Cuboid Bones with a Portion of the Astragalus.—The following operation by Bradford, of Ky., Brigade Surgeon U.S.A., resulted in a useful limb:—

"An incision was made on the outer margin of the tendo-achillis, commencing about an inch above the external malleolus, and extending downwards to the lower and outer part of the heel, to a point half an inch above the plantar border of the foot. From the termination of this incision another was made to extend along the outer aspect of the foot to within an inch of the posterior extremity of the fifth metatarsal bone. From the upper part of the first incision another was made directly across the lower part of the leg, terminating a little within the inner margin of the tendo-achillis, at its upper part; the two flaps thus formed were reflected, the outer from the external aspect of the os calcis, the inner from its internal surface, carefully protecting the posterior tibial artery and nerve as well as the adjoining tendons. The tendo-achillis was then divided, one fourth of an inch from its insertion, the external lateral ligaments cut asunder, and the joint between the astragalus and os calcis entered from behind. The os calcis was so completely disorganized, as to admit of but little leverage towards its separation from the astragalus and cuboid. The operation was thus far both tedious and difficult, it being with much difficulty that the interosseous ligament and the calcaneo-cuboid connexions were broken up. The greater part of the os calcis was removed in fragments; upon its completion, difficult and tedious as it was, it was found that the cuboid was involved. The incision upon the outer surface of the foot was extended up a little above the connexion of the fifth metatarsal bone with the cuboid. Portions of the cuboid which were disorganized were removed,

10*

fragment by fragment, and finally the remaining third of it in a body. Sponging and a careful examination of the surrounding bones, showed the commencement of the disease in the astragalus upon the outer and under surface where it joined and lay upon the os calcis. This fortunately was but slight, and was clipped off with the bone nippers, and the suspicious part dusted with pulverized caustic."

Resection of the Calcaneum and Cuboid Bones, the Proximal Extremity of the Fifth Metatarsal Bone, and of the articulating surface of the Astragalus.—The resection of these bones by Walter, of Pittsburgh, Pa., resulted in a perfectly useful limb. It was begun by an incision, commencing over the insertion of the tendo-achillis into the os calcis, downwards along the longitudinal axis of the os calcis to its articulation with the tarsal bones in the sole of the foot; from hence cross cuts were carried to each side of the foot; two large lateral flaps were thus formed on the sole of the foot, which were reflected, by dissections, from the sides of the os calcis, and held upwards; the calcaneum was next separated from its articulation with the cuboid, and raised by dissection from the astragalus from before backwards; the cuboid being found carious, was excised, with the posterior articulation of the fifth metatarsal bone; the articulation of the astragalus was also removed.

Resection of the Calcaneum and Astragalus.—Wakley performed the following operation, and a useful foot resulted (Fig. 232):—"The patient being put under chloroform, the diseased foot (the left) having been drawn forward, so as to be free from the table, an incision was made from malleolus to malleolus, directly across the heel. A second incision was next carried along the edge of the sole, from the middle of the first to a point opposite the astragalo-scaphoid articulation, and another on the opposite side of the foot, from the vertical incision to the situation of the calcaneo-cuboid joint. These latter incisions enabled the operator to make a flap about two inches in length from the integument of the sole. In the next place a circular flap of integument was formed between the two malleoli posteriorly, the lower border of the flap reaching to the insertion of the tendo-achillis. This flap being turned upwards the tendon was cut through, and the os calcis, having been disarticulated from the astragalus and cuboid bones, was removed, together with the integument of the heel included between the two incisions. The lateral ligaments connecting the astragalus with the tibia and fibula were next divided, and the knife was carried into the joint on each side,

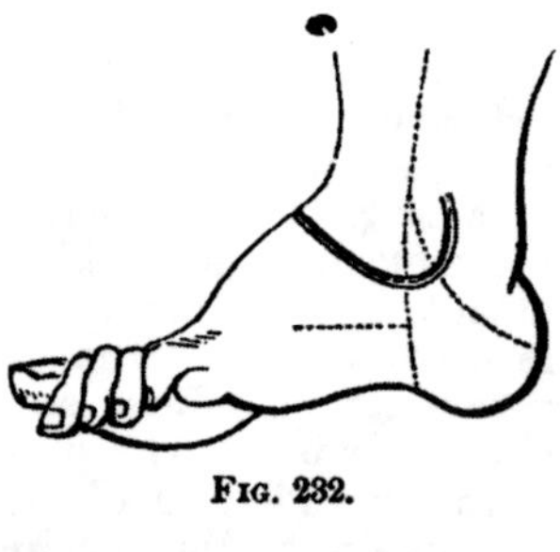

FIG. 232.

extreme care being observed to avoid wounding the anterior tibial artery, which was in view. The astragalus was then detached from the soft parts in front of the joint and from its articulation with the scaphoid bone, and the malleoli were removed with the bone-nippers. The only artery requiring ligature was the posterior tibial."

Resection of the Cuboid, Adjacent Articular Surface of the Calcaneum, Posterior Extremity of the Fourth and Inside of the Extremity of the Fifth Metatarsal Bones.—Moreau, sr., removed these bones at a single operation, and the patient recovered with a useful limb. An incision had been made to open an abscess between the third and fourth metatarsal bones. He extended his incision, according to Malgaigne, on the inside of the foot, from the posterior third of the fifth metatarsal bone, to above the anterior apophysis of the calcaneum; a transverse incision was then made, which united the incision into the abscess with that just made, thus forming a quadrilateral flap; this being reflected, the bones were removed.

Resections of the Fibula.—The fibula may be resected in whole or in part.

Resection of the Lower Extremity of the Fibula.—The lower extremity of the fibula articulates through the malleolus externus with the astragalus; the malleolus gives attachment by its extremity to the external lateral ligaments, three in number. The fibula also articulates with the tibia by a convex surface, the joint being continuous with that of the ankle. The ligaments of this articulation are, the interosseous, which passes between the two bones, and is continuous above, with the interosseous membrane; the anterior inferior ligament, a flat triangular band extending between the two bones, anteriorly; the posterior inferior ligament occupying the same position posteriorly; and the transverse ligament extending from the external malleolus to the tibia. On the posterior border of the bone are grooves for the passage of the tendons of the peroneus longus and brevis muscles.

Operation.—(Fig. 233.) A straight incision should be made over the bone the entire length of the diseased part; the soft parts are separated, the chain saw passed, and bone divided; the fragment is then seized with the forceps, and the disarticulation effected with the point of the knife.

Modifications.—Moreau added a transverse incision.

Resection of the Shaft of the Fibula.—The shaft of the fibula gives attachment to muscles by all its surfaces, and by its internal border to the interosseous membrane.

Operation.—The bone is exposed by a straight incision, the chain saw passed, and the shaft divided at proper points above and below the diseased part, and the exsection readily completed.

Resection of the Upper Extremity of the Fibula.—The upper extremity of the fibula articulates with the external part of the head of the tibia; this articulation communicates with the knee-joint; its ligaments are the anterior superior ligament, two or three flat bands, which pass obliquely upwards from the head of

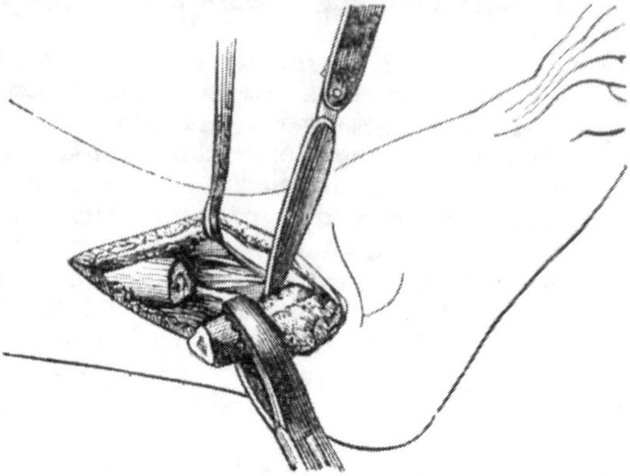

FIG. 238.

the fibula to the outer tuberosity of the tibia, and the posterior superior ligament, a single thick and broad band which passes from the back part of the head of the fibula to the back part of the outer tuberosity of the tibia.

Operation.—The exsection of the upper extremity is effected by the straight incision; the bone is divided with the chain saw, the diseased part is raised with the forceps, and the dissection is effected with the point of the knife.

Malgaigne states that he removed the upper third of the fibula, disarticulating it at its upper joint, which offers but little difficulty; but it requires great care not to wound the anterior tibial artery which passes around its neck.

RESECTION OF THE ENTIRE FIBULA.—An incision should be made parallel with the bone its entire length, the soft parts are separated, and the bone divided in the centre with the chain saw; each fragment is now separately disarticulated.

Resections of the Tibia.—The tibia, the principal bone of the leg, has also been removed in its entire extent, as also partially:—

RESECTIONS OF THE LOWER EXTREMITY OF THE TIBIA.—The lower extremity of the tibia forms the upper and internal part of the ankle joint; it is closely invested with tendons, and upon its postero-internal border the posterior tibial artery and nerve pass to the foot.

Operation.—A straight or crucial incision may be made along the posterior border of the bone, extending below the point of the malleolus; the bone is then divided at the proper point, and exsection effected by carefully dislodging the tendons from their grooves.

RESECTION OF THE SHAFT OF THE TIBIA.—The anterior and inner part of the tibia being subcutaneous, exsection of portions of its shaft is a comparatively simple operation; on the posterior part it gives attachment to muscles, and along its external border is attached the interosseous ligament connecting it to the fibula.

Operation.—A long curved incision is made in the length of the bone, having its convexity backwards; this flap is dissected up and turned outwards, the bone divided at the proper points, and the fragment raised with forceps. As excision of the shaft of the tibia is generally undertaken for necrosis, the gouge is found useful in separating dead bone, and the mallet may be used freely; it is also frequently desirable to use the trephine.

The shaft of the tibia has a strong tendency to reproduction if the periosteum is left undisturbed, and it is, therefore, exceedingly important, when the entire shaft is removed, to separate this membrane carefully from its connexions with the bone, and allow it to remain in the wound.

RESECTION OF THE UPPER EXTREMITY OF THE TIBIA.—The upper extremity of the tibia is broad, and presents upon its upper surface two cup-shaped cavities for articulation with the condyles of the femur; the ligaments which are attached to it are, *anteriorly*, the ligamentum patellæ, *internally*, the internal lateral, *posteriorly*, the posterior ligament, or the ligamentum posticum Winslowii, and *within*, the anterior and posterior crucial ligaments.

Operation.—Velpeau remarks (*Op. Surg.*):—"The operative process in these cases is entirely subordinated to the degree, actual situation, and form of the disease; so that we have sometimes occasion for the crucial incision, or the elliptical or simple incision, and also for every variety of saws and osteotomes."

Chassaignac recommends a curved incision, its convexity downwards, division of the bone with a chain saw, below the limit of the disease, disarticulation of the upper portion, luxated by the forceps.

Velpeau gives the following method of Manee:—"Make an incision more than semicircular at the anterior part of the integuments, below the ligamentum patellæ; we raise them up, divide the ligament, and then the crucial ligaments, after which we detach the tissues adherent to the posterior part of the tibia and fibula, by directing the cutting edge of the instrument downwards and forwards, to avoid the popliteal artery and nerves. Then divide the periosteum circularly, and having drawn aside the tissues from the bones, by means of a linen bandage or band, complete the exsection."

Resections of the Lower Extremities of the Tibia and Fibula.—The malleoli or the extremities of both bones, alone, or with portions of the astragalus, may require excision.

RESECTION OF A MALLEOLUS.—Guérin made a straight incision along the posterior border of the malleolus, and joined it at right angles by another, extending to the tibialis anticus; the flap is raised, and, if the external malleolus, the bone is divided with forceps, if the internal, the chain saw is employed.

Velpeau operated for removal of caries of the internal malleolus, by making a semilunar flap, having its free border anteriorly.

Resection of the Ankle-Joint.—The following methods have been pursued.

Lateral Straight Incisions—Moreau first operated by this method. Roux adopted it, and the following are the details (*Bernard* and *Huette*):—(Fig. 234.) 1st. Make on the outer side of the fibula a longitudinal incision three inches in length, commencing over the external malleolus, and carry it down to the bone. From the lower part of this incision, make a transverse section of the skin as far forwards as the tendon of the *peroneus tertius.* Dissect up the triangular flap thus formed, and opening the sheath of the *peroneus longus* and *brevis,* push them aside, and avoiding the vessels and nerves, denude the fibula of the soft parts, insinuate a chain saw between the tibia and fibula, and saw the bone from within outwards. This being effected, make use of the extremity of the fibula as a lever while it is being disarticulated. 2d. To exsect the tibia, make a longitudinal incision from three to four inches in length, along the inner margin of the bone, commencing over the internal malleolus, and carry it down to the bone. From the lower part of this incision, make a transverse section of the skin as far forwards as the tendon of the *tibialis anticus.* Dissect up the flap, and isolate the bone from the extensor tendons and anterior tibial vessels, pass a slip of wood beneath it to protect the soft parts, and complete its division with a small straight-bladed saw. The chain saw can also be used to divide the bone without endangering the tendons. The tibia being sawn through, it is disarticulated in the same way as the fibula."

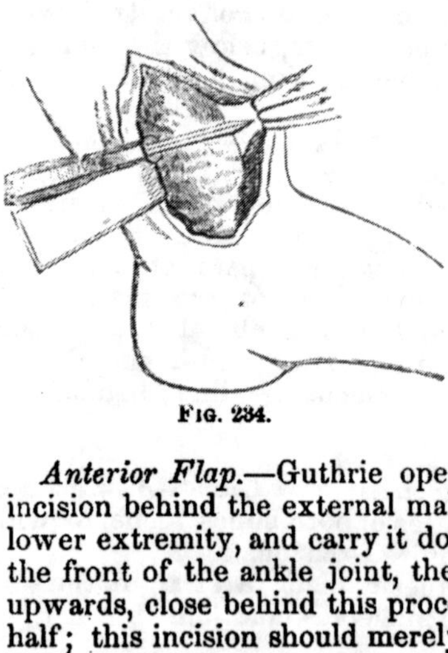

Fig. 234.

To raise the soft parts from the anterior face of the bones, a retractor is passed, and they are then readily thrown forwards. (Fig. 234.)

Anterior Flap.—Guthrie operated thus (Fig. 232):—Begin the incision behind the external malleolus, an inch and a half above its lower extremity, and carry it downwards and then forwards across the front of the ankle joint, then under the internal malleolus and upwards, close behind this process, to the extent of an inch and a half; this incision should merely divide the skin, and should not, on any account, wound the subjacent parts. Raise the flap thus made, and, placing the leg on its inside, detach and turn aside the peronei tendons from the groove behind the external malleolus. Cut through the external lateral ligaments of the ankle-joint, keeping the knife close to the end of the fibula; then, with the large bone-scissors or nippers, cut through the fibula from one-half to three quarters of an inch above its junction with the tibia, and, after dividing the ligamentous fibres connecting the two bones, remove the malleolus externus. Turn the leg on to its outer side, and cut through the internal lateral ligament close to the tibia, to avoid wounding the posterior tibial artery; this will allow the foot to be dislocated outwards, and the lower end of the tibia to be brought well out through the wound. An assistant keeping the foot and tendons out of the way, the lower end of the tibia is to be removed by a fine saw to the same extent as the fibula, or as high as the injury or disease requires. The articulating surface, or injured part of the astragalus, is then to be removed.

Resection of the Knee-Joint.—The knee is a hinge-joint having free motion in but two directions; it is supported principally by the lateral, the internal, and the posterior ligaments, and in front by the patella, and its ligamentous attachments; it has also a capsular ligament; the articular face of the tibia has a semilunar fibro-cartilage which deepens the articular surface for the condyles of the femur.

Operation.—Resection of the knee-joint has been performed by several different methods.

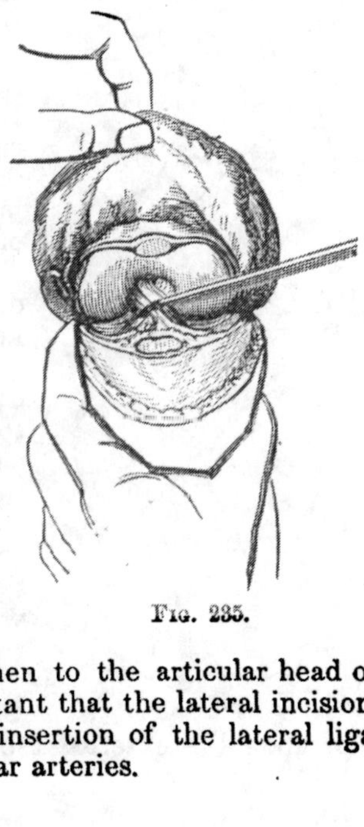

FIG. 235.

Semilunar Anterior Flap.—Wood, of New York, operates as follows:—The leg being flexed on the thigh, or straight, a curved incision is made commencing at the insertion of the internal lateral ligament into the inner condyle of the femur, and passing just below the lower extremity of the patella terminates at the same point on the external aspect of the joint; this flap is reflected upwards (Fig. 235), the patella removed, and the ligaments divided; a fold of cloth is then passed through the joint, and drawn firmly under the extremity of the bone to be sawn, thus completely isolating the soft parts behind; the saw is then applied, first to the extremity of the femur, and then to the articular head of the tibia (Fig. 236). It is very important that the lateral incisions should not be made lower than the insertion of the lateral ligaments, to avoid division of the articular arteries.

All diseased and degenerated tissues should be carefully removed,

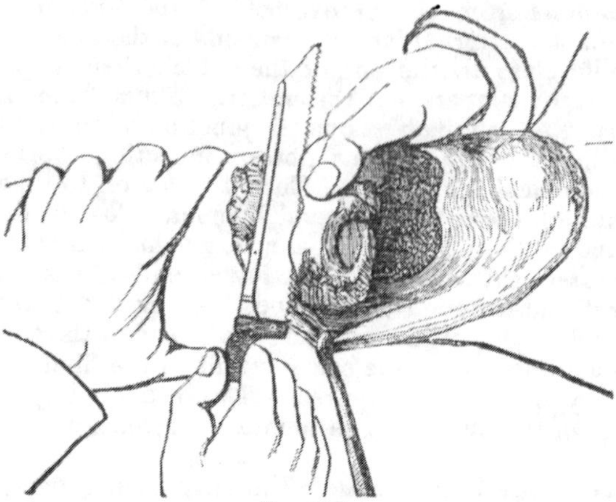

FIG. 236.

the wound cleansed, and the bones wired together. The wire selected should be the annealed iron-wire, and it should be inserted at two points corresponding to the insertion of the lateral ligaments.

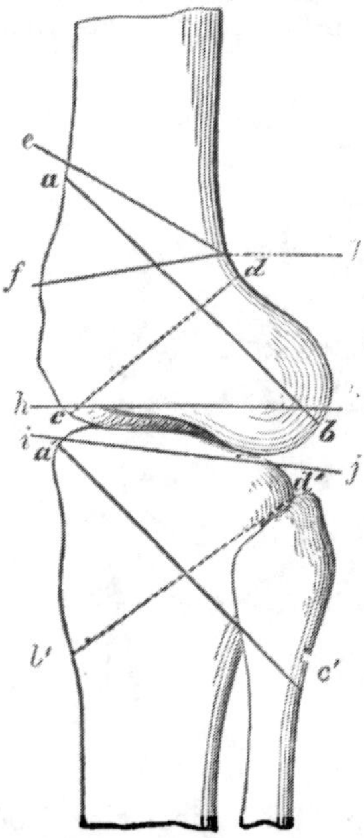

FIG. 237.

Modifications.—Mackenzie, of Edinburgh, made the flap extend downwards nearly to the tuberosity of the tibia; Buchanan, of Glasgow, made the incision above the patella; Jones, of Jersey, drew the ligamentum patellæ aside, and preserved it, the patella, and the tendon of the quadriceps extensor, uninjured.

Single Transverse Incision.—Watson, of Glasgow, operated as follows:—The knife was drawn across the front of the joint from a little below the inner condyle of the femur to the same point on the outside of the joint; the incision passed over the middle of the patella; this bone was removed.

Modification.—Bégin made the transverse incision first, entered the articulation, and made the lateral incisions upwards or downwards according to the particular bone involved in the disease.

Single External Lateral Incision.—Chassaignac directs a longitudinal incision upon the external aspect of the articulation, division of the neck of the fibula by the chain saw, and resection of its upper extremity; then removal by the same method of the lower extremity of the femur, and of the head of the tibia.

Elliptical Flap.—(Fig. 238.) Syme operated as follows:—First, Flex the leg at a right angle with the thigh; make a curved incision above the patella with its convexity upwards from one lateral ligament to the other, and carry it directly into the joint; a second curved incision should then be made below the patella, with its convexity downwards, and its extremities should join the angles of the first. An elliptical flap is thus formed, which removes the patella. The lateral and posterior ligaments are then to be divided, and carefully avoiding the popliteal vessels, separate the femur and tibia from the soft parts which surround them. Draw aside the soft parts with a split retractor, *e*, place a slip of wood or metal beneath the ends of the bones, *b*, *c*, and remove them with the saw, *d*.—*Bernard & Huette.*

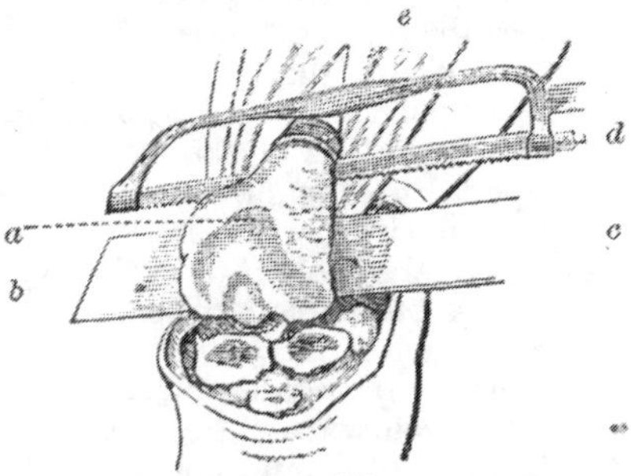

FIG. 238.

Oblique Transverse Incision.—Heyfelder proposed an incision, passing obliquely across the knee from the external to the internal side, commencing above and crossing the lower margin of the patella, the leg being in a flexed position; if the bone is large he joined this incision on either side with a vertical cut, making the following Ν: two flaps, an upper and lower, were thus raised, exposing the joint.

Crucial Incision.—Park made a crucial incision, the vertical cut extending from two inches above the patella to two inches below the transverse branch, being above the patella, and extending half the circumference of the limb; the tendons of the extensor muscles of the leg were then divided, the four flaps dissected and turned back, the patella removed, the lateral ligaments incised, the articulation opened; a knife was now passed through the joint, and the operator carefully separated the soft parts from the posterior surface of the bone; the bone was then sawn to the proper extent.

Quadrilateral Flap.—Moreau operated upon the knee as upon the elbow-joint, by making two lateral incisions a little in front of the borders of the ham; a third incision passes transversely from one lateral incision to the other below the patella; this quadrilateral flap is raised, the patella removed, if diseased, the soft parts dissected from the posterior surface of the femur, and the bone sawn; if the head of the tibia requires excision, the lateral incisions are prolonged, and a lower flap raised, which allows its section.

Remarks.—Section of the bones is to be made with reference to a true anchylosis at the knee; to render the limb most useful it is generally considered advisable to unite the bones at a slight angle anteriorly; the section of the bones should therefore be nearly in the lines, *h*, *k*, and *i*, *j* (Fig. 237).

Billroth suggests sawing the bones very obliquely when one portion of the shaft is diseased. Section of the femur and tibia may be made, *a*, *b*, and *a'*, *b'* (Fig. 237), when the anterior part of the lower portion of the femur is diseased, or *c*, *d*, and *c'*, *d'*, when the upper anterior part of the tibia is affected.

The propriety or necessity of removing the patella is a debatable question; the weight of authority is in favor of its removal; if diseased it is of course excised.

Exsection of Knee-joint for Anchylosis.—Buck, of New York, removed a triangular piece from a knee-joint anchylosed at right angles as follows:—"Preparatory to the operation, the tendons of the biceps, semi-tendinosus, semi-membranosus, and gracilis muscles had been divided five days before, in the usual manner, by two subcutaneous incisions, in doing which the peroneal nerve was unintentionally cut across, and was followed by numbness and pain extending to the foot; the punctures, however, had healed, and no inflammation remained in the ham. The tourniquet having been applied to the upper part of the thigh, an incision was made from the outer to the inner condyle, across the middle of the patella, and a second incision from the middle of this, perpendicularly downwards, to the tuberosity of the tibia. The included angles of integument were dissected down to a finger's breadth below and parallel with the margin of the articular surface of the tibia. The ligamentum patellæ and the fibro-ligamentous tissues on either side were cut through on the same level to the extent of nearly two-thirds of the circumference of the bone. With the amputating saw a section of the tibia was made at three-fourths of an inch below the joint anteriorly, and directed with a slight obliquity upwards, so as to terminate at the margin of the articular surface posteriorly. Two-thirds of this section was accomplished with the amputating saw. The second section was then commenced through the upper part of the patella, parallel with the first, and on a plane forming an angle with it, less than a right angle, and continued to about the same extent as in the first section with the same saw. The remainder of the section through the tibia, as well as through the condyles, was completed with a metacarpal saw and chisels. The included wedge-shaped portion of bone being removed, it was found the section had not been carried far enough backwards, the posterior portion of the condyles still remaining consolidated with the tibia. To conclude this a new section was undertaken, commencing upon the cut surface of the femur, three-fourths of an inch anterior to the angle at which the sections already made met, and directed backwards and upwards on a plane more oblique in reference to the axis of the femur. This new section being removed, the remaining points of connexion were ruptured by cautiously flexing the leg on the thigh, after which the irregular prominences were pared away with the bone forceps. An attempt was now made to extend the leg upon the thigh, when it was found that the bony surfaces could only be brought to within a finger's breadth of each other anteriorly. The soft parts in the ham being rendered tense and opposing great resistance to the extension, the attachments of the ligaments were dissected up posteriorly from the tibia while the leg was held in a state of extreme flexion, and, in addition to this, a further section of five-eighths of an inch thick was removed from the anterior two-thirds of the femur."

Resection of the Patella.—The patella, though in immediate relation with the knee-joint, has been excised with good results.

Operation.—A crucial incision is made, the transverse branch being over the base of the bone, or a second transverse incision may be made near the apex; the flaps are dissected off, and the bone or its fragments cautiously removed; the tendinous expansion surrounding the bone should be separated, and not divided, as far as possible.

Resections of the Femur.—The femur, like the humerus, has been excised in part, but never in its totality.

Resection of the Lower Extremity of the Femur.—Excision of the lower extremity of the femur, or any part of it, could be practised by some form of incision already given for excision of the knee-joint. Chassaignac recommends a long straight or slightly curved incision on the external aspect of the knee, isolation of the femur a little above the condyles, and section of the bone by the chain saw; the fragment is then made to protrude at the wound, and is seized with forceps and disarticulated.

Resection of the Shaft of the Femur.—Large fragments of the femur have been removed, and useful limbs have resulted by the reproduction of new bone. The body of the bone gives attachment to muscles throughout nearly its entire extent, and to reach it without injury to the soft parts, the muscular septa must be followed.

Operation.—Velpeau (*op. cit.*) remarks:—There are two modes of reaching these necroses in the thigh bone; one by election, represented by the antero-external region of the limb, and the other that of necessity, indicated by the seat of the disease. However few openings, therefore, or however little attenuation of the laminæ there may be on the convex portion of the femur, it is there nevertheless that we must endeavor to lay it bare to attack the disease. The curved incision and the semilunar flap would be of great advantage; raised up from without inwards, and from behind forwards, they would allow of laying bare the bone to a great extent. Barton removed a triangular portion of the shaft, *e*, *g*, *f* (Fig. 237), to straighten a limb anchylosed at the knee; he advised that there should not be a complete section of the bone at its posterior part, *g*; he also divided the shaft above the lesser trochanter for anchylosis at the hip-joint.

Rogers excised a small portion of the shaft to relieve anchylosis at the hip, by the following operation:—"An incision was made six inches in length in the course of the os femoris, beginning about an inch above the trochanter major. This was met about its middle by another from front, three inches in length. The flaps were turned off, and the soft parts easily detached from the bone, so that in a short time, and with much less difficulty than I had anticipated, my fingers were passed around the bone immediately above the trochanter minor. The division of the bone was attempted by the chain saw, but the instrument breaking, the section was completed with a saw recommended by Dr. Barton. Another section was made, and a wedge-shaped portion removed, the thickness of which at the outer part was about half an inch, and the less trochanter three-quarters of an inch."

Resection of the Trochanter Major.—The great trochanter gives attachment to the gluteus medius and minimus, and by its fossa to the external rotators.

Operation.—Velpeau directs the patient to be placed on the sound side, with the thigh in a state of semi-flexion during the incisions upon the skin—to be placed in complete flexion, with adduction and rotation inwards, at the moment of performing excision of bone. He operated with a T incision, the stem directed transversely, extending from the anterior border of the trochanter to two inches behind it towards the tuberosity of the ischium; the two flaps thus formed were reversed above and below; the wound being held apart, the bone was removed, lamina by lamina, with the concave rowel saw. He adds:—If the integuments are not degenerated to great depth, nor strongly adherent to the femur, a semilunar flap, having its base behind the great trochanter and its convex border in front, is preferable to any other kind of incision. Laying bare the whole bone on its external face and anterior border, it enables us to detach from it afterwards its posterior border and apex, without the necessity of changing the primitive form of the wound. The bone may be exsected by means of the hand saw or crested saw, directed from before backwards, from without inwards, and slightly from below upwards.

Fergusson directs:—"To effect the removal of disease in this process, a free crucial incision should be made through the skin and tendon of the gluteus maximus, and when the surface is sufficiently exposed, the gouge should be used to scoop the affected parts away. I should myself place most reliance on this instrument; but, if the disease prove extensive, should be inclined to divide the attachments of the glutei to the upper and fore part of the process, and then effect the removal of the entire trochanter by the united aid of a saw and forceps. A small Hey's saw would be more manageable here than any other."

Resection of the Upper Extremity of the Femur.—The upper extremity of the femur lies deeply enveloped with thick and powerful muscles, to many of which it gives attachment; the articular head is maintained in its position by the capsular ligament, and the ligamentum teres. Anteriorly the femoral vessels and nerves prevent approach to the articulation, and posteriorly the sciatic nerve, lying between the great trochanter and ischium, is to be carefully guarded from injury; the great trochanter, which is comparatively superficial, marks the point at which the upper extremity of the femur and its articular head may safely be exposed for resection. The following methods have been practised in the excision of this bone:—

Curved Incision.—(Fig. 239.) Chassaignac directs a curved incision, *a*, *c*, to be made, having its concavity forwards, and embracing the posterior part of the great trochanter; the bone, *b*, is next isolated at the point of section, the chain saw, *g*, passed with the needle, *d*, held in the right hand, *f*; the index finger of the left hand, *e*, is passed under the external side of the bone to liberate the point; the bone being sawn, the cut extremity, *a* (Fig. 240), is seized with forceps, or the tire-fond, *b*, and disarticulation is readily effected with the point of the knife, *c*.

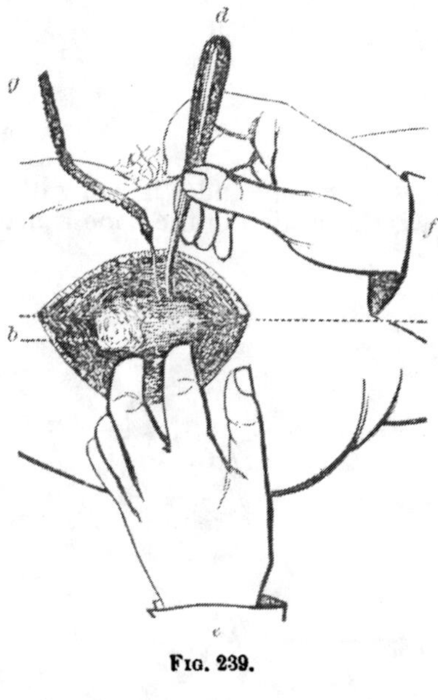

Fig. 239.

Straight Incision.—Several operators have recommended a straight incision, commencing about two inches above the great trochanter, and extending three inches below it; the tendons are divided; the capsule of the joint exposed and opened, and the head of the bone dislocated by pressing the knee inwards; the bone is thus exposed and sawn at the proper point.

Semilunar Flap.—(Fig. 241.) Sédillot recommended a semilunar incision, *a*, *b*, *c*, having its convexity upwards, and surrounding the trochanter, *d*, except on its lower part; this flap is dissected downwards, the attachment of muscles severed, the capsular ligament laid freely open, the limb is then adducted and rotated inwards, causing luxation of the head of the bone; a flat piece of

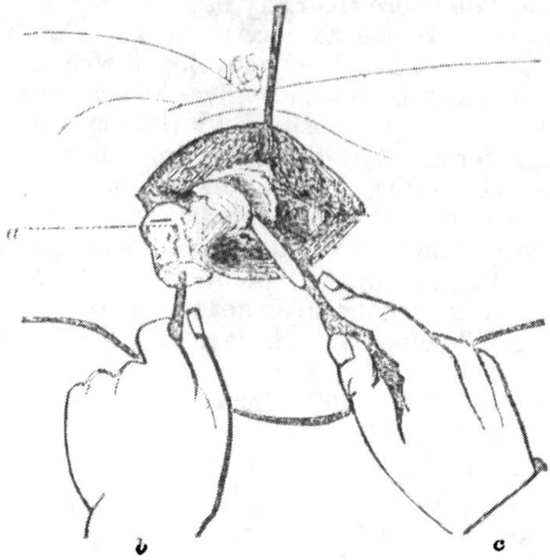

FIG. 240.

wood is passed under it, and with the chain saw, *f, f*, or a common saw, the section of the bone is made.

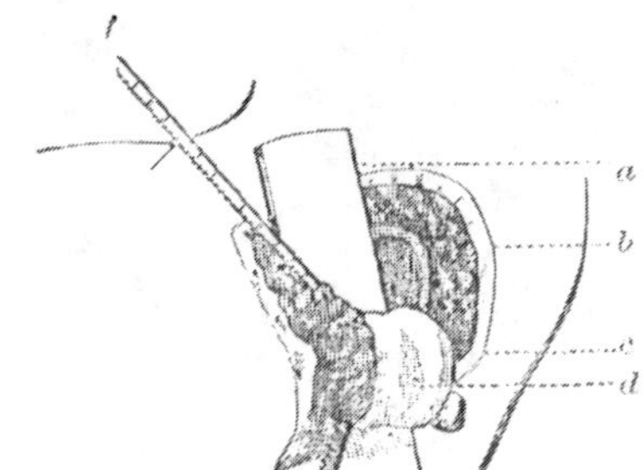

FIG. 241.

Modifications.—Gross makes the convexity of the flap downwards.

Curvilinear Incision.—Velpeau operated as follows (*Bernard* and *Huette*):—Make a curvilinear incision, extending from the anterior spinous process of the ilium to the tuberosity of the ischium, which will form a large flap with its convexity downwards. Raise up the flap, divide the posterior half of the articular capsule, adduct and flex the thigh, cut the round ligament, carry the knife between the head of the femur and the acetabulum, and divide the remainder of the capsular ligament. The head of the femur is then forced out and sawn off.

Oval Incision.—Textor made an oval incision (*South's Chelius*):—"He makes a cut beginning two inches above the great trochanter, carries it obliquely backwards and outwards, and ends it about an inch before the little trochanter. To this first cut follows a second, which, beginning on the front of the thigh opposite the point where the former ended, is carried obliquely outwards and upwards, and meets with it at a rather acute angle above the great trochanter. This second cut at first divides only the skin, but afterwards is continued down to the neck of the thigh bone. The soft parts are then separated from the great trochanter, the capsular ligament cut into with a strong scalpel from within outwards, following always the edge of the hip-socket, over half its extent, down to the head of the thigh bone; the knee being then bent inwards, the round ligament is divided with the scalpel, the head of the bone dislocated, fixed with the hand, and a knife carried round the part where the bone is to be divided, so that the track of the saw may be made easy, and then the bone cut through with the osteotome, or with a small bone or knife saw."

Triangular Flap.—Jaeger made a flap as follows (*South's Chelius*):—" A longitudinal cut beginning from two to two and a half inches above the great trochanter, and descending three inches below it, so as to make in the whole a cut from four and a half to five and a half inches long, from the upper end of which a second cut of four inches is carried backwards and downwards; this triangular flap is raised."

A Curved Transverse and Straight Vertical Incision.—Fergusson gives the following method:—" The body being placed a little to one side so as to elevate the hip, an incision with a strong bistoury should be carried in a semilunar course about two or three inches above the trochanter, its ends being so limited as not to interfere with the crural nerve in front, or the gluteal artery behind: from the centre of the concavity thus formed, a straight line of incision should be carried downwards over the trochanter, the two being each of a length proportioned to the bulk and depth of the parts. The knife should be carried deep, and one flap should be turned forwards and another backwards, so as to expose the upper part of the trochanter, neck of the bone, and capsular ligament—the three glutei, more especially the medius and minimus, being freely cut for the purpose. The capsule should next be opened on its upper aspect, when by twisting the thigh across its fellow, and rotating it outwards at the same time, the head of the bone will start from its socket: if the round ligament remains entire, which it probably will unless considerable force is used, it can be touched with a knife, and the articular surface of the femur will now be thoroughly exposed."

The T Incision.—Smith made the T incision which Erichsen approves, and cautions against making the transverse too far forwards lest the anterior crural nerve be wounded; nor too far backwards, lest a gluteal artery be injured.

RESECTIONS OF THE TRUNK.

Resection of the Coccyx.—Excision of the coccyx is occasionally required for necrosis or caries. It is composed of four small bones, the first, or upper, being the largest and separate, the lower united; it articulates above with the sternum, and gives attachment to the following muscles: at its apex to the sphincter ani, anteriorly to the levator ani, and posteriorly to the gluteus maximus.

Operation.—The patient is placed on the side, the thighs flexed, and the hips close to the edge of the bed; or the patient may be placed as for the operation for fistula in ano; the buttocks being separated, an incision is made in the median line, extending from the extremity of the coccyx upwards to the requisite extent; the bone is denuded of soft parts, and the diseased bone removed either with the gouge, or the burr drill of Isaacs (page 172), or the bone may be divided with the Hey's saw and removed with the proper forceps.

Modifications.—Onsenort first introduced the fore-finger of the left hand into the rectum, then made an incision from the base to the apex of the bone, in the median line, a transverse incision at its lower extremity enabled him to detach the soft parts on the inner side, and to disarticulate the bone.

Resection of the Sacrum.—Blackman exsected about one inch and three quarters of the upper and posterior walls of the sacrum by making a single large flap; the spinous process of the upper bone was removed with forceps and Hey's saw; a trephine was then applied, and an opening made, through which bone nippers were introduced, and the bone removed.

Resections of the Iliac Bones.—The crest of the ilium may be exsected to a limited extent by an incision along its border, and the separation of the soft parts externally and internally, with the common saw, or some form described, section of the bone may be made to the required extent. If the part is deeply situated, the method recommended by Chassaignac may be followed. This consists in exposing the bone externally and internally, and then perforating it with a drill (page 172), or what would answer a good purpose, the small trephine of Pope (page 172).

The tuberosity of the ischium and the pubes have been excised; Chassaignac remarks that in these resections the method of perforation with the drill is preferred to other modes.

Resections of the Vertebra.—The spinous processes of the vertebræ may be removed by a single longitudinal incision. The incision may be freely made at any point of the column; the bone being exposed, it is separated with the bone forceps.

Excision of the arch of the vertebra is much more difficult in the lumbar and dorsal than in the cervical region, owing to the

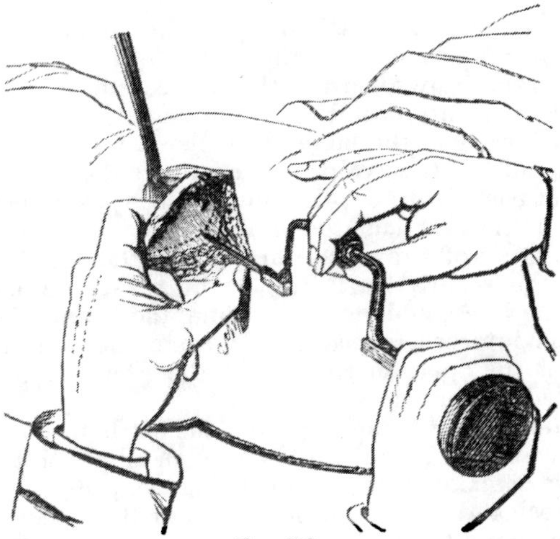

FIG. 242.

greatly increased size of the laminæ, and the covering of thick and powerful muscles.

Operation.—South (Chelius) describes the operation as follows: —the operation is tedious and tiresome, unless the muscles can be well drawn aside from the spine. A long incision should be made above the ridge of the spinous processes, the middle of which should be opposite the displacement, and from them all the muscles should be well cleared; divide all the attachments of the muscles to the articular processes, which gave plenty of room, as the one end of each muscular bundle being separated from its attachment, it retracted of itself, and needed little holding back with the finger. Generally, the saw or the nippers are sufficient to divide the vertebral arch; but, in an operation of this kind, the surgeon must be ready to use one instrument or another, according to the circumstances of the case. In sawing or cutting out the arch, it is always best to grasp the spinous process, if it be not broken, with a pair of stout tooth forceps; these are to be preferred to the elevator for lifting the detached bone from its natural connexions.

Cline advised the use of a small crowned trephine to cut through the vertebral arch; Tyrrell used Hey's saw; Goldsmith made a straight incision six inches in length, and at the extremities transverse incisions four inches long.

Resection of the Ribs.—The resection of the ribs may be

undertaken with much confidence, as this operation generally terminates successfully. The chief difficulty met with is the separation of the pleura.

Operation.—Place the patient upon the sound side, and expose the bone by an incision along the middle of the rib, or the incision may be curved downwards; the intercostal muscles are now divided, and the intercostal artery disengaged from its groove in the inferior border of the bone; the pleura is cautiously separated with the handle of the scalpel, or some similar instrument, and a thin piece of pasteboard or other substance is passed behind, and the bone sawn with the articulated or chain saw. Velpeau recommends to make section of the posterior part of the rib first; to avoid wounding the pleura "it is important to scrape carefully each border of the bone, and not to incline the point of the bistoury towards the intercostal space." In removing the false ribs, Velpeau advises the operator to support the free extremity while the rib is divided posteriorly.

Modification.—McClellan removed the sixth and seventh ribs for an enormous tumor (spina ventosa) by an elliptical incision.

Chassaignac makes a curved incision having its convexity downwards, exposing the diseased bone, two or three days before resection; after having cut the flap he passes two threads firmly united, by means of a curved needle along the internal face of the rib at the point where the bone is to be divided; these threads are replaced after twelve or twenty-four hours by a drainage tube; these tubes prepare the way for the passage of the chain saw; on the second or third day he saws the bone, and removes the fragment.

Resections of the Sternum.—Resections of this bone are performed with the gouge, or trephine; no special rules can be given for the operation. The incision is either crucial, or a vertical incision having transverse branches at both extremities.

Resection of the Pubic Bones.—Christoforis proposed subperiosteal resection of the pubic bones as a substitute for the Cæsarian section, alleging that the periosteum could be successfully separated, and that the bone would be reproduced. The first incision is across the mons veneris, between the crural arteries, about five inches long; the second extends from the upper margin of the commissure of the vulva horizontally one and a half inches, a third incision extends from the extremity of the latter to the middle of the tuberosity of the ischium; the periosteum having been separated, the horizontal and vertical branch of the pubes is divided on both sides with the chain saw. He also proposes to remove one or the other of the rami of this bone by the same method.

RESECTION OF THE BONES OF THE FACE.

Resection of the Bones of the Orbit.—Velpeau remarks that the os unguis, ascending process of the superior maxilla, and the ethmoid bone, have often been removed.

For the removal of the supra-orbitar arch he gives two methods, 1, by raising up on the forehead a semilunar flap from the eyelid; 2, by bringing down upon the eyelid a flap of the same form from the forehead. The bone could be removed with the bone forceps, or a small saw; he would not proscribe the gouge and mallet, in removing angular projections.

Resection of the Malar Bone.—Portions of the malar bone have been removed, as the processes and borders, by crucial and T incisions; the entire bone has been removed with the superior maxilla for necrosis.

Resections of the Superior Maxilla.—Malgaigne remarks of the anatomical relations of this bone:—"In attentively examining the face of the skeleton, we see that the superior maxillary bone is attached to the others in but three principal points. First, by its ascending process and articulations with the os unguis and ethmoid. Second, by the orbital border of the malar, as far as the spheno-maxillary fissure. Third, by the articulation of the two maxillary bones and palate bone with each other. There is a fourth point of contact behind with the pterygoid process and palate bone, which yields easily by simple depression of the maxillary bone into the interior of the mouth; in attacking these different points no large vessel is injured; the trunk of the internal maxillary artery may be easily avoided, or in any case tied after the removal of the bone: moreover, in case of unforeseen hæmorrhage during the operation, we have a resource in compression of the carotid. As for the nerves, only one important trunk need be divided, the superior maxillary; but it is easy to cut it before removing the bone, and so prevent any strain."

Resection of the Superior Maxilla below the Floor of the Orbit.—Guérin (Fig. 243) describes (*Elem. de Chir. Op.*) the following operation:—Make an incision slightly convex backwards commencing at the ala of the nose, and terminating at the corresponding commissure of the lip, following the naso-labial fold or furrow of the skin; dissect up the two flaps resulting from this incision until the nostril is exposed, and the malar process is completely denuded; with a small saw held in the right hand, *a*, the operator saws through the malar process from above downwards, and a little from within outwards; the soft palate having been detached from the posterior border of the palatine bone by a transverse incision made at the posterior border of the last great molar, and an incisor tooth having been extracted, the horizontal portion of the maxilla is divided from before backwards with Liston's forceps, *c*, one branch being in the mouth, and the other in the nares; a section of the bone is now made from the divided malar process to the nares by the forceps *b*; the bone is then seized with strong forceps, and removed, fracturing the pterygoid process.

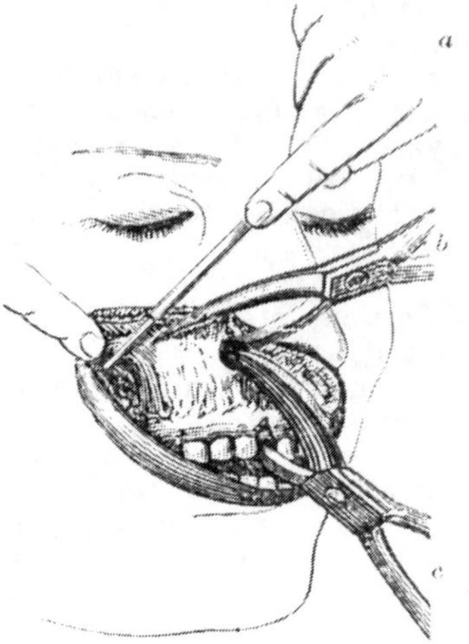

Fig. 248.

Resection of the Entire Superior Maxilla.—Gensoul's method was as follows (*Malgaigne, op. cit.*):—"The operator first makes a vertical incision, extending from the large angle of the eye to the upper lip, which he divides on a level with the canine tooth; from the middle of this incision, or rather almost on a level with the base of the nose, he makes a second, which he prolongs to half an inch in front of the lobe of the ear; and a third, extending from half an inch outside the external angle of the orbit to the point of termination of the second. The result is a quadrilateral flap, which is reflected back upon the forehead. The bone being thus laid bare, begin with a chisel and mallet the section of the external orbital arch, near the suture that unites the malar with the external orbital process of the frontal bone; then cut the zygomatic process of the malar. Then attack its upper and internal attachments, apply a large chisel below the internal angle of the eye, and cut through the inferior part of the os unguis and the orbital surface of the ethmoid; the ascending process is in like manner separated from the corresponding nasal bone: then detach with a knife all the soft parts that unite the ala of the nose to the superior maxilla: extract the first incisor tooth of the side operated on, and slip a chisel between the two bones, not directly from before backwards, but by the mouth, working it from side to side: lastly, to separate the articulation and adhesions to the pterygoid process, and above all to cut the superior maxillary nerve, pass a chisel flatly between the soft parts and floor of the orbit from above downwards and from before backwards, so as to cut the nerve well back, and at the same time to get a good purchase on the bone to depress it into the mouth. It only now remains to divide with the curved scissors or knife all the soft parts that still hold the bone, and especially the attachments of the velum of the palate to the palate bone, so as to leave the soft portion of this velum extended between the pterygoid process and the outer side of the mouth."

Modifications.—Velpeau modified this method as follows (Fig.

244) (*Bernard* and *Huette*):—"The patient being seated upon a low chair, with his head thrown backwards and supported upon the breast of an assistant, make an incision with its convexity

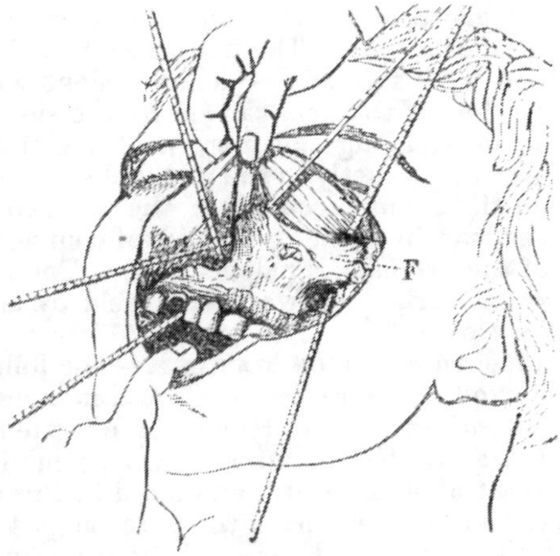

FIG. 244.

downwards, from the commissure of the lips to the temporal fossa. Dissect this large flap from below upwards, and turn it back upon the forehead. The maxillary bone being thus exposed, separate one after another its connexions with the other bones of the face. 1st, cut through with the cutting forceps the external orbitar process at its junction with the malar bone, the zygomatic arch, the os unguis, and the ascending nasal process of the upper jaw; 2d, divide the soft parts which connect the ala of the nose to the maxillary bone, and separate the two maxillæ in front with a chisel and mallet, or a small saw. Detach the soft parts from the floor of the orbit, and with flat cutting forceps, carried from above downwards, and from before backwards on the floor of the orbit, divide at once the superior maxillary nerve, and the connexions of the bone with the pterygoid process. Conclude the operation by cutting through with the bistoury, or curved scissors, the velum of the palate, and the remaining soft parts which still adhere to and retain the bone." The chain saw may be used to divide the processes, or the right and left saws (Figs. 202 and 203).

Syme directs two incisions to be made through the cheek, one extending from the inner angle of the eye directly downwards to the lip, the other beginning over the junction of the maxillary and malar bones and terminating at the angle of the mouth.

Liston operates as follows:—The point of the bistoury is entered over the external angular process of the frontal bone, is carried down through the cheek to the corner of the mouth, and is guided by the fore and middle fingers of the one or other hand, as may be placed in the cavity. A second incision made along and down to the zygoma falls into the other. Then the knife is pushed through the integument to the nasal process of the maxilla, the cartilage of the alæ is detached from the bone, and the lip is cut through in the mesial line. The flap thus formed is dissected up. Another method is thus given :—" The incisions were commenced at the inner canthus of the eye, carried by the side of and close to the alæ of the nose, along the margin of the nostrils, and then through the upper lip exactly in the middle line. Another incision was made from the commencement of the first, in a curved form, along the lower margin of the orbit, and, of course, in the direction of the fibres of the orbicularis palpebrarum. The flap thus formed was by dissection turned outwards and held by an assistant until the processes were cut."

Resection of both Superior Maxillæ.—The following methods have been followed in the resection of both maxillæ :—

Posterior Lateral Incisions.—Heyfelder operated as follows :—"The patient was seated in an arm chair; his head supported against the breast of an assistant, and fixed in this situation. The operator made two incisions from the outer angles of the eyes to the corner of the mouth, and pared all the softer parts away from the tumor to the inner angles of the eyes and the nasal bones. The flap thus formed being drawn upwards over the forehead, and the orbital margin being cleared down to the inferior ridge, he separated on both sides the junction between the jaw and cheek bone by means of a chain saw introduced through the inferior orbital fissure. In the same way, the separation of this bone with the nasal bone was effected. Then the bone and the other junctions still existing were divided by a bone forceps, and the soft palate separated from the hind edge of the hard palate. After that, pressure with a chisel upon the upper part of the tumor sufficed to dislocate the upper jaw bones out of the principal junctions, and so to finish the operation."—*Cooper's Surg. Dict.* (*New Edition.*)

Median Incision.—Dieffenbach made an incision from the root of the nose through the centre of the upper lip; if required, other incisions extend upwards on either side of the nose to the angles of the eyes; two flaps are thus formed, which are reflected, and the bones exposed.—*Ib.*

Resections of the Inferior Maxilla.—The lower jaw may be removed in part or whole.

Resection of the Central Portion of the Lower Jaw.—This portion of the inferior maxilla gives attachment anteriorly on either side of the symphysis to the levator menti, and more externally to the depressor labii inferioris, depressor anguli oris, and platysma myoides; internally, to the genio-hyoglossi and genio-hyoidei muscles; the fossa for the sublingual glands is more external, and below is the attachment of the digastric muscle.

Operation.—Dupuytren operated as follows (Fig. 245):—"Seat the patient in a slightly elevated chair, with his feet raised so that they will have no purchase on the floor. An assistant standing

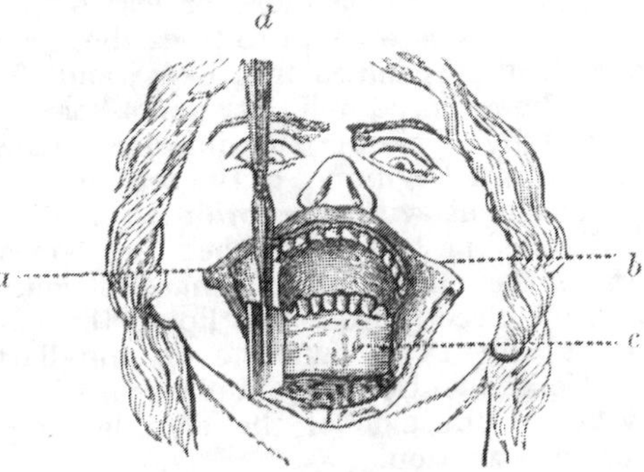

FIG. 245.

behind the patient holds his head firmly against his breast, and compresses at the same time the two facial arteries at the point where they cross the lower jaw. The surgeon, standing in front, seizes with his left hand one of the angles of the lower lip, while an assistant holds the other angle from the bone, and the whole in a state of tension. With a vertical incision he divides the lip through the median line at once to the bone, and afterwards prolongs it through the skin and subcutaneous cellular tissue down to the os hyoides. Keeping as close as possible to the bone, he then dissects back the two flaps, *a*, *b*, and the bone, *c*, being sufficiently denuded, incises the periosteum and extracts a tooth opposite to each point where it is to be sawn through. When dividing the bone, Dupuytren stood behind the patient and used a small Hey's saw, *d*; if the chain saw is used, the surgeon stands in front of the patient. The bone being sawn through on both sides, an assistant pushes back the tongue with a spatula, to protect it from the knife, and the surgeon holding the bone with his left hand, with a probe-pointed bistoury, held perpendicular, divides the muscles attached to it, as closely as possible to their insertion, carrying the knife along its concave surface. After the division of its attachments, the tongue will sometimes fall backwards, threatening suffocation. This is to be remedied by holding the head forwards, when the tongue will naturally fall into the same position."—*Bernard and Huette.*

Modifications.—If the portion of bone to be excised were so large as to require the removal of a portion of integuments, Dupuytren recommended two incisions, one on each side of the lip, and extending down to the os hyoides in the form of the letter V.

Malgaigne (*op. cit.*) remarks on the different modifications:—"If the longitudinal incision does not suffice on account of the extent of the disease, make it crucial by drawing another along the base of the bone. When you remove only a small portion of bone you may saw perpendicularly; but when the piece to be removed is large, in order to bring the fragments better together, it is well for the section to be more or less oblique, according to the thickness. In this case begin to trace the groove for the saw, by four or five small perpendicular strokes; and afterwards, incline it so as to have the required obliquity; in all cases, a firm support may be obtained by applying the inferior against the superior maxilla, at least in the beginning of the section.

"Gensoul finds fault with the ordinary method, because the cicatrix is in the median line; and when the bones no longer support the skin of the chin, a line of hard fibrous inodular tissue results, extending directly from the lip to the os-hyoides, which tends to retract and draw down the lip and flatten the newly-formed chin. Consequently Gensoul places his incision so that the cicatrix may be on one side of the chin, leaving the latter free from consecutive retraction.

"I do not know what may be the real value of this precaution, which, however, we may use without inconvenience; but with the method of Gensoul there remains also a very disagreeable cicatrix on the lip at the bottom of the face. Reux tried to avoid, at least in part, this deformity; and in a case which did not allow of doing more (the disease extending from the right incisors to near the last left molar), he succeeded in leaving the edge of the lip untouched, by means of a curved incision, which, starting from the depression under the chin, descended towards the hyoid region to again ascend below the left molar eminence, and circumscribed a flap which was dissected upwards. Velpeau cites this method as one that may be applied to lesions of the centre of the bone; but in trying it on the dead subject it will be very soon seen, that to expose the disease completely, and to apply the saw conveniently, the two ends of the incision must mount so high on the face that the deformity is replaced by another quite as disagreeable.

"I have tried on the subject a method which is free from all these objections. It consists in detaching the lower lip from above downwards, incising at the bottom of the groove between the bone and gums, and grazing the bone as far as the chin and some lines below it, to the extent of the lip itself. This dissection made, turn down, leaving a sufficient space at the inferior angle, to place there a little mêche of lint; and favor, if necessary, the escape of the pus."

Complications.—A serious complication is very liable to occur on the division of the attachments of the tongue; in many instances it has immediately fallen backwards, depressing the epiglottis upon the larynx, and threatening instant suffocation. The tongue may be seized and held with McCay's forceps (Fig. 246). Delpech recommended that the tongue be seized with a double tenaculum before the division of its attachments. After the operation he included the frænum in the suture. Wood, of New York, passes a strong ligature through the tip of the tongue at the commencement of the operation, and subsequently fastens it to the cheek with an adhesive strip. Chelius, however, says:—"It is unnecessary to draw the tongue forwards and fix it; its retraction depends on the contraction of the m. sterno-hyoideus, after the separation of the m. mylo-hyoideus and genio-hyoideus, if the head be drawn back; and, therefore, if the head be bowed towards the chest, the tongue resumes its proper place, and the choking ceases."

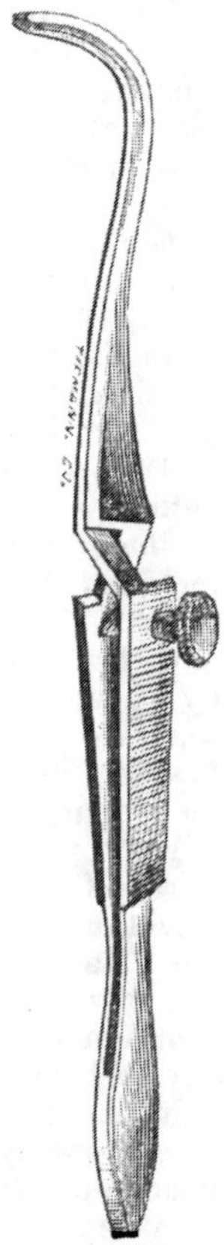

FIG. 246.

RESECTION OF HALF THE HORIZONTAL PORTION OF THE LOWER JAW.—The body of the lower jaw gives attachment on its internal surface to the mylo-hyoideus muscle, beneath which is the fossa for the submaxillary gland; on its external surface along its lower margin is the attachment of the platysma myoides muscle, and along its alveolar margin the buccinator; the facial artery mounts over its lower border, just anterior to the insertion of the masseter muscle.

The following operations have been practised for its removal:—

One Inferior Flap.—Cloquet made a horizontal incision, commencing at the commissure of the lips, and terminating at the distance of one or two lines beyond the ramus of the jaw; two vertical incisions join this: one descending from the free edge of the lip to the base of the bone, and the second parallel to this, but descending behind the ramus of the jaw several lines below the angle; the flap is dissected downwards, the soft parts separated from the internal surface of the bone, and the bone sawn at the proper points.

Modifications.—Liston divided the cheek by thrusting a long, narrow bistoury through it at the anterior edge of the masseter muscle, and then cut forwards to the angle of the mouth; from each extremity of this incision another is made downwards, the anterior inclining forwards, the posterior backwards.

ONE SUPERIOR INTERNAL FLAP.—Mott tied the carotid, and then made an incision curved downwards, commencing in front of the ear, on a level with the condyle, passing under the labial commissure and terminating near the chin; this flap was raised and reflected on the face; a second incision was made, beginning at the same point as the first, one inch long, close to the lobe of the ear, and terminating at the edge of the mastoid muscle. The bone was sawn through, first in front, and then behind, and the diseased part removed; if the operation is above a certain point the inferior maxillary nerve should be divided before the bone is withdrawn; the lingual branch of the fifth pair is to be avoided.

Modifications.—Malgaigne proposed, if the disease extended far behind, and less in front, a semilunar incision along the ramus and base of the bone from the ear to the chin, so as to have one superior internal flap, and no cicatrix on the face. Fergusson prefers also not to cut the lip at all, believing that any part of the lower jaw or even the whole bone may be removed without cutting the margin of the lip; Skey makes a similar incision along the base of the jaw; Wood made the incision under the base of the jaw terminating from a quarter to half an inch below the symphysis menti.

One Superior External Flap.—Lisfranc made a vertical incision from the free edge of the lip to a point below the chin; a second incision was carried from the latter point along the base of the jaw two lines beyond the angle; this flap was dissected upwards, and reflected on the face; the bone was then sawn in front and behind.

Modification.—Liston proposed, if the part to be removed was included between the lateral incisor and last molar teeth, to extract them, and make a semilunar incision along the base of the jaw, the extremities extending upwards over the spaces occupied by these teeth; the flap should be dissected up, the soft parts separated, and the bone divided with strong pliers, having been first notched with Hey's saw; Fergusson turns the horizontal incision upwards behind the angle of the jaw.

Resection of the Entire Horizontal Portion of the Lower Jaw.—Two methods have been proposed of accomplishing this resection. 1. Make an incision along the base of the jaw, extending it a little beyond the angle; now dissect the flap upwards, and saw the bone at the proper points. 2. In addition to the horizontal incision make a perpendicular one through the lower lip, thus raising two flaps.

Resection of one Half of the Lower Jaw.—The rami terminate in two processes, one for articulation, and the other to give attachment to the temporal muscles; the articulation is supported by an external and internal lateral ligament, and the capsular; the stylo-maxillary passes from the styloid process to the angle of the jaw. The internal maxillary artery passes behind the neck of the condyle in such proximity as to render care necessary to avoid wounding it in disarticulation of the jaw.

Semicircular Flap.—Mott operated as follows:—An incision commenced in front of, and about opposite the meatus auditorius externus, was carried downwards behind the angle of the jaw, and thence along the lower part of the tumor, in a semicircular direction, and was brought suddenly upwards by a short curve, and terminated upon the chin, within an inch of the inner margin of the lower lip, so as to open into the mouth opposite the second incisor tooth; the soft parts were separated from the body of the bone, the chain saw passed, and the bone divided; the dissection was continued upwards, the temporal muscle detached from the coronoid, and the disarticulation effected.

Quadrilateral Flap.—The following method is given by Bernard and Huette (Fig. 247):—1. Make a horizontal incision along the inferior border of the bone, extending from the symphysis to the angle of the jaw; make a vertical section at each extremity of this incision; the internal, dividing the lower lip, through the median line; the external, carried from the zygomatic arch behind the ramus of the jaw. This makes a quadrilateral flap, which is to be dissected and turned up, *f*, *a*, *b*. Saw through the jaw at the median line, *d*, and keeping close to the bone, detach with the bistoury all the soft parts adhering to its posterior surface as far as the angle of the jaw. Carry a probe-pointed bistoury beneath the zygomatic arch, and behind the coronoid process, and with it divide the tendon of the temporal muscle while depressing the bone to disengage the process and luxate the condyle. Pull the bone strongly outwards, *c*, as far as possible from the vessels, in order to avoid especially the internal maxillary artery, *e*, and complete the operation by dividing the pterygoid muscles and the articular ligaments.

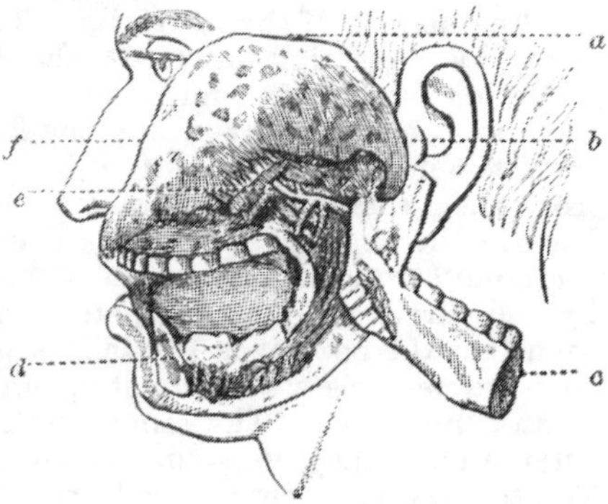

Fig. 247.

Single Curved Incision.—Wood, of New York, operated as follows:—The patient was placed on the operating table, with her head and shoulders elevated, and her face turned towards the left side. The external incision commenced midway between the angle and condyle of the right side, and extended along and under the base of the jaw, terminating one quarter of an inch below the symphysis menti. The soft parts were next divided, and the periosteum carefully separated from the bone. A chain saw was then passed under the jaw into the mouth, half an inch to the right of the symphysis, and the bone sawn through. The saw was again passed under the jaw, at its angle, for the purpose of dividing the bone at this point, but, unfortunately, on attempting to work it, the chain broke. He now seized the bone at this point with Liston's forceps, and endeavored to divide it, when it was readily discovered, in this attempt, that the jaw was necrosed to its articulation. He then endeavored, with the forceps, to remove the jaw entire upon the right side, and succeeded, with considerable effort, in completely enucleating it from its periosteal covering.

Resection of the Entire Lower Jaw.—Carnochan operated as follows: "The patient being seated on a chair, and the assistants properly arranged, an incision was first made, commencing opposite the left condyle, passing downwards towards the angle of the jaw, ranging at about two lines in front of the posterior border of the ramus, and extending thence along the base of the jaw, to terminate by a slight curve on the mesial line, half an inch below the free margin of the lower lip. The bone was now partially laid bare, by dissecting upwards the tissues of the cheek, and by reflecting downwards, for a short distance, the lower edge of the incision. The tissues forming the floor of the mouth, and situated upon the inner surface of the body of the bone, were separated from their attachments from a point near the mesial line, as far back as the angle of the jaw. The attachments of the buccinator were next divided. The facial artery, the sub-mental and the sub-lingual, already cut, were then secured by ligature. It was now seen that the bone was partially separated at the symphysis, and that the necrosis was complete from that point to the inferior portion of the ramus. The ramus itself was found diseased; the periosteum externally was inflamed, and in some parts easily detached. The tongue was now grasped and held forwards, while the attachments of the genio-hyo-glossi muscles were divided. A double ligature was passed through the anterior part of the root of the tongue, and intrusted to an assistant, in order to prevent its retraction upon the superior orifice of the larynx. A slight force exercised upon the left half of the body of the jaw, broke the connexion of the symphysis and at the angle, and this part was easily removed. The next step consisted in the removal of the left ramus. The external surface of the branch of the jaw, and of the temporo-maxillary articulation, were exposed, by dissecting the masseter upwards, as far as the zygomatic arch. Seizing the ramus in order to pull the coronoid process downwards below the zygoma, it was found that the temporal muscle was rigidly and permanently retracted. This circumstance presented an unexpected difficulty, which was increased by the unusual development of this apophysis, and by the retraction also of the pterygoid muscles. Passing the forefinger along the inner aspect of the ramus, the situation of the internal and external carotids was sought for and recognised. The insertion of the pterygoideus internus was then felt and cut, grazing the bone in doing so; the lingual nerve, here in close proximity, being carefully avoided. Passing still higher up, the orifice of the dental canal, indicated by an osseous projection, could be felt; and the instrument, still guided by the finger, divided the dental artery and nerve. The knife was thus made to separate the tissues attached to the inner face of the bone, as high up as a point situated about a line below the sigmoid notch, between the condyle and the coronoid process. On a level with this point, at the posterior margin of the ramus, the transverse facial, internal maxillary and temporal arteries form a kind of tripod, the two last named branches of which should not be divided, if possible. It now became necessary to detach the tendon of the temporal muscle. As the coronoid process could not be depressed, I proceeded cautiously, by dividing the lower attachments of the tendon, by means of blunt curved scissors; and by using them and a probe-pointed bistoury, alternately—keeping close to the bone—a considerable portion of the tendon was divided. Deeming it not prudent to use freely a sharp cutting instrument, deep in the temporal fossa, where the coronoid process was situated, I made use of a pair of bone scissors, curved flatwise; and by passing the blades of this instrument over the process, as far as its position would permit, the temporal muscle was detached; a small portion of the apex of the coronoid process being cut through. The ramus, now movable, could be made use of as a lever to aid in the disarticulation of the bone.

"In order to effect safely the disarticulation of the condyle, I began by penetrating into the joint, by cutting the ligaments from *before backwards* and from *without inwards.* The articulation was thus opened sufficiently to allow the condyle to be completely luxated. Blunt scissors were now used to cut carefully the internal part of the capsule and the maxillary insertion of the external pterygoid muscle; and by a slow movement of rotation of the ramus upon its axis, the condyle was detached, and the operation was completed on this side. To effect the removal of the other half of the lower jaw, the same incision was made on the opposite side, so as to meet the first on the mesial line. The dissection was also similar; and by disarticulating the second condyle in the same manner as had been observed for the first, I was successful again in avoiding lesion of the temporal and internal maxillary arteries.

"The object I had in view, in shaping the external incisions, in such a way that an inverted V should be formed in front of the insertion of the genio-hyo-glossi muscles, was to leave a portion of integument so fashioned, that the suture-pins could be passed through the integument, and, at the same time, through the root of the tongue, at the point where its muscles had been detached from the inner surface of the jaw."

RESECTIONS OF THE BONES OF THE CRANIUM.

Instruments.—The instruments required for resection of the bones of the cranium are the trephine and the saw. The ordinary trephine (Fig. 248) is a circular saw with a sliding pin in the centre, by which it is fixed in position. The handle is generally fastened to the shaft by a screw, with a button affixed to the end of the shaft; in the handle represented in Fig. 249, A. B. Mott, of New York, has attached the screw to one end of the handle; when the handle is placed on the shaft this screw is tightened, and its extremity reaches the shaft and fastens it firmly in its place. The advantage of this arrangement is that the upper surface of the handle is smooth, and the palm of the hand is not bruised as it is by the metallic button on the handle of the old instrument.

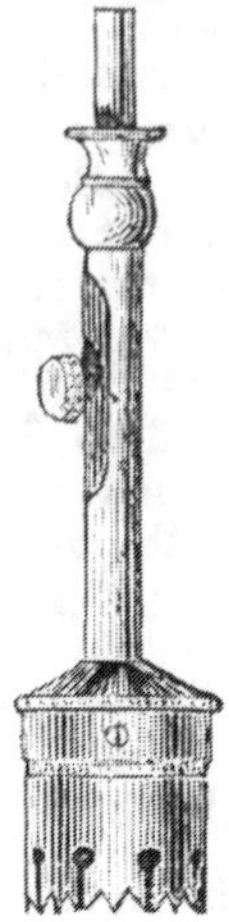

Fig. 248.

The conical trephine (Fig. 250) of Galt, of Va., is, in many respects, a great improvement upon the old trephine. The peculiar advantage of this trephine consists in dividing the cranial walls without any danger of wounding the membranes of the brain. In consists of a truncated cone, with spiral peripheral teeth, and oblique crown teeth; when applied, the peripheral teeth act as wedges so long as counteracting pressure exists on the crown teeth;

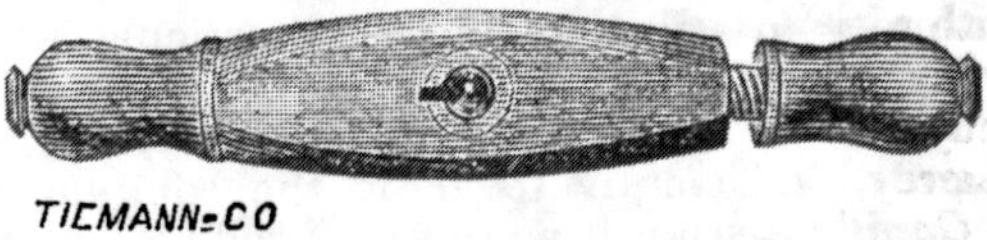

Fig. 249.

upon removal of that pressure of the cranial walls its tendency is to act on the principle of a screw; but owing to its conical form and the spiral direction of its peripheral teeth its action ceases. In the construction of this instrument, the inventor alleges that it is important to preserve the precise relative shape of the cone given in the illustration, the size, of course, of the peripheral teeth being the same. Upon this condition alone depends the complete success of the instrument. In repeated trials the membranes of the brain have not been injured.

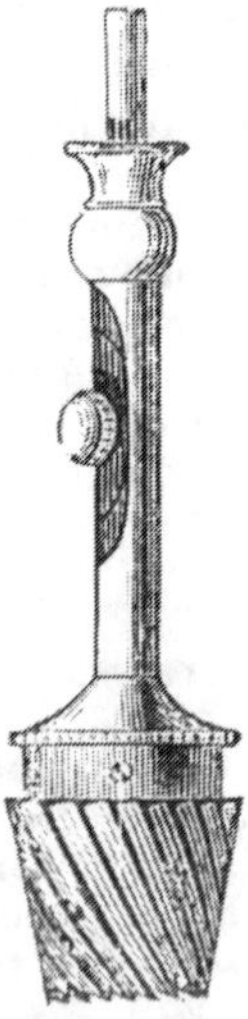

Fig. 250.

The anatomical peculiarities to be noticed in the application of the trephine to the skull are thus pointed out by Malgaigne (*op. cit.*):—

"1. When we trepan on the temporal fossa, Sabatier advises making a V-shaped incision, the base upwards, in order to respect the fibres of the temporalis muscle. Velpeau very properly remarks, that by so doing we cut, just the same, all the fibres comprised in the base of the flap. To respect these fibres as much as possible, we would advise making two incisions in the direction of the muscular fibres, and reuniting them inferiorly by a transverse incision, so as to form a V incision reversed, and cut off at the top; on the one hand, the division of these fibres, and the cicatrix that results, are less extensive; and on the other, the transverse incision, affecting more or less the deep aponeurosis on which most of its fibres terminate; we should divide really less muscular fibre.

"2. When we have to traverse the frontal sinus, the internal table of the bone not being on the same plane as the external, in performing the operation as usual, the dura mater would be torn at one point before the second table was cut through at the opposite. To cut the second table, then, a smaller crown should be used than that employed in sawing the first.

"3. When we trepan on the sagittal suture, or opposite the venous sinuses, we run a great chance of opening them; the hæmorrhage generally stops of itself, or yields to a little plugging.

"4. Lesion of the middle meningeal artery is more serious, on which account it has long been forbidden to trepan, at the anterior inferior angle of the parietal bone, under which the artery lies. If hæmorrhage occurs, it may be compressed with a bit of lint placed inside the cranium, and retained by a thread outside (Physick); or with a plate of lead, bent so as to embrace both surfaces of the bone; or it may be plugged with a bit of wax, if it is shut in a complete bony canal; or touched with a steel probe heated to whiteness (Larrey); or even tied, in which Dorsey once succeeded."

Operation.—The patient being placed in the recumbent position, with the head slightly raised, an incision is made down to the bone, having the form of a V, T, or +, or it may form a semicircle; the bone being scraped, the operator seizes the handle of the trephine with his right hand, and fixing the perforator by its screw, so that it protrudes slightly beyond the teeth, he places the perforator in the centre of the bone to be removed; the instrument is now worked alternately backwards and forwards, until the teeth have cut a groove sufficiently deep to receive them; the perforator is then loosened and slid up in the shaft and fixed, to avoid wounding the membranes; great care should be taken to maintain the instrument in a position perpendicular to the part operated upon, in order to avoid its penetrating more deeply on one side than the other, and thus suddenly and unawares wounding the cerebral membranes. It is important to examine the depth of the groove frequently with a toothpick, to ascertain how nearly the instrument has completed the section of the bone; the teeth of the trephine may occasionally require cleaning with a small brush or wet sponge. The disc of bone should be raised with the elevator (Fig. 207), and the edges smoothed with the lenticular knife at the other end of the elevator.

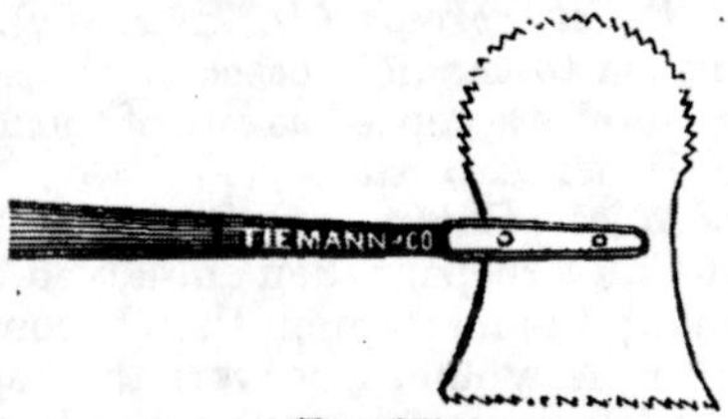

FIG. 251.

In fractures with depression there are frequently projecting points of bone which it is desirable to remove; this may be done with the bone nippers (rongeur), or with a Hey's saw (Fig. 251).

CHAPTER VI.

ON GUNSHOT WOUNDS.

GUNSHOT WOUNDS IN GENERAL.

Instruments.—A large number of instruments have been devised for the removal of balls, lodged in the track of gunshot wounds. The following list comprises some of those preferred by army surgeons, as also some of the more recent inventions:—

Double Crossing Forceps.—(Fig. 252.) This instrument, when closed, is a probe; in contact with the ball the blades are opened, and the ball seized by two very firm points, and readily withdrawn.

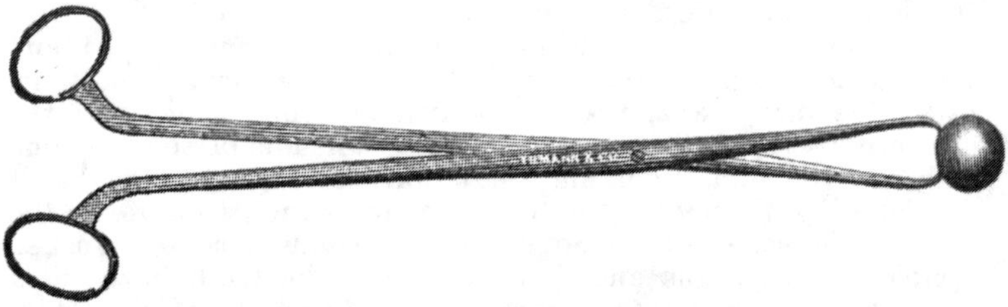

FIG. 252.

This forceps is generally received by army surgeons, as one of the most useful yet invented.

Bullet Forceps (U. S. Army).—(Fig. 253.) This forceps is furnished to the field cases of the surgeons of the U. S. Army, and is generally accepted as one of the most useful instruments of the kind.

Bullet Extractor.—(Fig. 254.) This instrument is the invention of Moses, Surgeon U. S. Army, and consists of a tube containing a sliding forceps; when employed, the forceps are withdrawn into the tube; the instrument then becomes a probe, which being introduced into the wound discovers the ball; when in contact with the body the forceps are gently pushed forwards, and expanding, embrace the ball, and the whole is withdrawn. The old bullet screw (Fig. 255), now little used, may also be adapted to this instrument, and being guided to the ball by the tube, can readily be made to penetrate it.

Flexible Bullet Extractor.—(Fig. 256.) Military surgeons have always regarded it as a desideratum to have an instrument for the extraction of balls which had a flexible tube, enabling it to follow a tortuous canal, and still have power when in contact with the foreign body to grasp it so firmly as to enable the operator to remove it. This object seems to have been accomplished by Mr. Stohlman, of

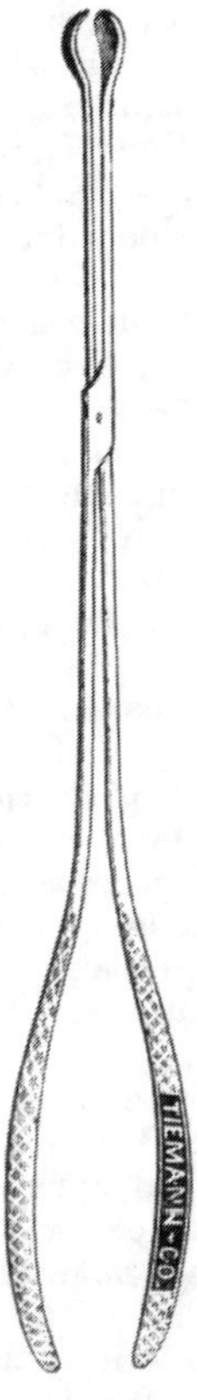

Fig. 253.

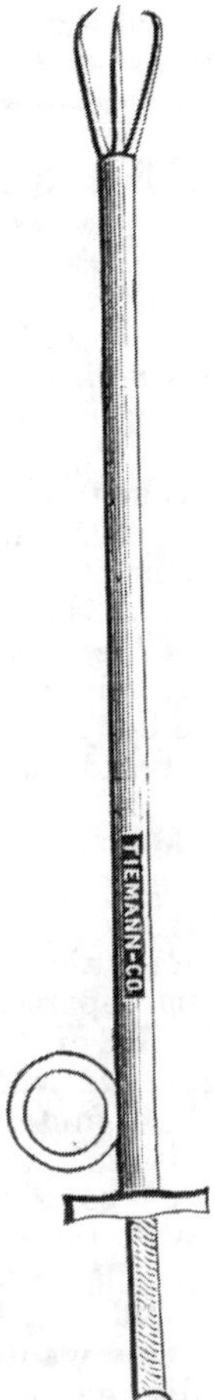

Fig. 254.

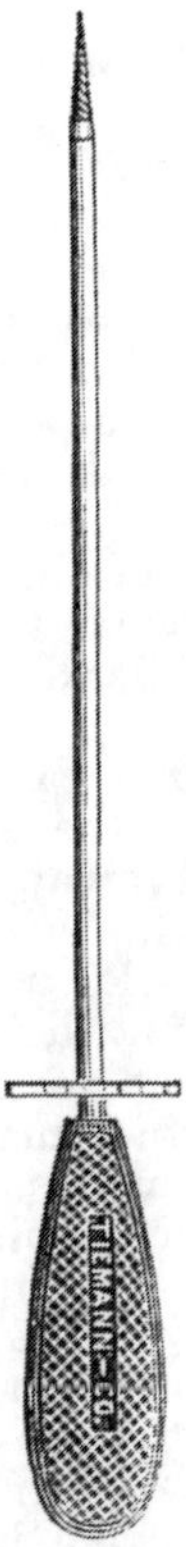

Fig. 255.

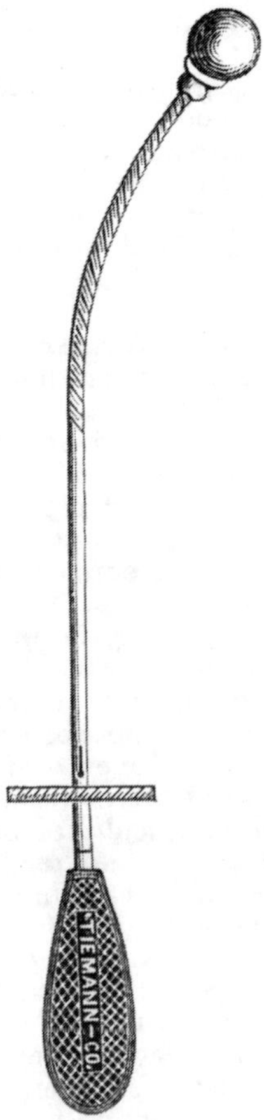

Fig. 256.

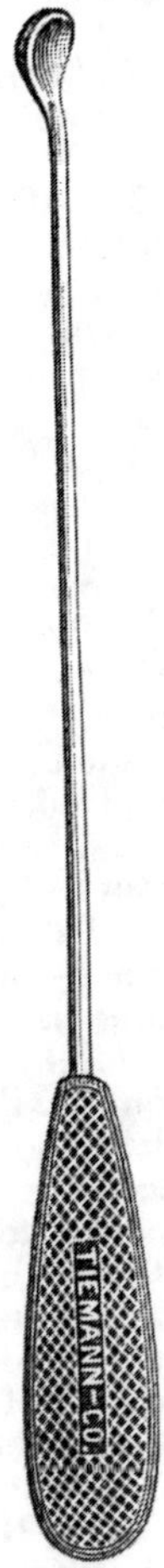

Fig. 257.

this city, in the flexible bullet extractor. The tube or canula consists of spiral flattened wire, so arranged as to give the required firmness, and at the same time a large degree of flexibility. The tube carries a concealed forceps of two prongs, like Moses's instrument, with which the ball is seized and withdrawn.

Bullet Scoop.—(Fig. 257.) This instrument was long used, either separately, or with the screw; it is still preferred by some surgeons.

The study of gunshot wounds belongs exclusively to the military surgeon. Without, therefore, presuming to discuss these subjects from the stand-point of civil practice, we present the following condensation of an article on *Gunshot Wounds*, communicated to *A System of Surgery*, recently published in London, by PROF. LONGMORE, Professor of Military Surgery in the English Military School at Fort Pitt, and the latest and most reliable writer on this subject.

1. **Character of Gunshot Wounds.**—When a cannon-ball at full speed strikes in direct line a part of the body, it carries away all before it. If the head, chest, or abdomen are exposed to the shot, an opening corresponding with the size of the ball is effected, the contiguous viscera are scattered, and life is at once extinguished. If it be part of one of the extremities which is thus removed, the end remaining attached to the body presents a stump with nearly a level surface of darkly contused, almost pulpified tissues.

2. In ricochet firing, or in any case where the force of the cannon-shot is partly expended, the extremity or portion of the trunk may be equally carried away, but the laceration of the remaining parts of the body will be greater; the surface of the wound will be less even. Muscles will be separated from each other, and hang loosely, offering at their divided ends little appearance of vitality; spiculæ of bone of larger size will probably be found among them; and the shaft may be found shattered and split far above the line of its transverse division.

3. If the speed be still further diminished, so that the projectile becomes what is termed a "spent ball," there will not be removal of the part of the body struck, but the external appearance will be limited usually to ecchymosis and tumefaction, without division of surface; or even these may be wanting, notwithstanding the existence of serious internal disorganization.

4. Should the cannon-ball strike in a slanting direction, the external appearances of the wound will be similar to those just described, according to its velocity, modified only in extent by the degree of obliquity with which the shot is carried into contact with the trunk or extremity wounded.

5. Large fragments of heavy shells generally produce immense laceration and separation of the parts against which they strike, but do not carry away or grind, as round shot. Ordinarily, the line of direction in which they move forms an obtuse angle with

the part of the body wounded. When they happen to strike in a more direct line, so as to penetrate, the external wound is mostly much smaller than the fragment itself, from the projectile not having had force enough to destroy the vitality and elasticity of the soft parts through which it entered.

6. Small projectiles, with force enough to penetrate the body, leave one or more openings, the external appearances of which also vary according to their form and velocity.

7. When the musket-ball strikes at a distance from the weapon by which it was propelled, but still preserves great velocity, the appearances of the wound are changed. An opening is observed, irregularly circular, with edges generally a little torn; and the whole wound is slightly inverted. There may be darkening of the margin, of a livid purple tinge, from the effects of contusion, or it may be simply deadlike and pale. Should the ball have passed out, the wound of exit will be probably larger, more torn, with slight eversion of its edges and protrusion of the subcutaneous fat, which is thus rendered visible. These appearances are the more easily recognised, the earlier the wound is examined. They are more obvious if a round musket-ball has caused the injury than when it has been inflicted by a cylindro-conoidal bullet.

8. A musket-ball ordinarily causes either one wound, as when after entering it lodges, or, as sometimes happens, from its escaping again by the wound of entrance; or two wounds, from making its exit at some point remote from the spot where it entered; but occasionally leads to a greater number of openings. This last result may happen from the ball splitting into two or more portions within the body, and causing so many wounds of exit.

9. The number of wounds made by one ball may be increased by its traversing two adjoining extremities of the same person, or even distant parts of the body from accidental relative position at the time of the injury.

10. The two openings made by one ball may hold such a relative situation as to lead to the mistake of their being supposed to be caused by two distinct balls. Length of traverse, and consequent distance between the two openings, parts of the body brought into unusual relations from peculiarities of posture, and peculiar deflections of the ball, may all be sources of this error.

11. The appearances of wounds resulting from penetrating missiles of irregular forms, as small pieces of shells, musket-balls flattened against stones, and others, differ from those caused by ordinary bullets in being accompanied with more laceration, according to their length and form; being usually projected with considerably less force than direct missiles, such projectiles ordinarily lead only to one aperture, that of entrance.

12. **Symptoms of Gunshot Wounds.**—A gunshot wound by musket-shot is attended with an amount of pain which varies very much in degree according to the kind of wound, condition of

mind, and state of constitution of the soldier at the time of its infliction. Sometimes the pain from the shot is described as a sudden smart stroke of a cane; in other instances as the shock of a heavy intense blow. Occasionally the pain will be referred to a part not involved in the track of the wound. When a ball does not penetrate, but simply inflicts a contusion, the pain is described to be more severe than where an opening has been made by it.

13. As a general rule, the graver the injury, the greater and more persistent is the amount of "shock." A rifle-bullet which splits up a long bone into many longitudinal fragments, inflicts a very much more serious injury than the ordinary fracture effected by the ball from a smooth-bore musket, and the constitutional shock bears like proportion. When a portion of one or of both lower extremities is carried away by a cannon-ball, the higher towards the trunk the injury is inflicted, the greater the shock, independent of the loss of blood. The practical experience of every army surgeon teaches him that where a ball has entered the body, though its course be not otherwise indicated, the continuance of shock is a sufficient evidence that some organ essential to life has been implicated in the injury.

14. When a part of the body is carried away by round shot or shell, the arteries are observed to be nearly in the same state as they are found to be in when a limb is torn off by machinery. The lacerated ends of the middle and inner coats are retracted within the outer cellular coat; the calibre of the vessel is diminished, and tapers to a point near the line of division: it becomes plugged within by coagulum; and the cellulo-fibrous investing sheath, and the clot which combines with it, form on the outside an additional support and restraint against hæmorrhage. When large arteries are torn across, and their hæmorrhage thus spontaneously prevented, they are seldom withdrawn so far but that their ends may be seen protruding and pulsating among the mass of injured structures; yet, though the impulse may appear very powerful, further hæmorrhage is rarely met with from such wounds. There is more danger of continued hæmorrhage from wounds by pieces of shell, as the arteries are liable to be wounded without complete transverse section of their coats. Primary but indirect hæmorrhage, in consequence of a gunshot injury, usually occurs as a complication of fractured long bones, the sharp points and edges of which, extensively torn up as they now are by conical bullets, are well calculated to cause such injuries.

15. **Provisional Treatment.**—When the circumstances of a battle admit of the arrangement, the wounded should receive surgical attention preliminary to their being transported to the regimental or general field hospitals in the rear. The provisional treatment should be of the simplest kind, and chiefly directed to the prevention of additional injury during the passage to the hospital, where complete and accurate examination of the nature

of the wound can alone be made, and where the patient can remain at rest after being subjected to the required treatment. The removal of any missiles or foreign bodies which may be readily obvious; the application of a piece of lint to the wound; the arrangement of any available support for a broken limb; protection against dust, cold, or other objectionable circumstances likely to occur in the transit; if "shock" exist, the administration of a little wine, aromatic ammonia, or other restorative, in water—need little time in their execution, and may prove of great service to the patient.

16. **Diagnosis.**—On arrival at the hospital, the following are the points to be attended to by the surgeon: firstly, examination of the wound with a view to obtaining a correct knowledge of its nature and extent; secondly, removal of any foreign bodies which may have lodged; thirdly, adjustment of lacerated structures; and fourthly, the application of the primary dressings.

17. One of the earliest rules for examining a gunshot wound is to place the patient as nearly as can be ascertained, in a position similar to that in which he was, in relation to the missile, at the time of being struck by it. In almost every instance the examination will be facilitated by attention to this precept.

18. When only one opening has been made by a ball, it is to be presumed that it is lodged somewhere in the wound, and search must be made for it accordingly. But even where two openings exist, and evidence is afforded that these are the apertures of entrance and exit of one projectile, examination should still be made to detect the presence of foreign bodies. Portions of clothing, and other harder substances, are not unfrequently carried into a wound by a ball; and, though it itself may pass out, these may remain behind, either from being diverted from the straight line of the wound or from becoming caught and impacted in the fibrous tissue through which the ball has passed. The inspection of the garments worn over the part wounded may often serve as a guide in determining whether foreign bodies have entered or not, and, if so, their kind.

19. Of all instruments for conducting an examination of a gunshot wound, the finger of the surgeon is the most appropriate. By its means the direction of the wound can be ascertained with least disturbance of the several structures through which it takes its course. The index finger naturally occurs as the most convenient for this employment; but the opening through the skin is sometimes too contracted to admit its entrance, and in this case the substitution of the little finger will usually answer all the purposes intended. When the finger fails to reach sufficiently far, owing to the depth of the wound, the examination is often facilitated by pressing the soft parts from an opposite direction towards the finger-end.

20. It does not often happen that it is necessary to enlarge

the openings of wounds to remove balls, although a certain amount of constriction of the skin may be expected from the addition of the instrument employed in the extraction; but if much resistance is offered to their passage out, it is better to divide the edges of the fascia and skin to the amount of enlargement required than to use force. In removing fragments of shells or detached pieces of bone, the fascia and skin have almost invariably to be divided to a considerable extent.

21. Where the finger is not sufficiently long to reach the bottom of the wound, even when the soft parts have been approximated by pressure from an opposite direction, and when the lodgment of a projectile is suspected, a long silver probe, that admits of being bent by the hand if required, is the best substitute. Elastic bougies or catheters are apt to become curled among the soft parts, and do not convey to the sense of touch the same amount of information as metallic instruments do. The probe should be employed with great nicety and care, for it may inflict injury on vessels or other structures which have escaped from direct contact with the ball, but have returned, by their elasticity, to the situations from which they had been pushed or drawn aside during its passage. The above directions for examining wounds apply more particularly to such as penetrate the extremities, or extend superficially in other parts of the body; where a missile has entered any of the important cavities, search for it is not to be made, but the surgeon's attention is to be directed to matters of more vital importance to be hereafter noticed.

22. **Treatment.**—As soon as the presence of a ball or other foreign body is ascertained it should be removed. If it be lying within reach from the wound of entrance, it should be extracted through this opening by means of some of the various instruments devised for the purpose. Instruments of two blades, or scoops, with ordinary hinge action, dilate the track of the wound injuriously before the ball can be grasped by them. The way to the removal of a bullet may often be smoothed by judiciously clearing away the fibres, among which it is lodged, during the examination by the finger; and sometimes, by means of the finger in the wound, and external pressure of the surrounding parts, the projectile may be brought near to the aperture of entrance, so that its extraction is still further facilitated. Such foreign substances as pieces of cloth can usually be brought out by the finger alone, or by pressing them between the finger and a silver probe inserted for the purpose. Sometimes a long pair of dressing forceps, guided by the finger, is found necessary for effecting this object. Caution must be used in employing forceps, where the foreign substance is out of sight, and of such a quality that the soft tissues may be mistaken for it.

23. In instances where the foreign body has not completely penetrated, but is found lying beneath the skin away from the

wound of entrance, an incision must be made for its extraction. Before using the knife, the substance to be removed should be fixed *in situ*, by pressure on the surrounding parts. In the instance of a round ball, the incision should be carried beyond the length of its diameter; an addition of half a diameter is usually sufficient to admit of the easy extraction of the ball. In removing conical balls, slugs, fragments of shells, stones, and other irregularly-shaped bodies, the surgeon cannot be too guarded in arranging that the fragment is drawn away with its long axis in line with the track of the wound. By proper care in this respect, much injury to adjoining structures may be avoided.

24. If balls are impacted in bone, as happens in the spongy heads of bones, in bones of the pelvis, and occasionally, though rarely, in other parts of long bones, they should be removed. This can be effected by means of a steel elevator, of convenient size; or, should this fail from the ball being too firmly impacted, a thin layer of the bone on one side of the ball may be gouged away, so that a better purchase may be obtained for the elevator, in effecting its removal. The fact is now fully established that, although in a few isolated cases balls remain lodged in bones without sensible inconvenience, in the majority the lodgment leads to such disease of the bony structure as often to entail troublesome abscesses, and in some instances eventually to necessitate amputation.

25. Should there be reason for concluding that a ball or other foreign body has lodged, but after manual examination, and observation as well by varied posture of the part of the body supposed to be implicated as by indications derived from the patient's sensations, effects of pressure or injury to nerves, and all other circumstances which may lead to information, should the site of the lodgment not be ascertained, the search should not be persevered in to the distress of the patient. Neither, although the site of lodgment be ascertained, if extensive incisions are required, or if there is danger of wounding important organs, should the attempts at extraction be continued. Either during the process of suppuration, by some accidental muscular contraction, or by gradual approach towards the surface, its escape may be eventually effected; or, if of a favorable form, and if not in contact with nerve, bone, or other important organ, it may become encysted, and remain without causing pain or mischief.

26. Extensive experience has shown that not only is the risk of subsequent ill results greater in those cases where foreign bodies remain lodged than when they have been cut out, but also that the advantages of a second opening for the escape of the necessary sloughs and discharges greatly preponderate over the disadvantages connected with it, as regards the additional extent of injured surface.

27. When a gunshot wound has been accompanied with much laceration and disturbance of the parts involved in the injury, it is necessary, after the removal of all foreign substances that can be

detected, to readjust and secure the disjointed structures as nearly as possible in their normal relations to each other. The simplest means—strips of adhesive plaster, light pledgets of moist lint, a linen roller, favorable position of the limb or part of the body wounded—should be adopted for this purpose. Pressure, weight, and warmth should be avoided as much as possible in these applications, consistent with the end in view. It must not be forgotten, in thus bringing the parts together, that the purpose is not to obtain union by adhesion, which cannot be looked for, but simply to prevent avoidable irritation and malposition of parts, during the subsequent stages of cure by granulation and cicatrization.

28. In all gunshot wounds, much discomfort to the patient is prevented by carefully sponging away all blood and clot from the surface adjoining the wound, and by adopting measures to prevent its spreading again in consequence of oozing. This can be readily done with the aid of a little warm water, and arrangement when the wound is first dressed, but can only be accomplished with considerable inconvenience after the thin clots have become hard and firmly adherent to the skin.

29. When the parts of a lacerated gunshot wound have been brought into apposition, as in simple penetrating wounds, the only dressing necessary is moistened lint. It should be kept moist either by the renewed application of water dropped upon it, or by preventing evaporation by covering it with oiled silk. The sensations of the patient may be consulted in the selection of either of these, and climate and temperature will be often found to determine the choice. Velpeau and other French surgeons have strongly recommended the use of linseed-meal poultices, above all wet linen applications. Charpie is still extensively employed in French military hospitals. M. Baudens and Dr. Stromeyer have strongly recommended the topical application of ice placed in bladders; others, the continued irrigation of the wound with tepid water. When much local inflammation has set in, and when there is much constitutional fever even without unusual local irritation, the non-evaporating or warm applications will be found to be the most advantageous.

30. When suppurative action has been fully established, the surgeon must be guided by the general rules applicable to all other such cases. Care must be taken to prevent the accumulation of pus, lest it burrow, and sinuses become established—not an unfrequent result of want of sufficient caution in this regard. If much tumefaction of muscular tissues beneath fasciæ occurs, or abscesses form in them, free incisions should be at once made for their relief.

31. In wounds where the communication between the apertures of entrance and exit is tolerably direct, occasional syringing with tepid water may be useful, by removing discharges and any fibres of cloth which may be lying in the course of the wound. Weak astringent solutions are occasionally employed in a similar

way, with a view to improving the tone of the exhalants and exciting a more vigorous action in the process of granulation.

32. The strictest attention to cleanliness and the complete removal of all foul dressings are essentially necessary, not merely for the comfort of the patient, but to prevent the accumulation of noxious effluvia, and also to obviate the access of flies to the wounds. Cloths dipped in weak solutions of creasote or disinfecting fluids, laid over the wound, are found necessary for this purpose when insects abound in great numbers.

33. The constitutional treatment in an ordinary gunshot wound, uncomplicated with injury to bone or structures of first importance, should be very simple. The avoidance of all irregularity in habits tending to excite febrile symptoms or to aggravate local inflammation, attention to the due performance of the excretory functions, and support of the general strength, are chiefly to be considered. Bleeding, with a view to prevent the access of inflammation in such cases, is now never practised, as formerly, by English surgeons. The diet should be nutritious, but not stimulating. A pure fresh atmosphere is a very important ingredient in the means of recovery. If from previous habits of the patient, or from circumstances to which he is unavoidably exposed, the local inflammation has become aggravated—indicated by pain, increased swelling, and redness about the wound—topical depletion by leeches or cupping, bleeding from the arm, saline and antimonial medicines, and strict rest in the recumbent position, must be had recourse to, the extent being regulated by the circumstances of each case.

34. When the inflammation has become diffused, the purulent secretion is not confined to the track of the wound, but is liable to extend among the areolar connexions of the muscles; and if the cure be protracted, attention will be necessary to prevent the formation of sinuses. If stiffness or contractions result, attempts must be made to counteract them by passive motion and friction, with appropriate liniments; if a tendency to œdema and debility remain in a limb after the wound is healed, the cold-water douche will be found to be one of the most efficient topical remedies.

35. In French practice, the administration of a chalybeate tincture,* as a tonic, or diluted, as an injection, in wounds threatening to assume an unhealthy character, is very highly praised. It is stated that under the conjoined employment of this remedy internally and externally, in wounds of a pallid, unhealthy aspect, accompanied by nervous irritability and symptoms of approaching pyemia, the granulations have resumed a red and healthy appearance, and the general state of health become rapidly favorable.

* Perchlorure de fer, thirty drops, two or three times daily as a tonic, and diluted with six parts of water as an injection.

GUNSHOT WOUNDS IN SPECIAL REGIONS OF THE BODY.

Gunshot Wounds of the Head.—Injuries of this class, the most slight in appearance at their onset, not unfrequently prove most grave as they proceed, from encephalitis and its consequences, or from plugging of the sinuses by coagula, leading to coma, paralysis, or pyemia. Mr. Guthrie has laid down as a rule, that injuries of the head, of apparently equal extent, are more dangerous on the forehead than on the side or middle portion, and still more so than those on the back part; and that a fracture of the vertex is infinitely less important than one at the base of the cranium. When the injuries are caused by rifle balls, however, these considerations are rarely of much avail.

WOUNDS OF THE SCALP AND PERICRANIUM.—These wounds are usually inflicted by projectiles which are brought into contact at a very acute angle, so that little direct injury to the brain or its membranes is inflicted, and the surgeon's attention need only be directed to the same considerations as must occur in any contused wounds of the scalp from other causes than gunshot. But even in these accidents, though appearing to be simple flesh wounds, serious cerebral concussion and other lesions are occasionally met with.

Treatment.—The treatment of an ordinary gunshot wound of the scalp should be very simple. Cleansing the surface of the wound, removing the hair from its neighborhood for the easier application of dressings, lint moistened with clean water, very spare diet, and careful regulation of the excretions, are the only requirements in most cases. The patient must be closely watched, so that measures may be taken to counteract inflammatory symptoms in their earliest stages. Even after one of these wounds has healed, and the patient to all appearance has quite recovered, it is necessary to enjoin continued abstinence from excesses of all kinds.

WOUNDS COMPLICATED WITH FRACTURE, BUT WITHOUT DEPRESSION ON THE CEREBRUM.—In these injuries there may be a simple furrowing of the outer table, without injury to the inner; or there may be fissure extending to a greater or less degree of length, or radiating in several lines; or both tables may be comminuted in the direction the ball has traversed in such small portions that they lie loosely on the dura mater without much alteration in the general outline of the cranial curve. The chief and only means, in many cases, of concluding that no depression upon the cerebrum has taken place is the absence of the usual symptoms of compression; such injuries are very likely to be followed by inflammation, and not improbably abscess, between the internal table and dura mater; and further, as a consequence of the vascular supply being stopped, and perhaps also partly from the effects of the original contusion by necrosis of the inner table itself.

Fissured fractures, when the fissure extends through the skull, usually result from injuries by shell. The passage of a ball may fracture and very slightly depress a portion of the outer table of the cranium, and then the line of fracture will very closely simulate fissured fracture extending through both tables, and the diagnosis between them be excessively doubtful. Fissures often extend to long distances. They may occur at a part remote from the spot directly injured.

The cases where comminution has resulted from the track of a ball across the skull generally present less unfavorable results than those where a single fissured fracture, extending through both tables, exists; the small, loose fragments can be removed.

WOUNDS COMPLICATED WITH FRACTURE AND DEPRESSION ON THE CEREBRUM.—Such wounds are most serious, and the prognosis must be very unfavorable. They must not be judged of by comparison with cases of fracture with depression caused by such injuries as are usually met with in civil practice. The severe concussion of the whole osseous sphere by the stroke of the projectile, the bruising and injury to the bony texture immediately surrounding the spot against which it has directly impinged, as well as the contusion of the external soft parts, so that the wound cannot close by the adhesive process, constitute very important differences between gunshot injuries on the one side, and others caused by instruments impelled solely by muscular force on the other. So, also, the injury to the brain within, and its investments, is proportionably greater in such injuries from gunshot.

WITH PENETRATION OF THE CEREBRUM.—It is obvious that, where a projectile has power not only to fracture, but also to penetrate the cranium, it will rarely be arrested in its progress near the wound of entrance. Either splinters of bone, or the ball, or a portion of it, will be carried through the membranes into the cerebral mass. Sometimes a ball, if not making its exit by a second opening in the cranium, will lodge at the point of the cerebral substance opposite to that of its place of entrance; but the course a projectile may follow within the cranium is very uncertain.

Treatment.—Modern surgeons generally have made use of the trephine only when there was reason for concluding that depressed bone was leading to *permanent* interruption of cerebral function, or that an abscess had formed within reach, and was capable of evacuation. Preventive trephining has been proved to be useless, as well as dangerous, and is no longer an admissible operation. The tendency of the most recent experience has been to limit the practice of trephining to the narrowest sphere.

Where irregular edges, points, or pieces of bone are forced down and penetrate—not merely press upon—the cerebral substance, or where abscess manifestly exists in any known site, or a foreign substance has lodged near the surface, and relief cannot be afforded by the wound, trephining may be resorted to for the purpose; but the application of the operation, even in these cases, will be very much limited if certainty of diagnosis be insisted upon. In all other cases, it seems now generally admitted that much harm will be avoided, and benefit more probably effected, by employing long-continued constitutional treatment.

Gunshot Wounds of the Spine.—Gunshot wounds of the spine are closely associated with similar injuries of the head. In both classes corresponding considerations must be entertained by the surgeon in reference to the important nerve-structures, with their membranes, which are likely to be involved in the injury to their osseous envelope; in both, the effects of concussion, compression, laceration of substance, or subsequent inflammatory action, chiefly attract attention.

Treatment.—In injuries of the vertebral column and spinal cord occurring in military practice, the mischief is usually so complicated and extensive, and the medulla itself so bruised, that the cases must be very rare indeed in which the operation of trephining, if justifiable in any case, can offer the slightest prospect of benefit.

Gunshot Wounds of the Face.—Wounds of the face from musket-shot, grape, and small fragments of shell are usually more distressing from the deformity they occasion than dangerous to life; the vascularity of this region leads to danger both of primary and especially secondary hæmorrhage—a circumstance which, in all deep wounds of this region, must be looked for as a not improbable complication. The other complications of these gunshot wounds are lesions of the organs of special sense, injury to the base of the skull, paralysis from injury to nerves, wounds of glands, their ducts, and of the lachrymal apparatus.

Treatment.—In the treatment of gunshot wounds of the face where the bones are splintered and torn, the surgeon should always retain and replace as many of the broken portions as possible. It is often surprising how small connexions with neighboring soft parts will suffice to maintain vitality and lead to restored union in this region.

Gunshot Wounds of the Chest.—Gunshot wounds of the chest may conveniently be divided into two classes, viz. *non-penetrating* and *penetrating*. NON-PENETRATING wounds become subdivided into simple contused wounds of the soft parietes; contused and lacerated wounds; the same accompanied with injury to bones or cartilage; and, lastly, those complicated with lesion of some of the contents of the chest, the pleura remaining unopened, or, if opened, without a superficial wound. PENETRATING wounds may exist without wound, or with wounds of one or more of the viscera of this cavity. Among the more serious complications with which the latter may be accompanied is the lodgment of the projectile or other foreign bodies, as of fragments of bone, within the chest. As wounds of the heart and great vessels are almost invariably at once fatal, and as the organs of respiration occupy the greater part of the cavity of this region, it is in reference to the latter that the treatment of chest wounds is chiefly concerned.

NON-PENETRATING WOUNDS.—In the simpler wounds, in which the soft parietes only are involved, the healing process is often prolonged by the natural movements of the ribs to which the wounded structures are attached, especially when the ball has taken a circuitous course beneath the skin, and the surgeon must be on his guard to watch for pleuritis arising as an occasional consequence of these injuries.

When the force has been great, as when fragments of shell or rifle-balls strike at full speed against a man's breast-plate, not only may troublesome superficial abscesses and sinuses follow, but the lungs may have been compressed and ecchymosed at the time of the injury, and hæmoptysis be one of the symptoms presented.

When the projectile has been of large size, although no opening of the parietes or fracture exists, death sometimes ensues by suffocation as the direct result of pulmonary engorgement. The danger of pleuritis or pneumonia will be greater when the injury has been so severe as to cause division of bone or cartilage, and the subsequent suppuration and process of exfoliation will not unfrequently prove very tedious and troublesome. Although the pleura has not been opened, the lung may be lacerated either by the force of contusion or by the edges of the fractured ribs, which may afterwards return to their normal relative positions, so as to leave no indication during life of the means by which the lung had been wounded. Such an injury would be rendered much more probable by the existence of old adhesions, connecting the pulmonary and costal pleuræ opposite to the site of injury.

Notwithstanding a projectile has not penetrated the parietes of the chest, a pleural cavity may be opened, as in injuries from other causes, and the lung wounded by the sharp edges of fractured ribs. This will be indicated by emphysema, pneumothorax, hæmoptysis, probably signs of internal hæmorrhage, and inflammation. Such wounds will generally be the result of injuries from fragments of shell.

PENETRATING WOUNDS.—These wounds, especially when the lung is perforated or the projectile lodges, are necessarily exceedingly dangerous. Fatal consequences are to be feared, either from hæmorrhage, leading to exhaustion or suffocation; from inflammation of the pulmonary structure or pleuræ; from irritative fever accompanying profuse discharges; or from fluid accumulations in one or both of the pleural sacs.

When the chest has been opened by a projectile, the following signs may be expected in addition to the external physical evidences of the injury: a certain amount of constitutional shock; collapse from loss of blood; and, if the lung be wounded, effusion into the pleural cavity, hæmoptysis, dyspnœa, and an exsanguine appearance.

The shock of penetrating wounds of the chest, apart from the collapse consequent on hæmorrhage, is not generally so great as happens in extensive injuries to the extremities or in penetrating wounds of the abdomen.

When loss of blood occurs without the lung being wounded, the hæmorrhage is probably proceeding from a wound of one of the intercostal arteries, which has been torn by the sharp ends of fractured bone.

When blood is effused in any large quantity into the pleural sac —as indicated by the exsanguine appearance of the patient, increasing dyspnœa, occasional hæmoptysis, and the stethoscopic signs on auscultation—the inference is, that the lung has been opened, and that it is from its structure the blood is flowing.

Hæmoptysis indicates injury to the lung, but does not give assurance that this organ has been penetrated. Dyspnœa is a frequent accompaniment of wounds penetrating the lung, but not a constant symptom before inflammatory action has set in. When dyspnœa is great in the early period, it will often be found to depend upon the injuries to the parietes, and on the pain caused on taking a full inspiration. If air and frothy mucus with blood escape by the wound, there can be no doubt of the nature of the injury. Emphysema is not common in penetrating gunshot wounds, but occasionally happens.

Treatment.—The object of the surgeon's care must be in the first place to arrest hæmorrhage; afterwards, to remove pieces or jagged projections of bone, or any other sources of local irritation. Although the shock may happen to be considerable, attempts to rally the patient, if any be made, should be conducted very cautiously; the prolongation of the depressed condition may be valuable in enabling the injured structures to assume the necessary state for preventing hæmorrhage. Hæmorrhage from vessels belonging to the costal parietes should be arrested by ligature, as in other parts, if the source from which it proceeds can be ascertained, and if the flow of blood be so free as not to be controlled by the ordinary styptics. Hæmorrhage from the lung itself must be treated on the general principles adopted in all such cases; the application of cold to the chest, perfect quiet, the administration of opium, and, if the patient be sufficiently strong, bleeding from a large opening until syncope supervenes. When blood has accumulated in any large quantity, and the patient is much oppressed, the wound should be enlarged, if necessary, so as, with the assistance of proper position, to facilitate its escape. If the effused blood, from the situation of the wound, cannot be thus evacuated, and the patient be in danger of suffocation, then the performance of paracentesis must be resorted to.

The extensive bleedings formerly recommended in all penetrating gunshot wounds of the chest are now practised with much greater limitations—indeed, should never be employed simply with a view to prevent mischief from arising. Venesection carried to a great extent does harm by lessening the restorative powers of the frame.

To remove splinters of bone, and readjust indented portions of the ribs, the finger should be introduced into the wound, and care taken that in doing so no pieces of cloth or fragments be separated and projected into the pleural sac. Notice must at the same time be taken of any bleeding vessel requiring to be secured. A pledget of lint should be laid over the wound, and a broad bandage placed round the chest, just tight enough to support the ribs and in some degree to restrain their movements, but with an opening over each wound large enough to permit the ready access of the surgeon to it if necessary. If the patient's comfort admits of it, he should be laid with the wound downwards, with a view to prevent accumulation of fluid in the pleura; and if there be two openings, as will be most frequently the case in rifle-ball wounds, one wound should be thus placed, and the upper one kept covered. In gunshot wounds, closure of the parietes by adhesion is of course not to be looked for.

If the presence of a ball within the cavity be ascertained, efforts should be made for its removal. But any attempt to determine where the ball has lodged should be made very cautiously, as more harm may result from the interference than from the lodgment of the foreign body.

WOUNDS OF THE HEART seldom come to the military surgeon's notice, as they ordinarily prove fatal on the battle-field.

Gunshot Wounds of the Neck.—Gunshot wounds of this region do not appear to be so fatal as might be anticipated from the large vessels and important canals leading to the thorax and abdomen, which at first sight appear to be so exposed and unprotected. Where the large vessels happen to be divided, death must follow almost immediately.

Superficial wounds of the neck offer no peculiarities. The larynx and trachea being the organs most prominent, and most frequently injured, are those which chiefly attract the surgeon's notice in warfare.

The liability to concussion of the cervical portion of the vertebral column, and to injury of the deep cervical and other nerves, must not be overlooked. Wounds of the neck are often accompanied by more or less loss of power in one of the upper extremities; and more extensive paralysis occasionally succeeds, although there was no primary evidence of the spine being implicated in the injury.

Gunshot Wounds of the Abdomen.—Gunshot wounds of the abdomen are divided into *non-penetrating* and *penetrating.*

NON-PENETRATING WOUNDS.—If, although the viscera have been contused, the injury does not amount to being mortal, the patient should be subjected to perfect quiet, extreme abstinence, and, only when inflammation arises, to the necessary treatment for its control. If the parietes have been much contused, abscess or sloughing may be expected; and a tendency to visceral protrusion must be afterwards guarded against.

When portions of the pelvic parietes are fractured by heavy projectiles, very protracted abscesses generally arise, connected with necrosed bone.

Penetrating Wounds.—A penetrating wound of the abdomen, whether viscera be wounded or not, is usually attended with a great amount of "shock." The prognosis will be extremely unfavorable, if there is reason to fear the projectile has lodged in the cavity of the peritoneum; and in all cases the danger will be very great from inflammation of this serous investment. The liability to accumulation of blood in the cavity, from some vessel of the abdominal wall being involved in the wound, must not be forgotten.

When, in addition to the cavity being opened, viscera are penetrated, and death does not directly ensue from rupture of some of the larger arteries, the shock is not only very severe, but the collapse attending it is seldom recovered from up to the time of the fatal termination of the case. This is sometimes the only symptom which will enable the surgeon to diagnose that viscera are perforated. The mind remains clear; but the prostration, oppressive anxiety, and restlessness are intense; and, as peritonitis supervenes, pain, dyspnœa, diffused tenderness, irritability of the stomach, distension, and the other signs of this inflammation are superadded.

In ordinary wounds from musket-shot, scarcely any matter will escape from the opening of the parietes, the margin of which becomes quickly tumefied; but if any escape, it will probably indicate what viscus has been wounded. If the stomach has been penetrated, there will probably be vomiting of blood from the first. If the spleen or liver be wounded, death from hæmorrhage is likely to follow quickly. If the small intestines have been perforated, and death follows soon after from peritonitis, the bowels usually remain unmoved, so that no evidence is offered of the nature of the wound from evacuations; but in any case of penetrating wound of the abdomen, when the opportunity is offered, steps should be taken—a matter not unlikely to be omitted under the circumstances of camp hospitals full of patients—to isolate and examine all evacuations which may follow. If the kidneys or bladder are penetrated, the escape of urine into the abdomen is almost a certain cause of fatal result. The latter viscus may, however, be penetrated without the peritoneal cavity being opened; and the wonnd is then by no means of a fatal character. Musket-balls sometimes lodge in the bladder; in all such cases it is probable that the bladder has been penetrated at some part uncovered by peritoneum, so that the cavity of the abdomen has not been opened; or, if otherwise, the foreign body has found its way in by ulceration, after adhesions had been established, and thus circumscribed the openings of communication.

When the abdominal parietes have been opened by shell or passage of large shot, protrusion of omentum and intestines will probably be one of the results; this does not always happen. Sometimes a wound caused by a large projectile, which was at first not penetrating, will indirectly become so, from the severe contusion and consequent sloughing to such an extent as to denude the viscera. Curious instances are recorded in which balls have passed directly through the abdomen without perforating any important viscus, as proved by examination after death.

Gunshot wounds of the colon, especially of the sigmoid flexure, appear to be less fatal, probably from structural causes, as well as circumstances of position, than wounds of the small intestine.

Wounds of the Diaphragm.—Musket-balls occasionally pass through the diaphragm; and Mr. Guthrie has remarked that these wounds, in instances where the patients survive, only become closed under rare and particular circumstances. Hence the danger of portions of some of the viscera of the abdomen, as the stomach or colon, passing into the chest, and thus forming diaphragmatic herniæ, and of these, eventually, from some cause becoming strangulated.

Treatment.—In the general treatment of penetrating wounds of the abdomen by gunshot, the surgeon can do little more than to soothe and relieve the patient by the administration of opiates, and to treat symptoms of inflammation when they arise on the same principles as in all other cases. The usual directions to attempt agglutination of the opposite portions of peritoneum by favorable posture cannot generally be carried out, the attempts being defeated by the restlessness of the patient. The collapse which attends such injuries may be useful in checking hæmorrhage; and the exhibition of stimulants is further contra-indicated by the risk of exciting too much reaction, should the wound not prove directly fatal. If the wound be caused by grape-shot, or a piece of shell, and intestine protrudes, it must be returned; if the intestine be wounded, sutures are inapplicable, as in an incised wound, without previously removing the contused edges. When the bladder is penetrated, care must be taken to provide for the removal of the urine, either by an elastic catheter, or, if this cannot be retained, by perineal incision.

Gunshot Wounds of the Perineum and Genito-Urinary Organs.—From the position of these parts of the body, uncomplicated gunshot wounds of them are comparatively rare. Perineal wounds are not unfrequently caused by shells bursting and projecting fragments upwards; but they are generally mixed with lesions of viscera of the pelvis, or fracture of its structure, or injuries about the upper parts of the thighs or buttocks.

GUNSHOT WOUNDS OF THE EXTREMITIES.

Gunshot wounds of the extremities divide themselves into flesh wounds and contusions, and those complicated with fracture of one or more bones. Flesh wounds may be simple, and these offer few peculiarities, whatever their site; or they may be accompanied with lesion to nerves or blood-vessels, or both, and these usually increase in gravity in proportion as they approach the trunk.

Upper Extremity.—Fractures of the bones of the arm are very much less dangerous than like injuries in the corresponding bones of the lower extremity. Unless extremely injured by a massive projectile, or longitudinal comminution exist to a great extent, especially if also involving a joint, or the state of the patient's health be very unfavorable, attempts should always be made to preserve the upper extremity after a gunshot wound.

In these injuries, where the bone is much splintered, the detached portions and any fragments which are only retained by very partial periosteal connexions, should be removed; projecting spicula sawn or cut off;* the wound being extended at the most dependent opening where two exist, or fresh incisions being made for this purpose, if necessary; light water-dressing applied; the limb properly supported; and the case proceeded with as in cases of compound fracture from other causes. The same general rules also apply in preserving as much of the hand as possible, in gunshot injuries. If the shoulder or elbow joint be much injured, but the principal vessels have escaped, the articulating surfaces and broken portions should be excised.

The results of excision practised in the shoulder and elbow joints, especially the former, after gunshot wounds, have been exceedingly satisfactory. These operations present no peculiarities in the mode of performance or their after treatment, as compared with similar resections in civil practice.

* Dupuytren made a division of the splinters of bone broken by gunshot into three classes, viz. primary sequestra, those directly and completely separated by the force of the projectile; secondary sequestra, those retaining partial connexions by periosteal, muscular, or other attachments, but afterwards thrown off during the suppurative process; and tertiary sequestra, or necrosed portions, produced by the effects of the contusion and prolonged inflammatory action in parts adjoining the seat of fracture. In accordance with this arrangement, the removal by the surgeon of the primary and secondary splinters has been regarded as simply anticipating nature in her work; but Dr. Esmarch states, as one result of the experience of the surgeons of the Sleswick-Holstein army, that, in the majority of comminuted fractures, the removal of splinters retaining any connexion with periosteum is unnecessary and often injurious, as is also the practice of sawing off the broken ends of the bone projecting from the comminuted part. By proper treatment and under favorable circumstances, he asserts, such splinters become impacted in callus, and in time unite with the other fragments of the bone, and in this manner a cure is completed without operative interference. It is a matter, however, of frequent observation that splinters which have thus become impacted in callus lead to mischief in various ways, or are subsequently discharged as if they were so many foreign bodies, while the removal of the jagged ends of the broken bones seems to be a valuable means of preventing irritation, and thus of favoring union between them; the English surgeons, therefore, generally pursue the practice above recommended.

Lower Extremity.—Gunshot wounds of the lower extremity vary much more greatly in the gravity of their results, as well as in the treatment to be adopted, according to the part of the limb injured, than happens in those of the upper extremity. As a general rule, ordinary fractures below the knee, from rifle balls, should never cause primary amputation; while, excepting in certain special cases, in fractures above the knee, from rifle balls, amputation is held by most military surgeons to be a necessary measure. The special cases are gunshot fractures of the upper third of the femur, especially where the hip-joint is implicated; for in these the danger attending amputation itself is so great that the question is still open, whether the safety of the patient is best consulted by excision of the injured portion of the femur, by simple removal of detached fragments and trusting to natural efforts for union, or by resorting to amputation. The decision of the surgeon must generally rest upon the extent of injury to the surrounding structures, the condition of the patient, and other circumstances of each particular case. If the femoral artery and vein have been lacerated, any attempt to preserve the limb will certainly prove fatal.

M. Legouest, in a recent essay in the *Memoirs of the Society of Surgery*, at Paris, maintains that amputation at the hip-joint should be reserved for cases of fracture with injury to the great vessels, and that where the vessels have escaped, resection should invariably be performed. He also inculcates, as a general principle, not to perform immediate *primary* amputation at the hip-joint in any case; but, even in the severest forms of injury, to postpone the operation as long as possible.*

With regard to gunshot fractures in the middle and lower third of the femur, the experience of the French and English armies in the Crimea has tended to confirm the doctrine of the older military surgeons, that many lives are lost which might be otherwise preserved, by trying to save limbs; and that, of the limbs preserved, many are little better than incumbrances to their possessors. In the late Italian battles, the practice of trying to save lower extremities, after comminuted fractures in these situations of the thigh, appears to have been abandoned.

In fractures of the leg, where neither the knee nor ankle joints are implicated, the results of conservative attempts have been more favorable. When the fracture is comminuted, and implicates the knee or ankle joint, opening the capsule, amputation is necessary. The knee-joint was once excised in the Crimea, but the patient died; as was the case in the only other instance where

* A committee was appointed by the Surgical Society of Paris to examine and report upon this essay of Dr. Legouest on Coxo-femoral Disarticulation for Gunshot Wounds. Baron Larrey drew up the report, which will be found in the 5th vol. of the Mémoires de la Société de Chirurgie, 1860. It confirms the principle laid down by Dr. Legouest, excepting only those cases of fracture where the mutilation of the limb from a heavy projectile has been so great as to partly separate it from the pelvis, and those in which there has been simultaneous lesion of the crural vessels and femur near the pelvis, with extensive laceration of the surrounding tissues.

this operation is known to have been performed for gunshot injury in the Sleswick-Holstein campaign. In the treatment of fractures of the leg, where it has been determined to seek union, the same remarks apply as to fractures in the upper extremity. In wounds of the foot it is especially necessary to remove as early as possible all the comminuted fragments of the bones injured, or tedious abscesses and much pain and constitutional irritation are likely to ensue.

AMPUTATION.

The greater success of primary amputation appears to be attributable to the facts, that a contused and mangled limb is a constant source of accumulating irritation; that the exciting circumstances connected with battle lead a man to bear with courage at an early stage what subsequent suffering and anxiety may render him less willing to submit to; that a soldier, when first wounded, is most probably in stronger health than he will be after hospital restraint and confinement; that though the amputation is a violence, it is one the patient is likely to submit to with resignation, knowing that it is performed to remove parts which, if unremoved, will destroy life; and lastly, because the operation takes away a source of dread which must weigh down the sufferer so long as it is impending.

In respect to the particular time at which primary amputation is to be performed, the general practice of the present day is, when the operation is inevitable, to perform it as soon as it can be done; provided the more intense effects of "shock," where it has supervened on the injury, have passed off; and this practice generally accords with the feelings of soldiers, who not unfrequently press the surgeon for an early turn in being relieved from the suffering resulting from a shattered limb. In the cases where primary amputation is to be performed, a further reason given by Dr. Scrive for the operation being done on the same day that the wound is received is, that chloroform acts then so much more benignantly and readily; while, on the following day, or day after, traumatic excitement becomes very energetic, and considerable resistance is offered to its influence by wounded men, and longer time and a much larger dose of the chloroform are required to produce the state of anæsthesia. If only a moderate amount of "shock" exist, this does not appear to be a sufficient reason for delaying amputation; for a moderate exhibition of stimulus and a few consolatory words will often remove this, and, even though some faintness, pallor, and depression remain, no ill consequences ensue. In the Crimea, primary amputations were repeatedly performed where shock had not wholly disappeared, and no harm resulted from the practice.

The introduction of chloroform, by its negative operation of preventing pain or alarm, and by its positive action as a stimulus, has done much to remove many of the objections which were urged by John Hunter against early amputations after gunshot wounds. If collapse be intense, more than is accounted for by the wound to the extremity, suspicion will be excited that some internal injury has been also inflicted, and delay will be necessary for further observation of the patient.

SECONDARY HÆMORRHAGE.

Army surgeons meet in practice with secondary more frequently than primary hæmorrhage in gunshot wounds. It may arise in several ways. Sometimes it results from the coagulum being forced out of an artery in which hæmorrhage had previously been spontaneously averted by the ordinary natural process, this accident being consequent upon muscular exertion or increased impulse of the circulating system from any cause. This occurrence in the bottom of a deep wound will be often found to be a very troublesome complication. Sometimes an artery which did not appear to be injured in the first instance ulcerates or sloughs; or, without direct injury, a vessel may become involved in unhealthy deterioration of the wound, and give way; or, in a granulating wound, general capillary hæmorrhage may be excited by stimulus of any kind, such as venereal excitement or excess in drinking; or the coats of the vessel may ulcerate under pressure from a detached fragment of bone or from some foreign body; or the artery may be accidentally penetrated by the end of a sharp spiculum. Secondary hæmorrhage has been said to arise from increased arterial action, from the first to the fifth day; from sloughing, the effects of contusion, from the fifth to the tenth; from ulceration, to any more distant date. M. Baudens has remarked that he has observed secondary hæmorrhage to be most frequent about the sixth day after the wound.

THE END.

INDEX.

Published by

Facsimile Publisher
Ashok Vihar, Delhi-110052 (India)
Website: www.facsimilepublisher.com

Distributed by

Gyan Books Pvt. Ltd.
5, Ansari Road, Daryaganj, New Delhi-110002 (India)
E-mail: books@gyanbooks.com, Website: www.gyanbooks.com

8 888000 397519